ADVANCES IN NONINVASIVE
ELECTROCARDIOGRAPHIC MONITORING TECHNIQUES

Developments in Cardiovascular Medicine

VOLUME 229

Advances in Noninvasive Electrocardiographic Monitoring Techniques

edited by

HANS-H. OSTERHUES
Department of Internal Medicine / Cardiology,
University of Ulm,
Ulm, Germany

VINZENZ HOMBACH
Department of Internal Medicine / Cardiology,
University of Ulm,
Ulm, Germany

and

ARTHUR J. MOSS
Medical Center,
University of Rochester,
Rochester, New York U.S.A.

KLUWER ACADEMIC PUBLISHERS
DORDRECHT / BOSTON / LONDON

A C.I.P. Catalogue record for this book is available from the Library of Congress

ISBN 0-7923-6214-4

Published by Kluwer Academic Publishers,
P.O. Box 17, 3300 AA Dordrecht, The Netherlands.

Sold and distributed in North, Central and South America
by Kluwer Academic Publishers,
101 Philip Drive, Norwell, MA 02061, U.S.A.

In all other countries, sold and distributed
by Kluwer Academic Publishers,
P.O. Box 322, 3300 AH Dordrecht, The Netherlands.

Printed on acid-free paper

TABLE OF CONTENTS

CHAPTER FOUR: Methods

CONTRIBUTORS LIST

M. Böhm / Dr O. Zolk
Klinik III für Innere Medizin, Universität zu Köln, Köln, Germany

D. De Buyzere / D. Clement
Dept of Cardiology – Hypertension, University Hospital UZ Gent, Gent, Belgium

P.F. Cohn
Cardiology Division, State University of New York, Health Sciences Center, Stony Brook, NY, USA

C. Droste / G. Kinne
Freiburg, Germany

H.-D. Esperer / A. Feldman / R. Cohen, Klinik für Kardiologie, Otto-v.-Guericke-Universität, Magdeburg, Germany

S. Erné / H.-P Müller
Zentrum für Biomedizinische Technik, Universität Ulm, Ulm, Germany

E. Fallen
Department of Medicine, Division of Cardiology, McMaster University Med. Centre, Hamilton, Ontario, Canada

M.R. Franz
Director of Electrophysiology, Nations Capital Veteran Affairs Medical Center, Washington DC, USA

V. Froelicher
Cardiology Division (111C), VA Palo Alto Health Care System, Palo Alto, CA, USA

J.R. Gonzàlez-Juanatey / C. González-Juanatey
Servicio de Cardiología y UCC, Complexo Hospitalario Universitario de Santiago de Compostela, c/ Galeras s/n, Santiago de Compostela, La Coruña, Spain

R. Haberl / P. Steinbigler
Medizinische Klinik I, Max.-Ludwig-Universität, München, Germany

R. Hainsworth
Institute for Cardiovascular Research, University of Leeds, Leeds, United Kingdom

H. Hayakawa \ H. Honma
First Dept. of Internal Medicine, Nippon Medical School, Tokyo, Japan

M. Höher
Dept. of Medicine II – Cardiology, Universität Ulm, Ulm, Germany

Th. Klingenheben
Department of Medicine, Division of Cardiology, J.W. Goethe Universität, Frankfurt-am-Main, Germany

V. Hombach / B. Scharf
Abteilung Innere Medizin II, Universität Ulm, Ulm, Germany

S. Juul-Möller / N. von Tarnava
Dept. of Cardiology, University of Lund, Malmö, Sweden

H. Kestler
Dept of Neural Information Processing, Universität Ulm, Ulm, Germany

M. La Rovere
Divisione di Cardiologia, Centro Medico Montescano, Fondazione "S. Mangeri" IRCCS, Montescano, Pavia, Italy

B. Lemmer
Institut für Pharmakologie und Toxikologie, Ruprecht-Karls-Universität
Heidelberg, Mannheim, Germany

E. Locati Heilbron / G. Bagliani
Sezione di Cardiologia, Università degli Studi di Perugia, Perugia, Italy

F. Lombardi
Divisione di Cardiologia, Instituto di Scienze Biomediche, Ospedale S. Paolo,
Milano, Italy

M. Mäkijärvi
First Dept. of Medicine, Cardiovascular Laboratory, Helsinki University Central
Hospital, Hyks, Finland

M. Malik / I. Savelieva
Dept. of Cardiological Sciences, St. George's Hospital Medical School, London,
United Kingdom

A. Malliani
Medicina Interna II, Ospedale L. Sacco, Universitá di Milano, Milano, Italy

W.J. McKenna / M.W. Norman
Dept. of Cardiological Sciences, St. George's Hospital Medical School, London,
United Kingdom

M. Meesmann
Medizin. Universitätsklinik Würzburg, Würzburg, Germany

A. Poletti / C. Rocco
Area di Emergenza, Ospedale Civile di Tolmezzo, Tolmezzo, Italy

A.J. Moss
Medical Center, University of Rochester, Rochester, NY, USA

T.J. Mullen
Harvard-MIT Division of Health Sciences and Technology, Cambridge, MA,
USA

J.M. Neilson
Dept. of Medical Physics, The Royal Infirmary of Edinburgh, Edinburgh, United Kingdom

H.-H. Osterhues
Abteilung Innere Medizin II, Universität Ulm, Ulm, Germany

J.L. Palma-Gàmiz
Service of Cardiology, Ràmon y Cajal University Hospital, Madrid, Spain

A.A. Quyyumi
Cardiology Branch, National Institutes of Health, Bethesda, MD, USA

U. Sechtem / C. A. Schneider
Abteilung Kardiologie, Robert-Bosch-Krankenhaus, Stuttgart, Germany

L. Sörnmo
Signal Processing Group, Dept. of Applied Electronics, Lund University, Lund, Sweden

P. Steinbigler
Medizinische Klinik I, Max.-Ludwig-Universität, München, Germany

J.S. Steinberg / R. Perera
Arrhythmia Service, Division of Cardiology, St. Luke's - Roosevelt Hospital Center, New York, NY, USA

S. Stern
Bikur Cholim Hospital, Jerusalem, Israel

P. Verdecchia
Unitá Operativa di Cardiologia, Ospedale R. Silvestrini, Località San Sisto, Perugia PG, Italy

R.L. Verrier
Institute for Prevention of Cardiovascular Disease, Beth Israel Deaconess Medical Center, Harvard Medical School, Boston, MA, USA

E. Vanoli
Dept. of Cardiology, Policlinico S. Matteo IRCSS, Pavia, Italy

A. Voss
Biosignalanalyse/Med. Informationsverarbeitung, Fachhochschule Jena, FB
Medizintechnik, Jena, Germany

K. Wasserman
Division of Respiratory and Critical Care Physiology and Medicine, Harbor-
UCLA, Medical Center, Torrance, CA, USA

W. Zareba
Heart Research Follow-Up Program, University of Rochester, Rochester, NY,
USA

PREFACE

It has been almost 100 years since the electrocardiogram was introduced by Einthoven, and the evolution of this technique during the 20th century can be divided into three periods. The initial 30-year period involved the development of a clinically useful recording technique, with focus on detection and analysis of cardiac arrhythmias, especially atrial fibrillation. In the next 30-year period, roughly from 1930 to 1960, the emphasis was on descriptive correlative associations between various disease entities, such as myocardial infarction and rheumatic valvular heart disease, with specific electrocardiographic patterns, and the establishment of normal electrocardiographic standards in clinically healthy subjects. In the last 40 years of the 20th century, clinical electrocardiography has involved the routine use of the 12-lead ECG, the ambulatory (Holter) ECG, and the exercise ECG. In addition, sophisticated digital-signal processing methods have been developed to further enhance the diagnostic potential of this remarkable, cost-effective, electrocardiographic procedure.

As the 20th century draws to a close, we now have available signal-averaged ECGs to identify low-amplitude, high-resolution signals in the P and QRS waves; heart rate variability techniques to evaluate modulated autonomic nervous system activity on the heart; microvolt T-wave recording methods for detecting non-visible T-wave alternans, T-wave lability, and other disturbances of ventricular repolarization; and magnetocardiography to more precisely identify the three-dimensional aspects of symptomatic and hibernating myocardial ischemia. Noninvasive electrocardiography provides a remarkable microscopic-type view of the intrinsic electrical and electrophysiologic activity of the heart in both normal and diseased states.

The maturation of electrocardiology did not occur in isolation. The fundamentals of electrocardiography were established by classical electrophysiologic studies involving human subjects, whole animals, and isolated-heart preparations, with a theoretic underpinning by dipole physics. The technique was further enhanced by the application of chip technology and digital-processing procedures to the analysis of recorded electrical signals from the heart. More recently, new insights have been obtained through patch-clamp studies of ion-channel currents across myocardial cell membranes and by the application of molecular-genetic techniques to patients with inherited disorders of the electrical activity of the heart. These molecular-genetic studies have provided fundamental insight into ion-channel structure and function that is responsible for the generation of myocellular action potential and the surface-recorded electrocardiographic signal.

As with any diagnostic procedure, the clinical usefulness and the relevance of the electrocardiographic technique are influenced by available therapy. Coronary and stent angioplasty and coronary artery bypass graft surgery have stimulated the need for more accurate diagnosis of coronary artery disease at earlier stages of the disease process, with increased interest in detecting silent ischemia in asymptomatic subjects. Pacemakers and implantable defibrillators have been the stimuli for improved identification of patients at risk for sinus node dysfunction, heart block, and malignant ventricular arrhythmias. Radiofrequency ablation techniques have highlighted the need for earlier identification of patients with paroxysmal supraventricular tachycardia, Wolff-Parkinson-White syndrome, and focal monomorphic ventricular tachycardia. Improved therapy begets the need for presymptomatic diagnosis of patients with high-risk cardiac disorders, and the newer electrocardiologic techniques are well suited to meet this challenge.

Classical 12-lead ECG, ambulatory (Holter) monitoring, and exercise stress testing are well-established, clinically-useful, diagnostic techniques that have been validated by extensive experience and appropriate studies. These diagnostic procedures have clearly stood the test of time. Newer electrocardiologic techniques continue to be introduced, actively investigated, and clinically validated. This never-ending progress in electrocardiology was the impetus for the establishment of the International Society for Holter and Noninvasive Electrocardiology (ISHNE) in 1988. The formation of this Society evolved from the first Congress on Holter Monitoring that Dr. Vinzenz Hombach organized in Cologne, Germany in 1984.

This book is an outgrowth of the scientific work presented at the Society's 8th Biennial International Congress on Holter and Noninvasive Electrocardiology that was held in Ulm, Germany in May 1998 when Dr. Hombach was President of the Society and Chairperson of the Congress. We were fortunate to have had the active participation of Professor Ronald W. F. Campbell (University of Newcastle upon Tyne, England) at that Congress. Professor Campbell, who died suddenly and unexpectedly within a month after the Congress, was a major player in electrocardiology. He was a member of the Board of Trustees of the Society, and he contributed many seminal publications in Holter monitoring, ventricular arrhythmias, atrial fibrillation, and QT dispersion, to name but a few of the electrocardiographic topic areas in which he excelled.

This book is intended for clinical cardiologists and internists who use electrocardiologic procedures in the management of their patients, for researchers actively involved in the field, and for students of electrocardiology who will continue to advance the science of electrocardiography into the next century. *Advances in Noninvasive Electrocardiographic Monitoring Tecniques* provides a clear and concise update of the status of electrocardiology at the close of the 20th century, with contributions by the established experts in the field. Dr. Hans-H. Osterhues and Professor Vinzenz Hombach join me in dedicating this book to our departed good friend and esteemed colleague, the late Professor Ronnie Campbell, whose warm-hearted personality and professional contributions to electrocardiology established a standard of excellence for all of us in the field.

Arthur J. Moss, M.D.
Professor of Medicine
University of Rochester Medical Center
Rochester, NY USA

INTRODUCTION

Noninvasive Electrocardiographic Monitoring is a fundamental part of cardiology.

Since the beginning of modern cardiology, the different forms of electrocardiographic monitoring have never lost their importance and are today indispensible for diagnosis and risk stratification of patients. This is due to continuous improvements and developments of new technologies in this area. On the other hand, the rapid progression of capabilities and technologies as well as the consecutive changing of diagnostic values of the methods force us to update our knowledge.

This book offers a comprehensive overview of the current state und future developments in the field of Noninvasive Electrocardiography Monitoring Techniques. It focuses on the various forms of Electorcardiography such as standard 12-lead ECG, high resolution ECG, ambulatory ECG, exercise ECG. Additionally, related domains such as magnetocardiography, newer signal detection and analysis techniques as well as ambulatory blood pressure monitoring are highlighted.

The individual contributions of the book were presented at the 8th International Congress on Holter and Noninvasive Electrocardiology, held in Ulm, Germany, on May 22/23 1998. An outstanding international faculty gathered under the auspices of the International Society for Holter and Noninvasive Electrocardiology (ISHNE) to discuss recent advances in this field.

The different methods are discussed with regard to methodological aspects, latest technical developments and clinical value of results. Furthermore, review articles focus on cardiovascular genetics, autonomic nervous system, monitoring of ischemic heart disease, quality control and standardization of monitoring techniques. The last section containing newer signal detection and analysis techniques opens our view to recently developed methods, e.g. non-linear dynamics and neural network analysis.

We are confident that this book serves as a useful and interesting source for clinical cardiologists as well as scientists in the field of Noninvasive Electrocardiographic Monitoring.

Ulm, Germany
Rochester NY, USA

Hans-H. Osterhues, Vinzenz Hombach and Arthur J. Moss

CHAPTER ONE: PHYSIOLOGY AND PATHOPHYSIOLOGY

SECTION ONE: BASIC RESEARCH / FROM GENE TO PHENOTYPE

1. CARDIOVASCULAR MOLECULAR GENETICS

MARK W. NORMAN, LEON G D'CRUZ, NIALL MAHON AND
WILLIAM J. MCKENNA

Over the last 10 years rapid advances in molecular biology have led to a much greater understanding of several important cardiac disorders. It is likely that over the next ten years great advances in management of these patients will occur as a result of further advances in molecular medicine. The moleculoar genetic basis of hypertrophic cardiomyopathy and some forms of dilated cardiomyopathy are known, as well as long QT syndrome and Marfans syndrome.

HYPERTROPHIC CARDIOMYOPATHY

Hypertrophic Cardiomyopathy is defined as a primary heart muscle disease, characterised by hypertrophy of the left and/or right ventricle. It is important to exclude secondary causes of hypertrophy such as hypertension or aortic valve disease when faced with a patient with cardiac hypertrophy.

Hypertrophy, typically involves the septum (asymmetric septal hypertrophy (ASH)), but, apical, concentric or other forms of hypertrophy may occur. Familial disease is present in approximately 90% of cases. Autosomal dominant transmission with variable penetrance is the commonest inheritance pattern described.

The prevalence of disease is thought to be 1 in 500 in young adults. Even before the molecular diagnoses it was recognised that expression of HCM is age related. Clinical manifestations typically occur during periods of growth; however, we now know with molecular diagnosis even adults may show partial

H.-H. Osterhues et al. (eds.),
Advances in Noninvasive Electrocardiographic Monitoring Techniques, 3–17.
© 2000 *Kluwer Academic Publishers. Printed in the Netherlands.*

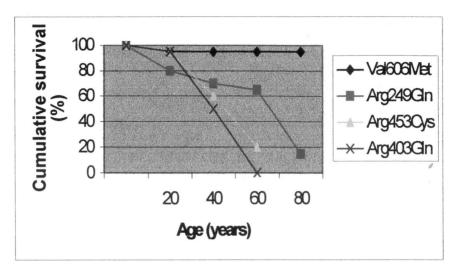

Figure 1. There is a different risk profile for HCM patients based upon the mutation present even within the same gene. Above shows a graphic representation of Kaplan-Meier survival for beta-myosin heavey chain mutations versus age. The Arg 403 Gin mutation is considered malignant in that a high proportion of people with this mutation have sudden death, whereas the Val 606 Met mutation is associated with better survival.

or incomplete expression as obligate carriers without clinical manifestations(1,2).

Clinical symptoms are variable and often paroxysmal, but typically include exercise-induced dyspnoea, chest pain, sustained palpitation and syncope or sudden death. Clinical examination may be unremarkable. Usually the apex beat is not displaced but there is a sustained imulse and a palpable atrial contraction.. The carotid upstroke is correspondingly brisk, with a double apical impulse if outflow obstruction occurs in mid-systole.

The ECG is usually abnormal (normal in less than 15%), with abnormal Q-waves, left ventricular hypertrophy, and ST- and T-wave abnormalities(3), although there is no typical ECG pattern. Arrhythmia is common : 25% have non-sustained ventricular tachycardia and 10% develop atrial fibrillation.

Echocardiography typically shows ventricular wall thickening, with the patterns described above. In 1/5th of cases additional features include narrowing of the outflow tract and systolic anterior motion of the mitral valve.

Gross pathology of hypertrophy of the ventricular muscle may not be helpful if there is a past history of hypertension or aortic valve disease. However, histology reveals characteristic myocyte disarray. Instead of myofibrils having a normal parallel arrangement, the myofibrils are seen to cross each other in a haphazard way. Myocytes are arranged in whorls around connective tissue, and fibrosis may be abundant.

It was not realised until the development of molecular genetic techniques that HCM represents the end result of several different genetic mutations in at least seven different contractile proteins. As all are sarcomeric protein elements many authors consider HCM as a disease of the sarcomere. The genetic heterogeneity is further complicated in that not only are there several different disease causing genes, different mutations within each of these genes have been described, some of which having important phenotypic differences from other mutations within the same gene.

Since a molecular sub-classification has become possible important genotype phenotype correlations have become apparent. Firstly, although HCM is defined as left ventricular hypertrophy >15mm, some genotypes are associated with significantly increased wall thickness while others may have subclinical or no detectable hypertrophy(4). For example patients with the beta myosin heavy chain mutations had an average wall thickness of 24mm, whereas those with Troponin T mutations are more typically associated with relatively mild hypertrophy (17mm)(5).

The importance of recognising HCM with mild hypertrophy has been aided by molecular medicine. Although the Troponin T mutations are associated with relatively milder degrees of hypertrophy, patients with these mutations are at a high risk of sudden death. The risk of sudden death has long been known to be sometimes independent of the degree and pattern of hypertrophy. Clinical indices have allowed risk stratification based upon risk factors but not based upon morphology. Those individuals with two risk factors or more have a 3% annual mortality. The clinical risk factors are history of familial sudden death, patients with syncope or episodes of ventricular tachycardia. Kaplan-Meier survival curves show some important differences in risk of sudden death with certain mutations (see figure 1). Some mutations in the beta-myosin heavy chain (i.e.Arg403Gln) are termed malignant in that they are associated with a high risk of premature sudden death as high as 50% mortality by age 40yrs(6). Others are termed benign (i.e. Val606Met or Arg403Trp) in that although they cause similar degrees of hypertrophy and result from mutations in the beta-myosin heavy chain gene they have a relatively good survival. Patients with Troponin T mutations are generally similar in survival terms as the high-risk β-myosin heavy chain groups(5). Therefore, correct identification of a particular mutation may provide important prognostic information and potentially influence management.

In addition different phenotypes are associated with different degrees of penetrance. For example, 95% of patients with the β-myosin heavy chain mutations have a high degree of expression as detected by echocardiography,

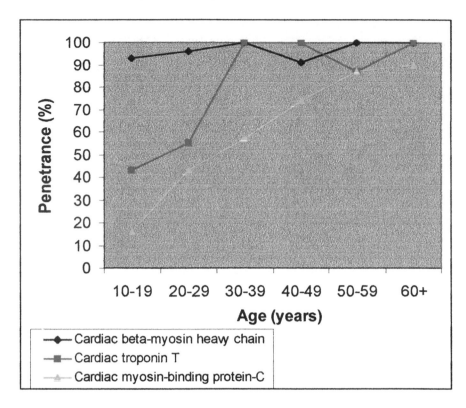

Figure 2. Age related penetrance for three different HCM genotypes. The most striking increase in age related penetrance is for the myosin binding protein-C variant which is associated with a low level of expression at a young age, but by age 50yrs almost 60% of persons with mutations in this gene have HCM disease expression.

whereas up to 1/3rd of Troponin T mutations have subclinical hypertrophy not detected by echocardiography.

An unusual form of late-onset HCM is the myosin binding protein C variant. An age related penetrance of the disease is seen in that 20-30% of 20yr olds with disease causing mutations have hypertrophy, but the expression of disease increases with age so that 58% of 50yr old patients have echocardiographic hypertrophy (see figure 2) (7). Previously this 'late-onset' form of HCM may have been misdiagnosed as hypertensive heart disease or hypertrophy of the elderly. The importance of molecular diagnosis with this late-onset variant is that there is a higher risk of sudden death or serious arrhythmia than with hypertensive heart disease, or hypertrophy of the elderly. Also there is a risk to offspring who may have earlier expression of the disease than their parents.

Table 1

Sarcomeric Protein	Annotation	Genetic locus
β-cardiac myosin heavy chain(11)	CMH1	14q11-12
Troponin T(12)	CMH2	1q3
α-Tropomyosin(12)	CMH3	15q2
Cardiac myosin binding protein-C(13)	CMH4	11p13-q13
Troponin I(14)	CMH5	
HCM associated with WPW(15,16)	CMH6	7q3
Ventricular myosin essential light chain	VMLC 1	12q23q24.3
Ventricular myosin regulatory light chain	VMLC 2	12q23q24.3

Some preliminary work at the level of the sarcomere has shown a difference in terms of the rate of contractility and the degree of force generation for some mutations. For example Lankford(8) has demonstrated two different mutations in the β-myosin heavy chain gene have depressed shortening velocity and reduced isometric force generation. Mutations in the gene encoding α-tropomyosin(9) lead to increased calcium sensitivity and increased contractility.

Modifier genes are thought to be important in expression of HCM, and the ACE genotype polymorphism has an effect on the degree of ventricular hypertrophy. Patients with the DD genotype have significantly more hypertrophy than those with either the II or ID genotypes(10). It is likely that other disease modifier genes and environmental factors have an important role in the degree of phenotypic expression. Ultimately the goal of molecular diagnosis is to clarify these issues and provide an effective treatment strategy to improve clinical symptoms and prognosis.

DILATED CARDIOMYOPATHY

Dilated Cardiomyopathy (DCM) is a myocardial disease characterised by dilatation and reduced contraction of the left ventricle, and sometimes the right ventricle.

Patients present with symptoms of cardiac failure, with fatigue, shortness of breath on exercise, reduced exercise tolerance, chest pain and presyncope. Physical examination may be normal or show signs typical of congestive cardiac failure. The blood pressure is typically low, with a narrow pulse pressure; there may be a diffuse and dyskinetic precordial impulse.

Clinical investigation may reveal an enlarged cardiac silhouette on chest X-ray. Echocardiography shows an increased end-diastolic volume of the left ventricle, with reduced fractional shortening. Electrocardiography is normal in less than 5%, with diffuse LV changes. One fifth of patients have established atrial fibrillation.

Treatment is non-specific, based upon standard anti-heart failure therapy. Namely, ACE inhibitors, diuretics, digoxin and beta-blockers. Anticoagulation is advised for both atrial fibrillation and those with a markedly reduced ejection fraction. Progressive deterioration may develop despite treatment and some patients require cardiac transplantation.

Pathologically DCM is recognised by dilated cardiac chambers. Histology is non-specific, with varying features such as perimyocyte and interstitial fibrosis, with myocyte hypertrophy and occaisonal inflammatory cells.

A familial basis to the disease is now established in over 50% of cases. Inheritance is predominantly autosomal dominant, but X-linked recessive(17) and autosomal recessive cases are reported.

As HCM has been defined in terms of a disease of the sarcomere; preliminary molecular studies suggest that DCM may be a disease of the myocardial cytoskeleton, which plays an essential role in maintaining cellular integrity and function of the myocardium. The cytoskeleton forms a network of intermediate filaments and microtubules, which may be disrupted by inflammatory processes. However, DCM is a more heterogenous disease than HCM and a number of factors are involved in the pathogenesis of DCM including alcohol, viral infections, toxins, and the immune system.

Molecular genetic studies of DCM with firstly linkage has found some genotype phenotype differences. As with hypertrophic cardiomyopathy clinical differences are recognised with several different genetic markers One particular form of DCM is associated with progressive cardiac conduction defects in the 20's and 30's with development of DCM in the 40's[20]. Another form of DCM with bradycardia as an early disease manifestation maps to a different chromosome(19). It is likely that as with hypertrophic cardiomy-

Table 2. showing the molecular differences within DCM families have been described in terms of linkage.

Author	Locus	Clinical Features
Kass et al (1994(20))	1p1-1q1	DCM + progressive cardiac conduction disease
Olson et al (1996)(19)	3p22-25	DCM + bradycardia
Durand(21)	1q32	Autosomal dominant DCM
Krajinovic et al (1995)(22)	9q13-q22	Autosomal dominant DCM
Bowles et al (1996)(23)	10q21-23	DCM + mitral valve prolapse

opathy a degree of genetic heterogeneity within DCM subgroups will identify different disease characteristics and risk profiles. Some families with DCM are known to have a high-risk of arrhythmic death, but as yet the genetic basis of these differences is unknown.

Genetic defects of the cytoskeleton have been identified in only a few isolated cases. The first described was X-linked DCM associated with abnormalities in dystrophin. Subsequently, autosomal dominant DCM has been described. Clinical variation is recognised as with HCM but the degree of genetic subclassification is very limited as only a few mutations have been described in isolated cases. Mutations in cytoskeletal proteins such as metavinculin, alpha-dystroglycan, alpha- and gamma-sarcoglycan, and muscle LIM protein have been found to result in dilated cardiomyopathy, suggesting that cytoskeletal proteins play a central role in cardiac function(18). Recently, two families with DCM with two different mutations in the gene encoding actin have been described (19).

ARRHYTHMOGENIC RIGHT VENTRICULAR CARDIOMYOPATHY

Arrhythmogenic right ventricular cardiomyopathy (ARVC) is also known as arrhythmogenic right ventricular dysplasia (ARVD). As there is a genetic basis to the disease, the term cardiomyopathy is favoured.

ARVC is defined pathologically as fibro-fatty replacement of the ventricular myocardium with a marked predilection for the right ventricle(24).

Table 3

Genetic Locus	Annotation	Clinical Features
14q24.3	ARVD 1	Autsomal dominant ARVC(29)
1q32	ARVD 2	ARVC + frequent ventricular arrhythmia(30)
14q12-q22	ARVD 3	ARVC autosomal dominant(32)
2q32.1-q32.3	ARVD 4	Recurrent left ventricular involvement(31)

Initially the disease is thought to be patchy forming more confluent areas of fibro-fatty replacement. The fatty replacement extends from the epicardium inward, affecting the right ventricular myocardium resulting in right ventricular dilatation, aneurysms, and systolic dysfunction. The fatty tissue is electrically inert and can cause electrical conduction abnormalities resulting in life-threatening ventricular arrhythmias.

Clinical features include palpitation, syncope, sudden death and progressive systolic heart failure(25). Definitive diagnosis requires demonstration of both fat and fibrosis replacing the ventricular myocardium.

Clinical diagnosis has been improved with proposed diagnostic criteria (26)based upon assessment with electrocardiography, echocardiography, histological data and cardiac MRI. Family pedigree analysis is now well advanced with the majority of cases showing an autosomal dominant inheritance pattern with variable penetrance(27). One peculiar variant of ARVC found on the Greek Island of Naxos is associated with woolly hair and palmoplantar keratoderma. The inheritance pattern of this unusual disease is autosomal recessive with complete penetrance, and the disease locus is 17q12 (28).

To date five loci are associated with ARVC, four of which are autosomal dominant. Again in comparison with both dilated cardiomyopathy and hypertrophic cardiomyopathy clinical differences are recognised. The first locus for autosomal dominant ARVC was found as the result of a study involving 82 subjects from two Italian families. 19 family members were affected by ARVC. The genetic locus maps to 14q24.3, close to the region encoding α-actinin(29). A second locus close to the actinin-2 gene on chromosome 1q32 is associated with ARVC families with frequent ventricular arrhythmias(30). Three independent families with ARVC characterised by recurrent left ventricular fibrofatty involvement maps to chromosome2q32.1-q32.3(31). (See figure 3)

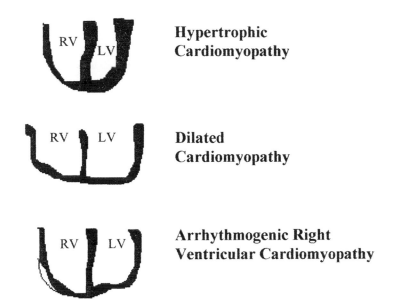

Hypertrophic Cardiomyopathy

Dilated Cardiomyopathy

Arrhythmogenic Right Ventricular Cardiomyopathy

Figure 3. the three different forms of cardiomyopathy. HCM Hypertrophic Cardiomypathy has left ventricular wall thickening and assymetric septal hypertrophy (ASH) DCM dilated cariomyopathy has biventricular enlargement in many but may initially only affect the left ventricle ARVC Arrhythmogenic Right Ventricular Cardiomyopathy typically has fibrofatty infiltration of the right ventricular free wall leading to arrhythmia and right ventricular enlargement although the left ventricle can also be affected.

THE LONG QT SYNDROME

The long QT syndrome is an inherited disorder that can result in sudden cardiac death from ventricular arrhythmias. The Romano-Ward syndrome is the classical autosomal dominant form(33), an autosomal recessive inheritance pattern associated with congenital neural deafness is eponymously known as the Jervell-Lange-Nielsen syndrome(34). Heterozygous mutations in the long QT syndrome genes result in the Romano-Ward syndrome, whereas homozygous mutations in a gene encoding I_{Ks} result in the Jervell and Lange-Nielsen syndrome.

Typically it affects young, apparently healthy people. Symptoms include syncope and seizures (may be misdiagnosed as idiopathic epilepsy). The proband within a family typically presents with syncope due to ventricular tachyarrhythmias or cardiac arrest precipitated by exercise or emotional stress.

Table 4

Chromosome	Annotation	Channel
11p15.5	KVLQT1 (LQT1)	Potassium inward stabilising current α-subunit (41)
7q35-36	HERG (LQT2)	Potassium inward rectifier current(42)
3p21-24	SCN5A (LQT3)	Sodium channel(37)
4q25-q27	LQT4	unknown
21q22.1-p22	MinK	Potassium inward stabilising current β-subunit

The diagnosis is based upon a QT interval corrected for heart rate (Bazetts formula: $QT_c = QT \div \sqrt{RR}$) longer than 0.44s for men and 0.46s for women. Classifications are both clinical and molecular. The clinical scoring system relates to both clinical symptoms and ECG findings. Individuals without symptoms and a corrected QT interval less than 0.41s are classed as unaffected.

Family screening is important as asymptomatic gene carriers can be identified. The mortality in untreated symptomatic cases can be as high as 60% over a 15yr period. Effective treatment with beta-blockers and pacing has reduced the mortality to 4% over a 10yr follow-up period. Recently long QT syndrome has been implicated as a cause of sudden infant death syndrome (SIDS). During an 8yr follow-up period of 34,442 Italian babies 34 died(35). Of these 24 were SIDS, and half of these had a prolonged QT interval.

Molecular genetic studies have linked the disease with five chromosomal markers on chromosomes 3, 4, 7, 11 and 21(36). Four long QT syndrome genes have been identified; all encode cardiac myocyte ion channels: SCN5A, a cardiac sodium channel on chromosome 3(37); HERG an inward rectifying potassium channel on chromosome 7(38); KvLQT1 the α-subunit of a potassium conducting channel on chromosome 11(39) and KCNE1, the β subunit of the potassium conduction channel on chromosome 21(40). To simplify the classification of each genotype a terminology for each mutation has been proposed: LQT1 on KvLQT1, LQT2 on HERG, LQT3 on SCN5A, LQT4 on chromosome 4, LQT5 on minK.

An interesting genotype/phenotype correlation is recognised with three known long QT syndrome genes in terms of morphology of the QT interval on ECG(43).

Most of the mutations in the LQT syndrome genes are distinctive mis-sense mutations. Few families have been described with a mutation that is in common; most are unique to each family. This degree of genetic heterogeneity underlies the clinical variation seen.

Further genotype/phenotype correlations show that different time and voltage current characteristics occur as a result of these mutations. Patients with LQT1 have arrhythmia especially on exercise. I_{Ks} is the predominant potassium current when there is high sympathetic activity especially when there are shorter cardiac cycle lengths. Therefore, reduced I_{Ks} leads to an inadequate action potential shortening and a high prevalence of arrhythmic events. LQT3 patients in contrast experience events during sleep or at rest; and they are able to shorten their QT interval during exercise. These patients may benefit from pacemakers to prevent bradycardia. With LQT3 mutations it has been proposed the presence of normal potassium currents allows a normal action potential shortening during exercise, but at rest inadequate inactivation of sodium inward currents will prolong the action potential plateau inward current.

Standard therapy for the long QT syndrome is beta-blocker. On the basis of molecular knowledge more specific therapy has been proposed. Mexiletene a sodium channel blocking agent has been shown to significantly shorten the QT_c of the LQT3 patients(44), but have only a mild effect on LQT1 and LQT2 both potassium channel related long QT syndrome. Also as the activity of HERG is dependent upon the extracellular potassium concentration, attempts to increase the extracellular potassium concentration have significantly shortened the QT interval and altered T-wave morphology in LQT2 patients.

As with HCM not all of the mutations responsible for the LQT syndrome have been found. As LQT is a disease of the ion channel it is likely that further forms of the disease are encode by cardiac myocyte ion channel abnormalities. LQT1 is the most frequently found form; LQT3 and LQT5 are rare. Recently some patients with typical drug-induced LQTS have been shown to have mutations on LQTS genes. It is thought the combination of a modest degree of channel blockade resulting from a 'silent mutation' and a variety of drugs, which may alter ionic currents, can result in early after-depolarisations and Torsades-de-Pointes.

MARFANS SYNDROME

Marfans syndrome is an autosomal dominant disorder with marked clinical variation; the age range of affected individuals can make detection difficult. There are established diagnostic criteria for Marfans syndrome, including aortic dilatation, aortic dissection in a young non-hypertensive person, ectopia lentis, dural ectasia, scoliosis, joint hypermobility, myopia and mitral valve prolapse.

The genetic basis of the disease is a mutation in the gene fibrillin-1(45). Fibrillin is a protein produced by fibroblasts, secreted into the extracellular matrix forming fibrillar aggregates, which are involved in the adhesion of connective tissue structures. Fragmentation and disorganisation of the elastic layer are pathological hallmarks of the disease.

The fibrillin-1 gene is mapped to chromosome 15q21.1, and over 100 mutations unique to each Marfans families have been detected. A second fibrillin gene FBN-2 on chromosome 5 is associated with congenital contractural arachnodactyly. A Marfan-like syndrome has been mapped to chromosome 3p24. Other important cardiovascular diseases with a connective tissue component and a genetic basis are Ehlers-Danlos syndrome and Pseudoxanthoma Elasticum.

CONCLUSIONS

Recent advances in molecular biology have made it possible to identify the functional abnormalities in cardiovascular diseases for which the underlying pathophysiology had been elusive.

In the future additional knowledge will be gained for the other cardiomyopathies, with increasing emphasis on gene identification, and genotype/phenotpye correlations. The ultimate aim is to provide a more effective means of therapy by an understanding of the direct molecular pathophysiological basis of cardiovascular disease.

REFERENCE LIST

1. Charron P, Carrier L, Dubourg O, Tesson F, Desnos M, Richard P, Bonne, Guicheney P, Hainque B, Bouhour JB, et al. Penetrance of familial hypertrophic cardiomyopathy. Genet.Couns. 1997;8(2):107-14.
2. Landing BH, Recalde AL, Lawrence TK, Shankle WR. Cardiomyopathy in childhood and adult life, with emphasis on hypertrophic cardiomyopathy. Pathol.Res.Pract. 1994;190(8):737-49.

3. Ryan MP, Cleland JF, French JA, Joshi J, Choudhury L, Chojnowska L, Michalak E, Al-Mahdawi S, Nihoyannopoulos P, Oakley CM. The standard electrocardiogram as a screening test for hypertrophic cardiomyopathy. Am.J.Cardiol. 1995;76(10):689-94.

4. Solomon SD, Wolff S, Watkins H, Ridker PM, Come P, McKenna WJ, Seidman, CE, Lee RT. Left ventricular hypertrophy and morphology in familial hypertrophic cardiomyopathy associated with mutations of the beta-myosin heavy chain gene. J.Am.Coll.Cardiol. 1993;22(2):498-505.

5. Watkins H, McKenna WJ, Thierfelder L, Suk HJ, Anan R, O'Donoghue A, Spirito P, Matsumori A, Moravec CS, Seidman JG, et al. Mutations in the genes for cardiac troponin T and alpha-tropomyosin in hypertrophic cardiomyopat. N. Engl. J. Med. 1995; 332(16):1058-64.

6. Anan R, Greve G, Thierfelder L, Watkins H, McKenna WJ, Solomon S, Vecchio C, Shono H, Nakao S, Tanaka H, et al. Prognostic implications of novel beta cardiac myosin heavy chain gene mutations that cause familial hypertrophic cardiomyopath. J.Clin.Invest. 1994;93(1):280-5.

7. Yu B, French JA, Jeremy RW, French P, McTaggart DR, Nicholson MR, Semsarian C, Richmond DR, Trent RJ. Counselling issues in familial hypertrophic cardiomyopathy. J Med Genetic 1998;35(3):183-8.

8. Lankford EB, Epstein ND, Fananapazir L, Sweeney HL. Abnormal contractile properties of muscle fibers expressing beta-myosin heavy chain gene mutations in patients with hypertrophic cardiomyopathy. J.Clin.Invest. 1995;95(3):1409-14.

9. Golitsina N, An Y, Greenfield NJ, Thierfelder L, Iizuka K, Seidman JG, Seidman CE, Lehrer SS, Hitchcock-DeGregori SE. Effects of two familial hypertrophic cardiomyopathy-causing mutations on alpha-tropomyosin structure and function. Biochemistry 1997;36(15):4637-42.

10. Yoneya K, Okamoto H, Machida M, Onozuka H, Noguchi M, Mikami T, Kawaguchi H, Murakami M, Uede T, Kitabatake A. Angiotensin-converting enzyme gene polymorphism in Japanese patients with hypertrophic cardiomyopathy. Am.Heart J. 1995;130(5):1089-93.

11. Geisterfer-Lowrance AT, Kass S, Tanigawa G, Vosberg H-P, McKenna W, Seidman CE, Seidman JG. A molecular basis for familial hypertrophic cardiomyopathy: A beta cardiac myosin heavy chain gene missense mutation. Cell 1990;62(5):999-1006.

12. Thierfelder L, Watkins H, MacRae C, Lamas R, McKenna W, Vosberg, Seidman JG, Seidman CE. Alpha-Tropomyosin and cardiac troponin T mutations cause familial hypertrophic cardiomyopathy: A disease of the sarcome. Cell 1994;77(5):701-12.

13. Watkins H, Conner D, Thierfelder L, Jarcho JA, MacRae C, McKenna WJ, Maron BJ, Seidman JG, Seidman CE. Mutations in the cardiac myosin binding protein-C gene on chromosome 11 cause familial hypertrophic cardiomyopathy. Nat.Genet. 1995;11(4):434-7.

14. Kimura A, Harada H, Park J-E, Nishi H, Satoh M, Takahashi M, Hiroi S, Sasaoka T, Ohbuchi N, Nakamura T, et al. Mutations in the cardiac troponin I gene associated with hypertrophic cardiomyopathy. Nat.Genet. 1997;16(4):379-82.

15. MacRae CA, Ghaisas N, Kass S, Donnelly S, Basson CT, Watkins HC, Anan, Thierfelder LH, McGarry K, Rowland E, et al. Familial hypertrophic cardiomyopathy with Wolff-Parkinson-White syndrome maps to a locus on chromosome 7q3. J.Clin.Invest. 1995;96(3):1216-20.

16. Shibata M, Yamakado T, Imanaka-Yoshida K, Isaka N, Nakano T. Familial hypertrophic cardiomyopathy with Wolff-Parkinson-White syndrome progressing to ventricular dilation. Am.Heart J. 1996;131(6):1223-5.

17. Muntoni F, Di Lenarda A, Porcu M, Sinagra G, Mateddu A, Marrosu G, Ferlini A, Cau M, Milasin J, Melis MA, et al. Dystrophin gene abnormalities in two patients with idiopathic dilated cardioyopathy. Heart 1997;78(6):608-12.

18. Towbin JA. The role of cytoskeletal proteins in cardiomyopathies. Current Opin Cell Biol 1998;10(1):131-9.

19. Olson TM, Keating MT. Mapping a cardiomyopathy locus to chromosome 3p22-p25. J Clin Invest 1996;97(2):528-32.

20. Kass S, MacRae C, Graber HL, Sparks EA, McNamara D, Boudoulas H, Basson CT, Baker IIP, Cody RJ, Fishman MC, et al. A gene defect that causes conduction system disease and dilated cardiomyopathy maps to chromosome 1p1-1q1. Nature Genetics 1994;7(4):546-51.

21. Durand J-B, Bachinski LL, Bieling LC, Czernuszewicz GZ, Abchee AB, Qun TY, Tapscott T, Hill R, Ifegwu J, Marian AJ, et al. Localization of a gene responsible for familial dilated cardiomyopathy to chromosome 1q32. Circulation 1995;92(12):3387-9.

22. Krajinovic M, Pinamonti B, Sinagra G, Vatta M, Severini GM, Milasin J, Falaschi A, Camerini F, Giacca M, Mestroni L, et al. Linkage of familial dilated cardiomyopathy to chromosome 9. Am J Hum Gen 1995;57(4):846-52.

23. Bowles KR, Gajarski R, Porter P, Goytia V, Bachinski L, Roberts R, Pignatelli R, Towbin JA. Gene mapping of familial autosomal dominant dilated cardiomyopathy to chromosome 10q21-23. J Clin Invest1996;98(6):1355-60.

24. Corrado D, Basso C, Thiene G, McKenna WJ, Davies MJ, Fontaliran F, Nava A, Silvestri F, Blomstrom-Lundqvist C, Wlodarska EK, et al. Spectrum of clinicopathologic manifestations of arrhythmogenic right ventricular cardiomyopathy/dysplasia: A multicenter study. J.Am.Coll.Cardiol. 1997;30(6):1512-20.

25. Marcus FI, Fontaine G. Arrhythmogenic right ventricular dysplasia/cardiomyopathy: A review. Pacing Clin.Electrophysiol. 1995;18(6):1298-314.

26. McKenna WJ, Thiene G, Nava A, Fontaliran F, Blomstrom-Lundqvist C, Fontaine G, Camerini F. Diagnosis of arrhythmogenic right ventricular dysplasia/cardiomyopathy. Br.Heart J. 1994;71(3):215-8.

27. Nava A, Canciani B, Thiene G, Scognamiglio R, Buja G, Martini B, Daliento L, Fasoli G, Stritoni P, Dalla VS. Analysis of the mode of transmission of right ventricular dysplasia. Arch.Mal.Coeur Vaiss. 1990;83(7):923-8.

28. Coonar A, Protonotarios N, Tsatsopoulou A, Needham S, Houlston R, Cliff S, Otter M, Murday V, Mattu R, McKenna WJ. Gene for Arrhythmogenic Right Ventricular Cardiomyopathy with diffuse nonepidermolytic palmoplantar keratoderma and woolly hair (Naxos Disease) maps to 17q21. Circulation 1998;97(20):2049

29. Rampazzo A, Nava A, Danieli GA, Buja G, Daliento L, Fasoli G, Scognamiglio R, Corrado D, Thiene G. The gene for arrhythmogenic right ventricular cardiomyopathy maps to chromosome 14q23-q24. Hum.Mol.Genet. 1994;3(6):959-62.

30. Rampazzo A, Nava A, Erne P, Eberhard M, Vian E, Slomp P, Tiso N, Thiene G, Danieli GA. A new locus for arrhythmogenic right ventricular cardiomyopathy (ARVD2) maps to chromosome 1q42-q43. Hum.Mol.Genet. 1995;4(11):2151-4.

31. Rampazzo A, Nava A, Miorin M, Fonderico P, Pope B, Tiso N, Livolsi B, Zimbello R, Thiene G, Danieli GA. ARVD4, a new locus for arrhythmogenic right ventricular cardiomyopathy, maps to chromosome 2 long arm. Genomics 1997;45(2):259-63.

32. Severini GM, Krajinovic M, Pinamonti B, Sinagra G, Fioretti P, Brunazzi, MC, Falaschi A, Camerini F, Giacca M, et al. A new locus for arrhythmogenic right ventricular dysplasia on the long arm of chromosome 14. Genomics 1996;31(2):193-200.

33. Tomita Y, Iijima M. Romano-Ward syndrome. Ryoikibetsu Shokogun Shirizu 1996;(12):211-4.

34. Aoki T. Jervell and Lange-Nielsen syndrome. Ryoikibetsu Shokogun Shirizu 1996;(12):188-91.

35. Schwartz PJ, Stramba-Badiale M, Segantini A, Austoni P, Bosi G, Giorgetti R, Grancini F, Marni E, Perticone F, Rosti D, et al. Prolongation of the QT Interval and the Sudden Infant Death Syndrome. N.Engl.J.Med 1998;338(24):1709-14.

36. Ackerman MJ. The long QT syndrome: Ion channel diseases of the heart. Mayo Clinic Proceedings 1998;73(3):250-69.

37. Wang Q, Shen J, Splawski I, Atkinson D, Li Z, Robinson JL, Moss AJ, Towbin JA, Keating MT. SCN5A mutations associated with an inherited cardiac arrhythmia, long QT syndrome. Cell 1995;80(5):805-11.

38. Satler CA, Walsh EP, Vesely MR, Plummer MH, Ginsburg GS, Jacob HJ. Novel missense mutation in the cyclic nucleotide-binding domain of HERG causes long QT syndrome. Am.J.Med Genet. 1996;65(1):27-35.

39. Neyroud N, Tesson F, Denjoy I, Leibovici M, Donger C, Barhanin J, Faure S, Gary F, Coumel P, Petit C, et al. A novel mutation in the potassium channel gene KVLQT1 causes the Jervell and Lange-Nielsen cardioauditory syndrome. Nat.Genet. 1997;15(2):186-9.

40. Duggal P, Vesely MR, Wattanasirichaigoon D, Villafane J, Kaushik V, Beggs AH. Mutation of the gene for IsK associated with both Jervell and Lange-Nielsen and Romano-Ward forms of Long-QT syndrome. Circulation 1998;97(2):142-6.

41. Donger C, Denjoy I, Berthet M, Neyroud N, Cruaud C, Bennaceur M, Chivoret G, Schwartz K, Coumel P, Guicheney P. KVLQT1 C-terminal missense mutation causes a forme fruste long-QT syndrome. Circulation 1997;96(9):2778-81.

42. Curran ME, Splawski I, Timothy KW, Vincent GM, Green ED, Keating MT. A molecular basis for cardiac arrhythmia: HERG mutations cause long QT syndrome. Cell 1995;80(5):795-803.

43. Moss AJ, Zareba W, Benhorin J, Locati EH, Hall WJ, Robinson JL, Schwartz PJ, Towbin JA, Vincent GM, Lehmann MH. ECG T-wave patterns in genetically distinct forms of the hereditary long QT syndrome. Circulation 1995;92(10):2929-34.

44. Priori SG, Napolitano C, Cantu F, Brown AM, Schwartz PJ. Differential response to Na+ channel blockade, beta-adrenergic stimulation, and rapid pacing in a cellular model mimicking the SCN5A and HERG defects present in the long-QT syndrome. Circ.Res. 1996;78(6):1009-15.

45. Keene DR, Jordan CD, Reinhardt DP, Ridgway CC, Ono RN, Corson GM, Fairhurst M, Sussman MD, Memoli VA, Sakai LY. Fibrillin-1 in human cartilage: developmental expression and formation of special banded fibers. J.Histochem.Cytochem. 1997;45(8):1069-82.

2. DILATED CARDIOMYOPATHY AND ARRHYTHMOGENIC RIGHT VENTRICULAR DYSPLASIA: FROM GENE TO PHENOTYPE

ANGELA POLETTI, CHIARA ROCCO, SNJEZANA MIOCIC AND
LUISA MESTRONI

DILATED CARDIOMYOPATHY

Dilated cardiomyopathy (DC) is characterized by dilatation and impaired contraction of the left or both ventricles. In the last few decades, it has been one of the most largely investigated heart diseases. Nevertheless, by now, its etiology still represents a challenge and the diagnosis is mainly based on the exclusion of any specific heart muscle disease, i.e. any disease associated with known cardiac or systemic disorder. Due to the scarce knowledge, the classification of the ethiologic factors is still tentative [1].

In the past, the presence of a familial aggregation of the disease was reported but certainly underestimated. In fact, in that studies the frequency of familiarity was less than 10%. With the growing interest for this problem and the evolution of molecular genetic techniques, prospective and finalized studies have been performed, demonstrating that genetic factors play a major role in the pathogenesis of the disease. The occurrence of a genetic transmission (familial DC or FDC) in controlled studies is detectable in about one third of patients with DC [2-4].

The research on the ethiology of FDC is complicated by the clinical and genetic heterogeneity. In our population, at least six different subgroups of FDC have been identified based on the patterns of inheritance, the clinical

19

H.-H. Osterhues et al. (eds.),
Advances in Noninvasive Electrocardiographic Monitoring Techniques, 19–26.
© 2000 *Kluwer Academic Publishers. Printed in the Netherlands.*

features and, when available, the genetic data[5] . The most common form in our population (56% of cases) was the autosomal dominant FDC, characterized by development of ventricular dilation and systolic dysfunction, with progressive heart failure and ventricular arrhythmia, and reduced and age-related penetrance. In the last few years, a disease locus has been identified on chromosome 9 [6] in italian kindreds with this form of FDC, while in a Utah family with similar clinical features, a second locus was localized on chromosome lq32 [7]. Finally, another locus has been reported on the short arm of chromosome 10 (l0q21-23) [8] in one large kindred, characterized by the association of DC with mitral valve prolapse and by high penetrance.

Autosomal recessive FDC was represented in the 16% of our patients. A peculiar and rare form of familial DC is a dominant cardiac conduction system disease with later development of dilated cardiomyopathy, named CDDC [9]. The affected family members manifest arrhythmias and atrio-ventricular block in the second to third decade of life, and a progressive cardiomegaly and heart failure in the fifth to sixth decade. In a large Ohio family, a first locus containing the disease gene was mapped in the centromere of chromosome 1 (lpl - lql) [10]. Recently, in another CDDC family of Swiss-German ancestry, linkage was found with the short arm of chromosome 3 (3p22-p25) [11].

The first known disease gene responsible for dilated cardiomyopathy was the dystrophin gene. Mutations or deletions of this gene cause the Duchenne and Becker muscular dystrophies as well as the X-linked dilated cardiomyopathy (XLDC or XLCM) [12,13]. XLDC is a rapidly progressive DC, presenting generally in young males as a congestive heart failure, in the absence of clinical signs of skeletal myopathy. Affected family members can have a mild increase of muscle creatine kinase (MM-CK). Manifesting female carriers have later onset of the disease, as well as a slower progression. This condition is characterized by the transmission of DC with the X chromosome (no male-to-male transmission), in a dominant fashion [14]. The identification of deletions in the region containing the muscle promoter - first muscle exon in two XLDC families [13, 15] suggested a critical role of the 5' end of the gene for the expression of dystrophin in the heart. This hypothesis was supported by the subsequent findings of two different point mutations in the same region of the gene in two further XLDC families[16, 17]. Finally, in-frame deletions in the region of the exon 48 of the dystrophin gene, previously described in patients with Becker muscle dystrophy associated with DC, can also lead to a typical XLDC phenotype [18]. It is therefore possible that different defects both within critical functional regions of the dystrophin protein, or defects in the regulation of the expression of the dystrophin mRNA could lead to the XLDC phenotype.

By analogy with dystrophin, other cytoskeletal proteins appear to be potential candidates for causing dilated cardiomyopathy. Deficiency of adhalin, a dystrophin-associated glycoprotein, has recently been described in a patient with DC associated with signs of muscle dystrophy [19]. A deficiency of transcription of meta-vinculin (the cardiac isoform of vinculin) has been shown in a patient with FDC [20]. Morcover, delta-sarcoglycan has been found to be the cause of the Syrian hamster cardiomyopathy [21]. Very recently variants of exons 5 and 6 of actin cardiac gene on chromosome 15ql4 have been demonstrated in two families with dilated cardiomyopathy.

The analysis of our families led to the isolation of another subgroup of families with subclinical skeletal muscle involvement resembling the one seen in XLDC, but with autosomal dominant pattern of transmission [18]: the main features of this group were the absence of overt signs of muscular dystrophy, frequent conduction defects and ventricular arrhythmia, inconstant mild increase of serum CK. Molecular genetic studies are being undertaken in the hypothesis that an altered protein of the cytoskeletal network could be responsible for this form.

Unclassifiable FDC include families with different pattern of disease such as left ventricular apical hypertrophy or associated retinitis pigmentosa; no data have been yet published on the genetic basis of these forms.

Finally, the possibility that mitochondrial DNA (mtDNA) defects may underlie DC has long been considered, in particular in families with suspected matrilineal transmission of the disease [22]. The development of cardiomyopathy with dilatation, dysfunction with or without hypertrophy, is a common clinical feature of several mitochondrial syndromes [23, 24], in which there is invariably a multi-organ involvement and a wide clinical variability due to heteroplasmy. If the causal role of deletions in DC is controversial, and seems to be related rather to the severity of the myocardial dysfunction and to the age, on the other hand, point mutations of the mtDNA could have a pathogenetic role in a subset cases with isolated DC [25].

The identification of a familial and a "sporadic" form of DC and of different subgroups of FDC led to the research of predictive factors of each form. Nevertheless clinical features able to distinguish between sporadic and familial and among the different familial forms couldn't be ascertained by now. In particular, arrhythmia have been demonstrated in all the forms and no data are available on being more represented in FDC in comparison to sporadic DC, and neither in a form of FDC in comparison to another. Moreover preliminary data on our population, suggest that there was no difference in mortality for sudden death versus heart failure in different subgroups.

ARRHYTHMOGENIC RIGHT VENTRICULAR DYSPLASIA

As defined by the Task Force of the Working Group of Myocardial and Pericardial Disease of the European Society of Cardiology, arrhythmogenic right ventricular dysplasia (ARVD) or cardiomyopathy is a heart muscle disorder of unknown cause that is characterized pathologically by fibro-fatty replacement of the right ventricular myocardium [26] The first cases were described in 1977 by Fontaine et al. [27], but until now, its real incidence is still unknown. Males seem to be more frequently affected than females, with a ratio of 2:1 and 3:1. According to some data its prevalence is estimated from 6/10000 to 4.4/1000 in some geographical areas appear to present a higher prevalence, estimated from 4.4/1000 up to 6/10000 individuals [28]. The few ethio-pathogenetic theories include inheritance, disontogenesis, a degenerative process, or inflammation due to both viral persistence or to an autoimmune reaction. More recently, the theory of "apoptosis", or programmed premature cell death, has been proposed [29].

ARVD was initially considered as a consequence of a developmental defect, although the late onset in some cases and the evidence of evolutivity of the disease during aging [30] do not support this theory. Data on the presence and significance of inflammatory infiltrates are still controversial: in particular, it is still non clear how an autoimmune response or an aspecific inflammation against other noxae could affect selectively some cardiac structures leading to a progressive fibrosis.

Some experimental data documented the development of right ventricular aneurysm in BALB/c rates after selective perimyocarditis due to Coxsackie virus [31]. However, studies on endomyocardial biopsies or on explanted hearts of affected patients failed to demonstrate enteroviral particles [32]. Furthermore, the incidence of organ-specific cardiac autoantibodies were the same in the relatives of ill patients as in the control group [33], and no other evidences of an autoimmune process were found in ARVD. These findings suggest that inflammation could represent an aspecific response to cell death.

On the other hand, the variability in prevalence of ARVD with a possible *founder effect* in some geographical areas as well as the frequent familial occurrence confirm the importance of a genetic background in this disease. The first familial forms were reported by Marcus in 1982 [34]. The frequency of the familial form of ARVD was estimated to be about 30% in non- controlled studies [26], with an autosomal dominant transmission and variable penetrance and clinical expression. However, the frequency of familiarity could be underestimated since prospective studies based on systematic family screening are still missing. The variability in the phenotype and in the age of onset

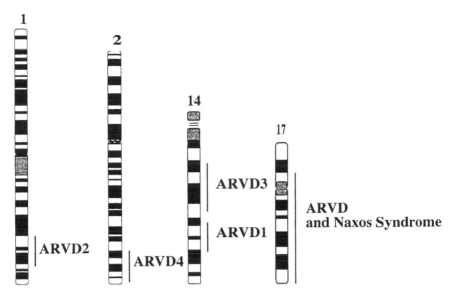

Figure 1. Known disease loci for arrhythmogenic right ventricular cardiomyopathy or dysplasia (ARVD).

suggest genetic heterogeneity which indicates that different genes could be responsible for the disease.

Recently, a relevant contribution was obtained in the study of ARVD by molecular genetics: using molecular genetic techniques and linkage analysis, in a large pedigree with over 80 family members, and in another small family, the first disease gene was mapped in the long arm of chromosome 14 (14q23-q24) [28]. Subsequently, other ARVD loci have been identified: one on chromosome 1 (1q42-q43) [35] in a single large kindred, and the other on chromosome 14 (14q12-q22) [36] in three unrelated families (locus D14S252). Finally, preliminary data of a linkage study on the Naxos syndrome (ARVD associated with palmoplantar keratoderma and woolly hair) suggest the existence of another ARVD locus on chromosome 17 (17plq3) [37] (Figure 1). These findings support the hypothesis of genetic heterogeneity. However, the disease genes are still unknown and are under investigation.

Conclusions: At present, both in familial DC and ARVD very little is known about the correlations between phenotype and genotype. In our patient population, we could not identify any significant difference in the clinical expression between sporadic and familial cases in both diseases. The definition of this important aspect will await the identification of the molecular basis of the disease.

REFERENCES

1. Report, of the 1995 World Health Organization/International Society and Federation of Cardiolgy Task Force on the Definition and Classification of Cardiomyopathies. Circulation 1996;93:841-842.
2. Michels VV, Moll PP, Miller FA, Tajik AJ, Chu JS, Driscoll DJ, Burnett JC, Rodeheffer RJ, Chesebro JH, Tazelaar H. The frequency of familial dilated cardiomyopathy in a series of patients with idiopathic dilated cardiomyopathy. NEngl JMed 1992;326:77-82.
3. Keeling PJ, Gang G, Smith G, Seo H, Bent SE, Murday V, Caforio ALP, McKenna WJ. Familial dilated cardiomyopathy in the United Kingdom. Br Heart J 1995;73:417-421.
4. Gregori D, Rocco C, Di Lenarda A, Sinagra G, Miocic S, Camerini F, Mestroni L. Estimating the frequency of familial dilated cardiomyopathy and the risk of misclassification errors. Circulation 1996;94:1-270.
5. Rocco C, Gregori D, Miocic S, Di Lenarda A, Sinagra G, Caforio AL, Vatta M, Matulic Mt Zerial T, Giacca M, Mestroni L. New insight into the gentic of dilated cardiomyopathy. Circulation 1997;96:I-696.
6. Krajinovic M, Pinamonti B, Sinagra G, Vatta M, Severini GM, Milasin J, Falaschi A, Camerini F, Giacca M, Mestroni L. Linkage of familial dilated cardiomyopathy to chromosome 9. Am J Hum Genet 1995;57:846-852.
7. Durand J-B, Bachinski LL, Bieling LC, Czernuszewicz GZ, Abchee AB, Yu QT, Tapscott T, Hill R, Ifegwu J, Marian AJ, Brugada R, Daiger S, Gregoritch JM, Anderson JL, Quinones M, Towbin JA, Roberts R. Localization of a gene responsible for familial dilated cardiomyopathy to chromosome lq32. Circulation 1995;92:3387-3389.
8. Bowles KL, Gajarski R, Porter P, Goytia V, Bachinski L, Roberts R, Pignatelli R, Towbin JA. Gene mapping of familial autosomal dominant dilated cardiomyopathy to chromosome 10q21-23. J Clin Invest 1996;98:1355-1360.
9. Graber HL, Unverferth DV, Baker PB, Rayan JM, Baba N, Wooley CF. Evolution of a hereditary cardiac conduction and muscle disorder: a study involving a family with six generations affected. Circulation 1986;74:325-327.
10. Kass S, MacRae C, Graber HL, Sparks EA, McNamara D, Boudoulas H, Basson CT, Baker III PB, Cody RJ, Fishman MC, Cox N, Kong A, Wooley CF, Seidman JG, Seidman CE. A gene defect that causes conduction system disease and dilated cardiomyopathy maps to chromosome lpl-lql. Nature Genet 1994;7:546-551.
11. Olson TM, Keating MT. Mapping a cardiomyopathy locus to chromosome 3p22-p25. J Clin Invest 1996;97:528-532.
12. Towbin JA, Hejtmancik F, Brink P, Gelb BD, Zhu XM, Chamberlain JS, McCabe ERB, Swift M. X-linked cardiomyopathy (XLCM): molecular genetic evidence of linkage to the Duchenne muscular dystrophy (dystrophin) gene at the Xp21 locus. Circulation 1993;87: 1854-1865.
13. Muntoni F, Cau M, Ganau A, Congiu R, Arvedi G, Mateddu A, Morrosu MG, Cianchetti C, Realdi G, Cao A, Melis MA. Deletion of the dystrophin muscle-promoter region associated with X-linked dilated cardiomyopathy. N Engl JMed 1993;329:921-925.
14. Berko B, Swift M. X-linked dilated cardiomyopathy. N Engl J Med 1987;316:1186-1191.
15. Yoshida K, Ikeda SI, Nakamura A, Kagoshima M, Takeda S, Shoji S, Yanagisawa N. Molecular analysis of the Duchenne muscular dystrophy gene in patients with Becker

muscular dystrophy presenting with dilated cardiomyopathy. Muscle & Nerve 1993;16: 1161-1166.

16. Milasin J, Muntoni F, Severini GM, Bartoloni L, Vatta M, Krajinovic M, Mateddu A, Angelini C, Camerini Г, Falaschi A, Mestroni L, Giacca M. Λ point mutation in the 5' splice site of the dystrophin gene first intron responsible for X-linked dilated cardiomyopathy. Hum Mol Genet 1996;5:73-79.

17. Ortiz-Lopez R, Li H, Su J, Goytia V, Towbin JA. Evidence for a dystrophin missense mutation as a cause of X-linked dilated cardiomyopathy (XLCM). Circulation 1997;95:2434-2440.

18. Mestroni LM, F.; Milasin, J.; Di Lenarda, A.; Sinagra, G.; Rocco, C.; Vatta, M.; Matulic, M.; Falaschi, A.; Camerini, F.; Giacca, M. Familial dilated cardiomyopathy with subclinical skeletal involvement. Circulation 1996;94:I-271.

19. Fadic R, Sunada Y, Waclawik AJ, Buck S, Lewandoski PJ, Campbell KP, Lotz BP. Brief report: deficiency of a dystrophin-associated glycoprotein (adhalin) in a patient with muscular dystrophy and cardiomyopathy. N Engl J Med 1996;334:362-366.

20. Maeda M, Holder E, Lowes B, Bies RD. Dilated cardiomyopathy associated with deficiency of the cytoskeletal protein metavinculin. Circulation 1997;95:17-20.

21. Nigro V, Okasaki Y, Belsito A, Piluso G, Matsuda Y, Politano L, Nigro G, Ventura C, Abbondanza C, Molinari AM, Acampora D, M. M, Hayashizaki Y, Puca GA. Identification of the syrian Hamster cardiomyopathy gene. Hum Mol Genet 1997;6:601-607.

22. Suomalainen A, Paetau A, Leinonen H, Majander A, Peltonen L, Somer H. Inherited dilated cardiomyopathy with multiple deletions of mitochondrial DNA. Lancet 1992;340: 1319-1320.

23. Santorelli FM, Mak S-C, El-Schahawi M, Casali C, Shanske S, Baram TZ, Madrid RE, DiMauro S. Maternally inherited cardiomyopathy associated with a novel mutation in the mitochondrial tRNA Lys gene (G8363A). Am J Hum Genet 1996;58:933-939.

24. Zeviani M, Gellera C, Antozzi C, Rimoldi M, Morandi L, Villani F, Tiranti V, DiDonato S. Maternally inherited myopathy and cardiomyopathy: association with mutation in mitochondrial DNA tRNA Leu(UUR). Lancet 1991;338:143-147.

25. Grasso M, Fasani R, Diegoli M, Bianchieri N, Porcu E, Concardi M, Pilotto A, Fortina P, Surrey S, Vigano' M, Arbustini E. Mitochondrial DNA base changes in sporadic and familial dilated cardiomyopathy (DCM) and in controls. J Mol Med 1995;73:A28.

26. McKenna WJ, Thiene G, Nava A, Fontaliran F, Blomstrom-Lunqvist C, Fontaine G, Camerini F. Diagnosis of arrhythmogenic right ventricular dysplasia/cardiomyopathy. Br Heart J 1994;71:215-218.

27. Fontaine GH, Guiraudon G, Franc R. Stimulation studies and epicardial mapping in VT: study of mechanisms and selection for surgery. In: Kulbertus H (ed.) Reentrant arrhythmias, Lancaster PA, MTP, 1977:334-350.

28. Rampazzo A, Nava A, Danieli GA, Buja G, Daliento L, Fasoli G, Scognamiglio R, Corrado D, Thiene G. The gene for arrhythmogenic right ventricular cardiomyopathy maps to chromosome 14q23-q24. Hum. Mol. Genet. 1994;3:959-962.

29. Mallat Z, Tedgui A, Fontaliran F, Frank R, Durigon M, Fontaine G. Evidence of apoptosis in arrhythmogenic right ventricular dysplasia. N Engl J Med 1996;335: 1190-6.

30. Daliento L, Turrini P, Nava A, Rizzoli G, Angelini A, Buia G, Sognamiglio R, Thiene G. Arrhythmogenic right ventricular cardiomyopathy in young versus adult patients: similarities and differences. J Am Coll Cardiol 1995;25:6555-664.
31. Matsumori A, Kawai C. Coxsackie virus B 3 perimyocarditis in balb-C mice: experimental model of cronic perimyocarditis in the right ventricle. J Pathol 1980; 131 :97- 106.
32. Thiene G, Corrado D, Nava A, Rossi L, Poletti A, Boffa GM, Daliento L, Pennelli N. Right ventricular cardiomyopathy: is there evidence of an inflammatory aethiology? Eur Heart J 1991;12:22-25.
33. Hoffmann R, Trappe HG, Klein H, Kemnitz J. Chronic (or healed) myocarditis mimicking arrhythmogenic right ventricular dysplasia. Eur Heart J 1993;14:717-720.
34. Marcus FI, Fontaine GH, Giraudon G, Franc R, Laurenceau JL, Mallergue C, Grosgogeat Y. Right ventricular dysplasia: report of 24 adult cases. Circulation 1982;65:384- 398.
35. Rampazzo A, Nava A, Erne P, Eberhard M, Vian E, Slomp P, Tiso N, Thiene G, Danieli GA. A new locus for arrhythmogenic right ventricular cardiomyopathy (ARVD2) maps to chromosome lq42-q43. Hum. Mol. Genet. 1995;4:2151-2154.
36. Severini GM, Krajinovic M, Pinamonti B, Sinagra G, Fioretti P, Brunazzi MC, Falaschi A, Camerini F, Giacca M, Mestroni L. A new locus for arrhythmogenic right ventricular dysplasia on the long arm of chromosome 14. Genomics 1996;31:193-200.
37. Coonar AS, Protonotarios N, Tsatsopoulou A, Needham EWA, Murady VA, Houlston RS, Cliff S, Otter MI, Mattu RK, McKenna WJ. A gene locus for arrhythmogenic right ventricular cardiomyopathy maps to chromosome 17pl-q3. J Am Coll Cardiol 1997;29:4A.

3. HEART FAILURE: FROM GENE TO THERAPY

OLIVER ZOLK, STEPHANIE BAUDLER, GEORG NICKENIG AND
MICHAEL BÖHM

Congestive heart failure is the final endstage of various cardiac diseases with varying pathologies resulting in impaired systolic and diastolic function, activation of neurohumoral pathways, and high morbidity and mortality. The pathogenic processes leading to altered structure of the heart in the development of heart failure with systolic dysfunction has been termed „ventricular remodeling". This concept relates to a complex of anatomical, physiological, histological and molecular changes of the myocardium in response to injury and increased wall stress (Fig. 1). Our understanding of ventricular remodeling has rapidly progressed from initial bedside observation of large hearts and edema in patients with heart disease to studies of the mechanical consequences of increased volumes, hemodynamic changes and wall stress in the failing left ventricle. Following the discovery of the neurohumoral activation in heart failure, more recently, attention has been attracted to the molecular and genetic alterations that promote further detoriation of the function of the heart and that determine the inexorable course to end-stage heart failure.

A mammalian organism contains about 100,000 different genes. Only a small fraction, approximately 15%, are expressed in each individual cell. It is the choice of which genes are expressed that determines all life processes, development and differentiation, homeostasis, response to insults, cell cycle regulation, ageing, and even programmed cell death. The course of normal development as well as the pathological changes that arise in syndromes such as heart failure, whether caused by a single gene mutation or a complex of multigene effects, are driven by changes of gene expression. Answering basic questions about cardiac muscle differentiation program, gene regulation, and

27

H.-H. Osterhues et al. (eds.),
Advances in Noninvasive Electrocardiographic Monitoring Techniques, 27–38.

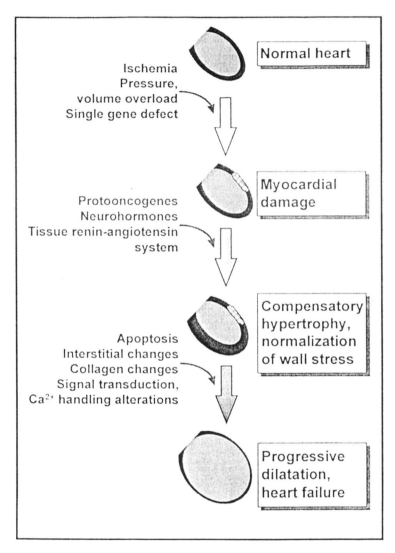

Figure 1. Pathogenic mechanisms operating in a patient undergoing myocardial damage. Changes in gene expression with reactivation of "fetal" genes and activation of neuroendocrine systems like the renin-angiotensin- or the β-adrenergic system, promote myocardial hypertrophy. Alterations in β-adrenergic signal transduction and Ca^{2+} handling may underlie progressive systolic and diastolic dysfunction. The end-result in many patients is progressive ventricular dilatation and advancing heart failure.

disease pathophysiology has become a prerequisite for identification of new targets and for developing new therapies for heart failure. There are several areas in which significant progress has been made: the genetic mechanisms of inherited cardiomyopathies, the identification of risk-genes and the characterization of changes in gene expression pattern in the failing myocardium.

FAMILIAR CARDIOMYOPATHY

Primary familiar cardyomyopathy was the first cardiovascular disease characterized by molecular genetics in 1990 (1,2). It was mapped to the chromosome 14q11-12 locus, which has been identified as the gene for the beta-myosin heavy chain (2). There is now a long list of cardiomyopathies for which the gene loci have been mapped and, for many, the genes have been fully characterized. In patients with hypertrophic cardiomyopathy due to beta myosin heavy chain alterations, over 40 mutations have been identified. Some of these mutations are associated with a high incidence of sudden cardiac death. However, various mutations were shown to have varying degrees of significance for prognosis and it has been suggested that besides genetic abnormality environmental factors exert a significant effect on the course of the disease. A detailed description of the genetic background of familiar cardiomyopathies is given in another article of this issue.

GENETIC RISK FACTORS IN HEART FAILURE

In 1988 Soubrier and coworkers (3) reported the sequence of human angiotensin converting enzyme (ACE) cDNA. Two years later a deletion/insertion polymorphism of the human ACE-gene was characterized by Cambien et al. (4). Depending on the incorporation of the ALU-repeat sequence into intron 16 of the ACE-gene, an individual has one of three possible ACE geneotypes: the homozygous genotypes II or DD, or the heterozygous genotype ID. In their first report on 80 subjects, about half of the interindividual variance in circulating ACE-activity was related to this polymorphism (4). More recently this polymorphism has been implicated in the pathogenesis of a variety of cardiovascular disorders, including left ventricular hypertrophy and heart failure (5). Studies analyzing the genotypes of patients with hypertrophic, dilated or ischemic cardiomyopathy showed that the DD-genotype was more common in these patients compared to normal individuals (6,7). However, whether the ACE DD genotype is a risk factor cannot be determined until larger population studies are completed. In addition to the DD ACE-genotype risk for cardiovascular disease, molecular variants of angiotensinogen and the angiotensin II type-1 (AT1) receptor now being

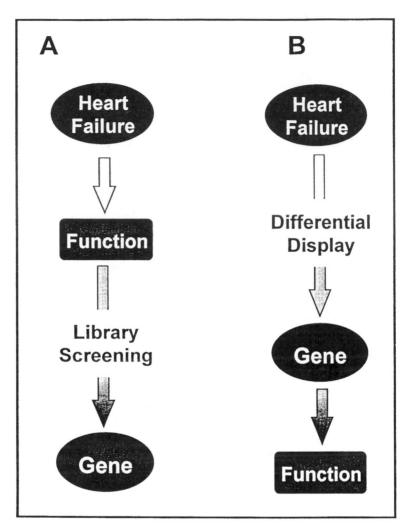

Figure 2. Strategies for identification of heart failure candidate genes. In general, two approaches for identification of genes associated with the pathogenesis of heart failure are possible: (i) The study of gene function precedes gene identification. Information about function are used for specific screening of cDNA- or expression-libraries. (ii) Genes which are differentially expressed in failing myocardium are identified by techniques like mRNA differential display, differential hybridisation or subtractive library screening. In a second step the function of these genes and their relevance for pathogenesis of heart failure is characterized.

identified as potential risk factors (8,9). From these examples, one can expect many genetic risk factors to be discovered within the next few years. These genes may be readily typed and developed into routine diagnostic tests, causing a great impact on the diagnostic and therapeutic practice in cardiology.

APPROACHES FOR IDENTIFICATION OF CANDIDATE GENES

Several methods have been developed in the last decade to identify candidate genes potentially involved in the pathogenesis of heart failure (Fig 2). mRNA differential display is found to be one of the most flexible and comprehensive method available for the detection of heart failure candidate genes. The principal strategy is to amplify partial cDNA sequences from subsets of mRNAs by reverse transcription and polymerase chain reaction. These short sequences are then displayed on a sequencing gel. Pairs of primers are selected so that each will amplify DNA from about 50-100 mRNA because this number is optimal for display on the gel (Fig 3). Individual bands differentially expressed can readily be cloned and used as probes for Northern (10) or Southern (genomic DNA) blotting or to isolate genes from genomic libraries. Furthermore, these cDNAs can be sequenced and compared with sequences in data banks. First successful applications of this novel technique indicate that major cytoskeleton proteins like titin are differentially expressed in pressure overload hypertrophy and heart failure (11).

The mRNA differential display has the advantage of high sensitivity and multiple side-by-side comparison of both up- and down-regulated genes. However, it has the disadvantage of high incidence of false positive results. An alternative strategy which combines recombinant cloning strategies and immunological analysis allows to rapidly screen for genes participating in autoimmune processes which may be involved in the pathogenesis of heart failure. Recently this technique has been applied to myocardial tissue isolated from a patient with dilated cardiomyopathy (DCM). A human DCM expression library was constructed and the expressed myocardial antigens were screened with the serum of the patient. Thereby, myocardial recombination signal binding protein-jκ (RBP-jκ) was identified as a gene potentially involved in the pathogenesis of human dilated cardiomyopathy (12).

CHANGES IN GENE EXPRESSION

A major field of recent investigation has been to describe changes in the expression of genes in heart failure. Because the cardiac β-adrenergic system plays a pivotal role in cardiac function and adaptation, investigations have focused on changes in the expression of proteins that are involved in β-

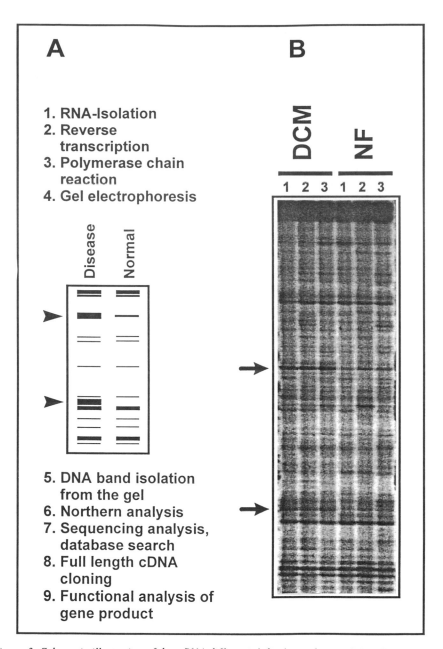

Figure 3. Schematic illustration of the mRNA differential display technique (A) and representative autoradiograph of differential display products for RNA isolated from hearts with dilative cardiomyopathy (DCM) and non-failing (NF) control myocardium (B). Arrows indicate genes that are depressed for their mRNA-expression in DCM-hearts.

adrenergic signal transduction processes and excitation-contraction coupling. In the failing human heart, the β-adrenergic system is characterized by a decreased responsiveness which is in part due to agonist-mediated down-regulation of β-adrenoceptors and an increased amount of Gi-proteins (10,13). The decreased β-adrenoceptor number has been shown to be specific for the β1-adrenergic receptor, which is the predominant subtype in human heart (14). Besides internalization and degradation by lysosomal enzymes, β-adrenoceptor downregulation is mediated via reduction of receptor synthesis by decreased levels of receptor mRNA (15). This in turn seems to be the consequence of alterations of the transcription rate and destabilization of the mRNA (16,17). Transient expression of luciferase reporter gene constructs indicates that the 5′flanking region consists of positive and negative transcriptional regulatory elements (17). However, the precise mechanism of transcriptional regulation is not yet characterized. In addition, it has been demonstrated that β-adrenoceptor mRNA expression is regulated via modulation of mRNA turnover (18). Agonist-mediated destabilization of β-adienosceptor mRNA has been associated with mRNA-binding proteins coupling to the 3′untranslated region of human β-adrenoceptor mRNA (16,19). Thus, mRNA destabilization may be a decisive mechanism leading to decreased β-adrenoceptor mRNA expression in heart failure.

Increased expression of the inhibitory G-protein is assumed to contribute to desensitization of adenylyl cyclase in heart failure. Increased Giα2 mRNA levels after prolonged in vivo β-adrenoceptor stimulation are caused by enhanced transcription of Giα2-mRNA in the ventricular myocardium of Wistar-Kyoto-rats, as shown in nuclear run on assays (20). Studies of the effects of cAMP on the Giα2 promotor activity by reporter gene assays in cultured cardiomyocytes indicate that increases in intracellular cAMP upregulates Giα promotor activity which probably represents a predominant mechanism of regulation (21). The promoter region of the Giα2 gene possesses a binding domain for activator protein-2 (AP-2), which is a cAMP-dependent transcription promoting factor (22).

Another area of investigation in the mechanisms of progression to heart failure involves changes in the expression of genes involved in intracellular calcium handling. Especially sarcoplasmic calcium proteins were studied extensively in the past years using conventional animal models, transgenic analyses, and gene targeting approaches (16,23,25). Calcium uptake by the sarcoplasmic reticulum is the main mechanism responsible for cardiac relaxation (26). Transport of calcium ions takes place against a concentration gradient mediated by the sarcoplasmic reticulum ATPase (27). Similar as myosin and actin, SERCA represents a multigene family (28). One of the isogenes, SERCA2, is alternatively spliced at its 3′end and one of the mRNAs, SERCA2a, is present in adult cardiac muscle (28). Most authors agree that a decrease in

SERCA2a steady state mRNA level occurs in conditions of hemodynamic overload and end stage heart failure (29). Obviously, the decrease in SERCA2a mRNA expression is not the result of an isoform switch. In contrast, the results regarding function and protein levels have been discussed more controversial. A decreased SERCA-activity resulting in reduced Ca^{2+} reuptake (27,29) and a decrease in SERCA2a protein quantity has been shown in large series of failing human hearts (30,32) whereas other studies indicate neither a reduced sarcoplasmic Ca^{2+} uptake (33) nor an alteration in SERCA2a protein (34).

Phospholamban inhibits SERCA2a with this inhibition being attenuated by phosphorylation. The role of phospholamban in the regulation of basal myocardial contractility has been recently elucidated through the generation of transgenic mice with different phospholamban protein expression levels ranging from 0% to 200% of the phospholamban levels present in wild-type mice (23,35,36). Phospholamban knockout mice display increased systolic function and increased rates of left ventricular relaxation (36), whereas expression of additional phospholamban molecules results in contractile dysfunction due to an inhibition of the sarcoplasmic Ca^{2+}-transport (23). These findings indicate that phospholamban acts as a critical repressor of basal myocardial contractility and may be a key phosphoprotein in mediating the cardiac contractile responses to β-adrenergic agonists. However, phospholamban mRNA or phospholamban protein expression is slightly if at all reduced in the failing human myocardium (27,30,34). Rather than alterations of phospholamban content, a reduced phospholamban phosphorylation in the failing myocardium seems to account for the diminished cardiac capacity to restore low resting Ca^{2+}-levels during diastole and diminished lusitropic and inotropic responses to β-agonists (37).

PERSPECTIVES

In recent years, the striking development of molecular biology and molecular genetics has brought completely new insights into the pathogenetic understanding of heart failure. Molecular changes in heart failure, as shown in this review, may be the consequence of primary gene defects, or altered gene expression as a consequence of transcriptional or posttranscriptional regulation processes. Understanding the molecular mechanisms of heart failure facilitates the discovery of novel and helps to optimize existing therapeutic strategies. The molecular cloning of target molecules and the development of in vivo heart failure assay systems in genetically manipulated animals has led to rapid throughout screening approaches to identify appropriate pharmaceutical agonists or antagonists (38). The forthcoming introduction of the first endothelin-receptor antagonists into clinical practise not more than one decade after the discovery of endothelin or the design of a β-adrenoceptor blocker with additional α1-adrenoceptor blocking and antioxidant properties like carvedilol may serve as a prime examples.

Recognizing the possible role that intrinsic cardiac genes may play in pathogenesis of heart failure, a systematic search for such genes needs to be conducted. One important strategy is the separation and identification of differentially expressed mRNAs in pairs of failing and non-failing hearts by means of the polymerase chain reaction (39). Such candidate genes may be further characterized, localized to specific cell types, and expressed in order to explore the protein of interest. Ultimately, transgenic overexpression or gene knock-out animal models may be engineered that may allow hypothesis testing for gene function and determination of the relevance of the candidate genes to heart failure. The technology needed to pursue all aspects of such strategies has been developed, and its use in the search for genes related to heart failure has begun. Once candidate genes are known, gene therapy strategies could be developed as a potential treatment for heart diseases (40,41). Currently, gene therapy remains experimental, with the majority of work having been performed in animal models (42). In vitro studies have shown that adenoviral gene transfer for the β-adrenoceptor or an inhibitor of the β-adrenoceptor kinase1 was able to restore β-adrenergic signaling deficiencies in failing ventricular cardiomyocytes (43). The gene transfer of SERCA2a to isolated rat myocytes has been shown to cause an abbreviated relaxation phase and enhanced contractility (44). These experiments gives an indication of the clinical potential that can be realized once the technical obstacles facing direct gene transfer have been overcome. Viral vectors are used as a vehicle to introduce the genes of interest into the living cells. However, the use of currently available transfer vector systems has been limited by low transfection efficiencies and/or immunogenecity they provoke in host tissues (41). As gene therapy vectors improve, they will become an important route by which the identification of candidate genes for heart failure can find direct clinical application.

REFERENCES

1. Geisterfer-Lowrance AA, Kass S, Tanigawa G, Vosberg HP, McKenna W, Seidman CE: A molecular basis for familial hypertrophic cardiomyopathy: a beta cardiac myosin heavy chain gene missense mutation. *Cell* 1990;62:999-1006

2. Solomon SD, Geisterfer-Lowrance AA, Vosberg HP, Hiller G, Jarcho JA, Morton CC, McBride WO, Mitchell AL, Bale AE, McKenna WJ: A locus for familial hypertrophic cardiomyopathy is closely linked to the cardiac myosin heavy chain genes, CRI-L436, and CRI-L329 on chromosome 14 at q11-q12. *Am.J.Hum.Genet.* 1990;47:389-394

3. Soubrier F, Alhenc-Gelas F, Hubert C, Allegrini J, John M, Tregear G, Corvol P: Two putative active centers in human angiotensin I-converting enzyme revealed by molecular cloning. *Proc.Natl.Acad.Sci.U.S.A.* 1988;85:9386-9390

4. Rigat B, Hubert C, Alhenc-Gelas F, Cambien F, Corvol P, Soubrier F: An insertion/deletion polymorphism in the angiotensin I-converting enzyme gene accounting for half of th variance of serum enzyme levels. *J.Clin.Invest.* 1990;86:1343-1346

5. Schunkert H, Hense HW, Holmer SR, Stender M, Perz S, Keil U, Lorell BH, Riegger GA: Association between a deletion polymorphism of the angiotensin- converting-enzyme gene and left ventricular hypertrophy. *N.Engl.J.Med.* 1994;330:1634-1638

6. Raynolds MV, Bristow MR, Bush EW, Abraham WT, Lowes BD, Zisman LS, Taft CS, Perryman MB: Angiotensin-converting enzyme DD genotype in patients with ischaemic or idiopathic dilated cardiomyopathy. *Lancet* 1993;342:1073-1075

7. Andersson B, Sylven C: The DD genotype of the angiotensin-converting enzyme gene is associated with increased mortality in idiopathic heart failure. *J.Am.Coll.Cardiol.* 1996;28:162-167

8. Raynolds MV, Perryman MB: The role of genetic variants in angiotensin I converting enzyme, angiotensinogen and the angiotensin II type-1 receptor in the pathophysiology of heart muscle disease. *Eur.Heart J.* 1995;16 Suppl K:23-30

9. Tiret L, Bonnardeaux A, Poirier O, Ricard S, Marques-Vidal P, Evans A, Arveiler D, Luc G, Kee F, Ducimetiere P: Synergistic effects of angiotensin-converting enzyme and angiotensin-II type 1 receptor gene polymorphisms on risk of myocardial infarction. *Lancet* 1994;344:910-913

10. Böhm M, Lohse MJ: Quantification of beta-adrenoceptors and beta-adrenoceptor kinase on protein and mRNA levels in heart failure. *Eur.Heart J.* 1994;15 Suppl D:30-34

11. Collins JF, Pawloski-Dahm C, Davis MG, Ball N, Dorn GW, Walsh RA: The role of the cytoskeleton in left ventricular pressure overload hypertrophy and failure. *J.Mol.Cell Cardiol.* 1996;28:1435-1443

12. Nickenig G, Wolff M, Böhm M: Enhanced expression and autoimmunity of recombinant binding protein-jκ in human dilated cardiomyopathy. *Circulation* 1998;98(suppl):I-406

13. Böhm M, Eschenhagen T, Gierschik P, Larisch K, Lensche H, Mende U, Schmitz W, Schnabel P, Scholz H, Steinfath M: Radioimmunochemical quantification of Gi alpha in right and left ventricles from patients with ischaemic and dilated cardiomyopathy and predominant left ventricular failure. *J.Mol.Cell Cardiol.* 1994;26:133-149

14. Stiles GL, Taylor S, Lefkowitz RJ: Human cardiac beta-adrenergic receptors: subtype heterogeneity delineated by direct radioligand binding. *Life Sci.* 1983;33:467-473

15. Ihl-Vahl R, Eschenhagen T, Kubler W, Marquetant R, Nose M, Schmitz W, Scholz H, Strasser RH: Differential regulation of mRNA specific for beta 1- and beta 2-adrenergic receptors in human failing hearts. Evaluation of the absolute cardiac mRNA levels by two independent methods. *J Mol Cell Cardiol.* 1996;28:1-10

16. Pende A, Tremmel KD, De MC, Blaxall BC, Minobe WA, Sherman JA, Bisognano JD, Bristow MR, Brewer G, Port J: Regulation of the mRNA-binding protein AUF1 by activation of the beta-adrenergic receptor signal transduction pathway. *J Biol.Chem.* 1996;271:8493-8501

17. Evanko DS, Ellis CE, Venkatachalam V, Frielle T: Preliminary analysis of the transcriptional regulation of the human beta 1-adrenergic receptor gene. *Biochem.Biophys.Res.Commun.* 1998;244:395-402

18. Danner S, Lohse MJ: Cell type-specific regulation of beta2-adrenoceptor mRNA by agonists. *Eur.J.Pharmacol.* 1997;331:73-78

19. Danner S, Frank M, Lohse MJ: Agonist regulation of human beta2-adrenergic receptor mRNA stability occurs via a specific AU-rich element. *J.Biol.Chem.* 1998;273:3223-3229

20. Müller FU, Boheler KR, Eschenhagen T, Schmitz W, Scholz H: Isoprenaline stimulates gene transcription of the inhibitory G protein alpha-subunit Gi alpha-2 in rat heart. *Circ.Res.* 1993;72:696-700

21. Eschenhagen T, Friedrichsen M, Gsell S, Hollmann A, Mittmann C, Schmitz W, Scholz H, Weil J, Weinstein LS: Regulation of the human Gi alpha-2 gene promotor activity in embryonic chicken cardiomyocytes. *Basic.Res.Cardiol.* 1996;91 Suppl 2:41-46

22. Weinstein LS, Spiegel AM, Carter AD: Cloning and characterization of the human gene for the alpha-subunit of Gi2, a GTP-binding signal transduction protein. *FEBS Lett.* 1988;232:333-340

23. Kadambi VJ, Ponniah S, Harrer JM, Hoit BD, Dorn GW, Walsh RA, Kranias EG: Cardiac-specific overexpression of phospholamban alters calcium kinetics and resultant cardiomyocyte mechanics in transgenic mice. *J.Clin.Invest.* 1996;97:533-539

24. Movsesian MA, Schwinger RH: Calcium sequestration by the sarcoplasmic reticulum in heart failure. *Cardiovasc.Res.* 1998;37:352-359

25. Lalli J, Harrer JM, Luo W, Kranias EG, Paul RJ: Targeted ablation of the phospholamban gene is associated with a marked decrease in sensitivity in aortic smooth muscle. *Circ.Res.* 1997;80:506-513

26. Wankerl M, Schwartz K: Calcium transport proteins in the nonfailing and failing heart: gene expression and function. *J Mol Med* 1995;73:487-496

27. Schwinger RH, Böhm M, Schmidt U, Karczewski P, Bavendiek U, Flesch M, Krause EG, Erdmann E: Unchanged protein levels of SERCA II and phospholamban but reduced Ca^{2+} uptake and Ca^{2+}-ATPase activity of cardiac sarcoplasmic reticulum from dilated cardiomyopathy patients compared with patients with nonfailing hearts. *Circulation* 1995;92:3220-3228

28. Wu KD, Lee WS, Wey J, Bungard D, Lytton J: Localization and quantification of endoplasmic reticulum Ca^{2+}-ATPase isoform transcripts. *Am.J.Physiol.* 1995;269:C775-C784

29. Flesch M, Schwinger RH, Schnabel P, Schiffer F, van Gilst W, Bavendiek U, Südkamp M, Kuhn-Regnier F, Böhm M: Sarcoplasmic reticulum Ca^{2+}ATPase and phospholamban mRNA and protein levels in end-stage heart failure due to ischemic or dilated cardiomyopathy. *J.Mol.Med.* 1996;74:321-332

30. Hasenfuss G, Meyer M, Schillinger W, Preuss M, Pieske B, Just H: Calcium handling proteins in the failing human heart. *Basic.Res.Cardiol.* 1997;92 Suppl 1:87-93

31. Mercadier JJ, Lompre AM, Duc P, Boheler KR, Fraysse JB, Wisnewsky C, Allen PD, Komajda M, Schwartz K: Altered sarcoplasmic reticulum Ca^{2+}-ATPase gene expression in the human ventricle during end-stage heart failure. *J.Clin.Invest.* 1990;85:305-309

32. Darvish A, Schomisch-Moravec SC: Decreased sarcoplasmic reticulum content in the failing human heart is associated with a decrease in the Ca^{2+} ATPase and phospholamban proteins. *Circulation* 1994;90:I-217(Abstract)

33. Movsesian MA, Bristow MR, Krall J: Ca^{2+} uptake by cardiac sarcoplasmic reticulum from patients with idiopathic dilated cardiomyopathy. *Circ.Res.* 1989;65:1141-1144

34. Movsesian MA, Karimi M, Green K, Jones LR: Ca^{2+}-transporting ATPase, phospholamban, and calsequestrin levels in nonfailing and failing human myocardium. *Circulation* 1994;90:653-657

35. Luo W, Wolska BM, Grupp IL, Harrer JM, Haghighi K, Ferguson DG, Slack JP, Grupp G, Doetschman T, Solaro RJ, Kranias EG: Phospholamban gene dosage effects in the mammalian heart. *Circ.Res.* 1996;78:839-847

36. Luo W, Grupp WL, Harrer J, Ponniah S, Grupp G, Duffy JJ, Doetschmann T, Kranias EG: Target ablation of the phospholamban gene is associated with markedly enhanced myocardial contractility and loss of β-agonist stimulation. *Circ.Res.* 1994;75:401-409

37. Bartel S, Stein B, Eschenhagen T, Mende U, Neumann J, Schmitz W, Krause EG, Karczewski P, Scholz H: Protein phosphorylation in isolated trabeculae from nonfailing and failing human hearts. *Mol.Cell Biochem.* 1996;157:171-179

38. Chien KR, Shimizu M, Hoshijima M, Minamisawa S, Grace AA: Toward molecular strategies for heart disease--past, present, future. *Jpn.Circ.J.* 1997;61:91-118

39. Liang P, Pardee AB: Differential display of eukaryotic messenger RNA by means of the polymerase chain reaction. *Science* 1992;257:967-971

40. Aoki M, Morishita R, Muraishi A, Moriguchi A, Sugimoto T, Maeda K, Dzau VJ, Kaneda Y, Higaki J, Ogihara T: Efficient in vivo gene transfer into the heart in the rat myocardial infarction model using the HVJ (Hemagglutinating Virus of Japan)--liposome method. *J.Mol.Cell Cardiol.* 1997;29:949-959

41. Smith LC, Eisensmith RC, Woo SL: Gene therapy in heart disease. *Adv.Exp.Med.Biol.* 1995;369:79-88

42. Franz WM, Mueller OJ, Hartong R, Frey N, Katus HA: Transgenic animal models: new avenues in cardiovascular physiology. *J.Mol.Med.* 1997;75:115-129

43. Akhter SA, Skaer CA, Kypson AP, McDonald PH, Peppel KC, Glower DD, Lefkowitz RJ, Koch WJ: Restoration of beta-adrenergic signaling in failing cardiac ventricular myocytes via adenoviral-mediated gene transfer. *Proc.Natl.Acad.Sci.U.S.A.* 1997;94:12100-12105

44. Hajjar RJ, Kang JX, Gwathmey JK, Rosenzweig A: Physiological effects of adenoviral gene transfer of sarcoplasmic reticulum calcium ATPase in isolated rat myocytes. *Circulation* 1997;95:423-429.

CHAPTER ONE: PHYSIOLOGY AND PATHOPHYSIOLOGY

SECTION TWO: AUTONOMIC NERVOUS SYSTEM

4. AUTONOMIC NERVOUS SYSTEM: PHYSIOLOGY AND PATHOPHYSIOLOGY

ROGER HAINSWORTH

The autonomic nervous system is concerned primarily with the unconscious regulation of bodily functions. Both afferent and efferent nervous impulses travel in both autonomic divisions and subserve reflexes that are important to the normal function of the various systems, including cardiovascular, respiratory, digestive and genito-urinary. Activity in the two divisions is often complementary. For example, as parasympathetic activity to the heart decreases, sympathetic activity increases. Changes in autonomic nervous activity occur frequently in disease processes and may be a cause, an effect or a modulating influence on the course of the disease.

RESPONSES TO EFFERENT STIMULATION OF CARDIOVASCULAR AUTONOMIC NERVES

Cardiac effects

The heart receives its efferent nerve supply from the two vagal (10th cranial) nerves, the preganglionic cell bodies of which are in the dorsal motor vagal nucleus and the nucleus ambiguus in the brain stem, and the sympathetic nerves with preganglionic cell bodies in the lateral grey horn of the spinal cord at level T 3-4. The vagal innervation is mainly to the sinu-atrial node and the atrio-ventricular conducting mechanism. There is also some innervation of the atrial myocardium but there is no physiological evidence of a substantial ventricular motor innervation. Sympathetic nerves, however, innervate all cardiac chambers as well as the pacemaker and conducting pathways.

The effect of vagal stimulation on the cardiac pacemaker cells is to cause hyperpolarization and to reduce the rate of depolarization. This can be very potent and high levels of vagal activity can cause asystole. The effect is also

H.-H. Osterhues et al. (eds.),
Advances in Noninvasive Electrocardiographic Monitoring Techniques, 41–49.

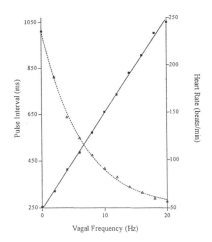

Figure 1. Effects of stimulation of vagus nerves at various frequencies in an anaesthetized rabbit • — • shows effects on pulse interval, Δ — Δ responses shown as heart rate. Pulse interval is linearly related to stimulus frequency, whereas heart rate shows a hyperbolic realtionship. Drawn from data obtained from ref.2.

extremely rapid with the maximum response to a single stimulus occurring in only 400 ms[1]. This means that the vagus can control heart rate on a beat-to-beat basis. The action of the vagus implies that it is actually the cardiac interval that is directly controlled rather than heart rate. This results in a linear relationship between interval prolongation and vagal stimulus frequency[2] and consequently a hyperbolic relationship between stimulus frequency and heart rate which is an inverse function of interval (Fig.1). This relationship may be important when considering vagal responses from different baselines. The response of heart rate to a given change in vagal activity is much greater at high than at low heart rates, whereas pulse interval responses are the same. At rest there is usually a tonic vagal discharge which slows the heart rate from the intrinsic pacemaker rate of 110–120 beats/min to normal resting levels of 60–80 beats/min.

The vagus nerves also innervate the atrio-ventricular conducting mechanism and stimulation slows conduction and may cause complete block. They also innervate atrial muscle and stimulation causes a negative inotropic response. The question of efferent ventricular innervation is controversial and apparent decreases in ventricular inotropic state may largely be due to the atrial response.

Sympathetic stimulation causes chronotropic effects by increasing the rate of pacemaker depolarization. The chronotropic effect of sympathetic activity is the mechanism by which heart rate increases to values above intrinsic rate and the high rates achieved during physical exercise imply a high level of sympa-

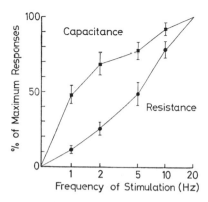

Figure 2. Capacitance and resistance responses in abdomianl circualtion of anaethetized dog to stimulation of sympathetic nerves at various frequencies. Values are means ± SEM from 14 days and show responses expressed as percentages of changes at 20 Hz. Note the preponderance of the capacitance responses at the lower stimulus frequencies (Modified from ref. 4).

thetic activity. At lower rates the actual heart rate depends on the balance between sympathetic and vagal activities with the two changing in a reciprocal fashion.

The other major effects of sympathetic nerves on the heart rate are to increase the rate of atrio-ventricular conduction and to cause positive inotropic effects on both atrial and ventricular muscle[3]. These effects are manifested as increased energy of contraction from any given myocardial fibre length and increased rate and decreased duration of cardiac contraction. These effects are essential for maximal cardiac performance during exercise In particular, the shortening of systole at high heart rates allows adequate preservation of diastolic filling time. This differs from abnormal tachyarrhythmias where diastole is not preserved and consequently cardiac output may fall catastrophically.

Sympathetic responses differ from those of the vagi in that they develop much more slowly requiring up to 20 seconds for maximal responses to develop. This implies that if an effect occurs in a substantially shorter time it cannot be sympathetically mediated.

Vascular effects

Arterial blood pressure is controlled mainly by the level of activity in the sympathetic nerves supplying the microscopic resistance vessels, the small arteries and arterioles. Poiseuille's equation reveals that for flow through a system of tubes, pressure is proportional to the flow but it is inversely proportional to the fourth power of the radius. This means that whereas to increase pressure by 50% requires an increase in flow of 50%, it requires only a 10% reduction in radius.

The state of contraction of vascular smooth muscle, and therefore the vessel radius, is dependent on the balance between vasodilator influences, largely products of metabolism, and neurally mediated vasoconstriction. Activity in sympathetic nerves also constricts capacitance vessels, which are essentially veins, particularly those within the splanchnic circulation[4]. In supine rest there is a very low level of sympathetic activity. This increases with standing and increases further during stresses and hypotension. Capacitance vessels are particularly sensitive to low levels of sympathetic activity (Fig.2) which means that during progressive stresses, the capacitance vessels would contract before there is a large change in resistance.

REFLEX CONTROL

Baroreceptors

Baroreceptors are stretch receptors in the walls of various arteries, particularly the aortic arch and carotid sinuses. We have recently described another group which responds to coronary artery pressure[5,6]. Baroreceptors are normally tonically stimulated and their discharge increases as blood pressure increases. They have phasic characteristics showing a burst discharge during the rising phase of pressure and silence as pressure decreases. They sense not only the absolute level of pressure but the rate of change and are thus able to detect changes in pulse pressure and therefore, indirectly changes in ventricular stroke volume. In animals baroreceptor responses may be studied using 'open loop' preparation where the stimulus is localised. In people, their function has been studied by changing blood pressure using vasoconstrictor or dilator agents[7], application of subatmospheric or positive pressures to the neck[8], or by analysis of transfer function of spontaneous changes in blood pressure and heart period[9].

Baroreceptors respond to increases in blood pressure by inducing reflex responses to restore the pressure (negative feedback). The most obvious immediate response is a slowing of the heart due to increased vagal activity. A stimulus to the carotid baroreceptors prolongs cardiac interval with a latency of only 0.75s and thus can maximally affect the next or next-but-one beat[10]. Cardiac sympathetic activity is inhibited leading to reductions in both rate and force of contraction, but with a longer latency. Sympathetic tone to peripheral blood vessels is also under baroreceptor control and this forms the main mechanism for stabilising blood pressure.

Baroreceptors interact with other reflexes. One prominent example is the effect of respiration where during inspiration the reflex is inhibited and this leads to a sinus arrhythmia[11].

Pathophysiological effects. Baroreceptors usually operate with the midpoint of their sigmoid stimulus-response relationship at the normal level of blood pressure. If pressure changes, baroreceptors 'reset' so that they continue to buffer increases and decreases in pressure[12]. In hypertension the changes become chronic and associated with a decrease in sensitivity. Baroreceptor sensitivity is also low in ischaemic heart disease and, depression is correlated with risk of arrhythmias[13,14]. It may be greater than normal in hypovolaemia[15] and high sensitivity is often associated with susceptibility to attacks of syncope[16].

Atrial receptors

These are specific vagal nerve endings, concentrated at the junctions of the great veins and the atria. They are slowly adapting stretch receptors and are stimulated as atrial filling increases. Because one of the factors influencing atrial filling is blood volume, atrial receptors are often referred to as 'volume receptors'.

Bainbridge[17] first described reflex tachycardia in response to rapid intravenous infusions and this was subsequently shown to have been due to stimulation of atrial receptors[18]. The efferent pathway of the reflex to the heart is unusual in that it involves solely the sympathetic nerves to the sinu-atrial node and not efferent vagal nerves or sympathetic nerves to the myocardium. Atrial receptors also do not control vascular resistance[19] (Fig.3), except to the kidney where they decrease renal nerve activity[20]. They also inhibit the release of vasopressin (ADH)[21]. Thus, an increase in stimulation of atrial receptors increases heart rate, causes a water diuresis through inhibition of ADH, and increases urinary salt and water excretion through inhibition of renal nerves.

Pathophysiological effects. The normal function of atrial receptors, which is to control heart rate and extracellular fluid volume, is impaired in chronic cardiac failure[22] and may contribute to causing fluid retention. This effect is at least partly due to desensitization of the receptors. In tachyarrhythmias the atria may become distended sometimes leading to an abnormal diuresis

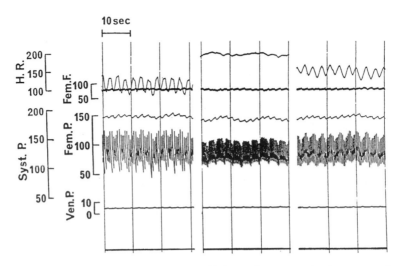

Figure 3. Response in a dog to stimulation of left atrial receptors by distension of small balloons at the pulmonary vein-atrial junctions. Traces show heart rate (beats/min); femoral perfusion flow (held constant, ml/min) and pressures in perfused femoral artery, systemic artery and femoral vein. Atrial receptor stimulation (centre panel) causes a large increase in heart rate, but little effect on vascular resistance (perfusion pressure nearly constant at constant flow). (From ref. 19).

Ventricular receptors

Most of the ventricular innervation is to the left ventricle and by nonmyelinated vagal afferents with no specific endings[23]. Some afferent fibres run in sympathetic nerves and these may have multiple endings often terminating in different cardiac chambers[24]. Ventricular receptors may be chemosensitive, mechanosensitive or both. Chemosensitive afferents do not respond to physiological changes in the blood such as hypoxia or hypercapnia but rather to injections of extraneous chemicals like veratridine and capsaicin, although they may be stimulated by chemicals released during injury, including bradykinin and prostaglandins[25]. Mechanosensitive endings may or may not have a cardiac rhythm and are stimulated by increases in ventricular systolic or diastolic pressures or inotropic state.

Chemical stimulation of ventricular receptors may elicit a profound brady-cardia and vasodilatation. This is the Bezold-Jarisch reflex and may sometimes be seen in response to intravenous and particularly intracoronary injections.

The effects of mechanical stimulation are very much smaller and tend only to be transient. It has not yet been established whether ventricular receptors have a role in normal cardiovascular regulation as responses only seem to be occur to extreme unphysiological stimuli[27].

Pathophysiological effect. Ventricular receptors may be stimulated during ischaemia or infarction partly as the result of released chemical stimulants and possibly partly by abnormal distension of the ischaemic region. The effects of ischaemia are complicated in humans by responses to pain and by buffering by baroreceptors. Inferior wall ischaemia may elicit depressor reflexes through vagal afferents[28], whereas anterior wall ischaemia tends to increase heart rate and blood pressure and redispose to arrhythmias, possibly through excitation of sympathetic afferent nerves[29].

Ventricular receptors were formerly thought to initiate vasovagal syncope as it had been shown that some receptors were excited when the ventricle contracted powerfully at a small volume[30]. However, experiments in animals have not confirmed this[31] and in patients, heart transplant did not prevent the response[32].

Other autonomic reflexes

Peripheral chemoreceptors in the carotid and aortic bodies, and central chemoreceptors in the medulla influence the cardiovascular as well as the respiratory system. Generally, hypoxia and hypercapnia cause vasoconstriction. Carotid chemoreceptors cause a primary bradycardia[33] although this may be masked by a secondary tachycardia resulting from an increase in respiratory activity. Receptors also exist in the pulmonary artery which, when stimulated by an increase in pressure, cause a reflex vasoconstriction[34].

Exercise causes very large autonomic changes[35]. At the start, heart rate increases in response to vagal withdrawal initiated by central command. Metaboreceptors in exercising muscle contribute to the vagal inhibition and sympathetic excitation and inhibit the baroreceptor reflex. The effects of exercise can be modified by training which causes increases in cardiac volumes and slowing of the heart at submaximal levels of exercise[36]. It does not influence the maximal heart rate which is more dependent on the subject's age.

This short review has outlined some of the mechanisms involving autonomic nerves to the cardiovascular system. It is important to remember, however, that both in health and in disease, reflexes do not operate in isolation and any resulting responses are dependent on background conditions and on complex interactions of very many diverse reflex control mechanisms.

REFERENCES

1. Levy MN, Martin PJ, Iano T. Effects of single vagal stimuli on heart rate and atrioventricular conduction. Am J Physiol 1970; 218: 1256-1262.
2. Parker P, Celler BG, Potter EK, McClosky DI. Vagal stimulation and cardiac slowing J Auton Nerv Syst. 1984; 11: 226-231.
3. Furnival CM,Linden RJ, Snow HM. Chronotropic and inotropic effects on the dog heart of stimulating the efferent cardiac sympathetic nerves. J Physiol. 1973; 230: 137-153.
4. Karim F, Hainsworth R. Responses of abdominal vascular capacitance to stimulation of splanchnic nerves. Am J Physiol. 1976; 231: 434-440.
5. Drinkhill MJ, Moore J, Hainworth R. Afferent discharges from coronary arterial and ventricular receptors in anaesthetized dogs. J Physiol. 1993; 472: 785-800.
6. Al-Timman JKA, Drinkhill MJ, Hainsworth R. Reflex responses to stimulation of mechanoreceptors in the left ventricle and coronary arteries in anaethetized dogs. J Physiol. 1993; 472: 769-784.
7. Smyth HS, Sleight P, Pickering GW. Reflex regulation of arterial pressure during sleep in man. A quantatitive method of assessing baroreceptor sensitivity. Circulation Res. 1969; 24: 109-121.
8. Kelly AP, El-Bedawi KM, Hainsworth R. An improved neck chamber for the study of carotid baroreceptors in humans. J Physiol. 1993; 467: 142P.
9. Pagani M, Lombardi F, Guzzetti S, et al. Power spectral analysis of heart rate and arterial pressure variabilities as a marker of sympatho-vagal interaction in man and conscious dog. Circulation Res. 1986; 59: 178-193.
10. Eckberg DL. Temporal response patterns of the human sinus node to brief carotid baroreceptor stimuli. J Physiol. 1978; 258: 769-782.
11. Eckberg DL, Kifle YT, Roberts VL. Phase relationship between normal human respiration and baroreflex responsiveness. J Physiol. 1980. 304: 489-502.
12. Chapleau MW, Abboud FM. Mechanisms of adaption and resetting of the baroreceptor reflex. In: Hainsworth R, Marks AL (Eds). Cardiovascular Reflex Control in Health and Disease. London, England: Saunders, 1993; 165-194.
13. La Rovere MT, Spechia G, Motara A, Schwartz PJ. Baroreflex sensitivity, clinical correlates, and cardiovascular mortality among patients with a first myocardial infarction: a prospective study. Circulation. 1998; 78: 816-824.
14. Farrell TG, Odemuyiwa O, Bashir Y, Cripps TR, Malik M, Ward DE, Camm AJ. Prognostic value of baroreflex sensitivity testing after acute myocardial infarction. Br Heart J. 1992; 67: 129-137.
15. Vatner SF, Boettcher DH, Heyndrickx GR, McRitchie RJ. Baroreflex sensitivity with volume loading in conscious dogs. Circulation Res. 1975; 37: 236-242.
16. El-Sayed H, Hainsworth R. Relationship between plasma volume, carotid baroreceptor sensitivity and orthostatic tolerance. Clin Sci. 1995; 88: 463-470.
17. Bainbridge FA. The influence of venous filling upon the rate of the heart. J Physiol. 1915; 50: 65-84.
18. Ledsome JR, Linden RJ. A reflex increase in heart rate from distension of the pulmonary vein-atrial junctions. J Physiol. 1964; 170: 456-473.

19. Carswell F, Hainsworth R,Ledsome JR. The effects of distension of the pulmonary vein-atrial junctions upon peripheral vascular resistance. J Physiol. 1970; 207: 1-14.
20. Sreeharan N, Kappagoda CT. Linden RJ. The role of renal nerves in the diuresis and natriuresis caused by stimulation of atrial receptors. Q J Exp Physiol. 1981; 66: 431-438.
21. Bennett KL, Linden RJ, Mary DASG. The effect of stimulation of atrial receptors on the plasma concentration of vasopressin. Q J Exp Physiol. 1983; 68: 579-589.
22. Zucker IH, Earle AM, Gilmore JP. The mechanism of adaption of left atrial stretch receptors in dogs with chronic congestive heart failue. J Clin Invest. 1977; 60: 323-331.
23. Coleridge HM, Coleridge JCG, Kidd C. Cardiac receptors in the dog, with particular reference to two types of afferent ending in the ventricular wall. J Physiol. 1964; 174: 323-339.
24. Banzett RB, Coleridge HM, Coleridge JCG, Kidd C. Multiterminal afferent fibres from the thoracic viscera in sympathetic rami communicantes in cats and dogs. J Physiol. 1976; 254: 57P.
25. Kaufman MP, Baker DG, Coleridge HM. Stimulation by bradykinin of afferent vagal C-fibers with chemosensitive endings in the heart and aorta of the dog. Circ Res. 1980; 46: 476-484.
26. Oberg B, Thoren P. Studies on left ventricular receptors signalling in non-medullated vagal afferents. Acta Physiol Scand. 1972; 85: 145-163.
27. Hainsworth R. Reflexes from the heart. Physiol Rev. 1991; 71: 617-658.
28. George M, Greenwood TW. Relation between bradycardia and the site of myocardial infarction. Lancet. 1967; 2: 739-740.
29. Webb SW, Adgey AA, Pantridge JF. Autonomic disturbance at onset of acute myocardial infarction.Br Med J. 1972; 3: 89-92.
30. Oberg B, Thoren P. Increased activity in left ventricular receptors during hemorrhage or occlusion of caval veins in the cat. A possible cause of the vaso-vagal reaction. Acta Physiol Scand. 1972; 85: 164-173.
31. Al-Timman JKA, Drinkhill MJ, Hainsworth R. Reflex vascular responses to changes in left ventricular pressure, heart rate and inotropic state in dogs. Exp Physiol. 1992; 77: 455-469.
32. Fitzpatrick AP, Banner N, Cheung A, Yacoub M, Sutton R. Vasovagal reactions may occur after othotopic heart transplantation. J Am Coll Cardiol. 1993; 177: 203-214.
33. Hainsworth R, Jacobs L, Comroe JH Jr. Afferent lung denervation by brief inhalation of steam. J Appl Physiol 1973; 34: 708-714.
34. Ledsome JR, Kan K. Reflex changes in hind limb and renal vascular resistances to distension of the isolated pulmonary arteries of the dog. Circulation Res. 1977; 40: 64-72.
35. Vatner SF, Pagani M. Cardiovascular adjustments to exercise: hemodynamics and mechanisms. Prog Cardiovasc Dis. 1976; 29: 91-188.
36. Saltin B, Blomqvist G, Mitchell JH, Johnson RL, Willenthal K, Chapman CB. Response to exercise after bedrest and after training. Circulation. 1968; 37 (supp 7): 1-55.

5. METHODS TO ASSESS BAROREFLEX SENSITIVITY AS A MEASURE OF THE ACTIVITY OF THE AUTONOMIC NERVOUS SYSTEM

MARIA TERESA LA ROVERE

Among the several methods which have been proposed for determination of sympathetic-parasympathetic interactions at the level of the sinus node, the assessment of baroreflex sensitivity (BRS) and the analysis of heart rate variability have been shown to carry prognostic information in ischemic heart disease (1). This article describes several quantitative approaches developed for evaluating BRS including the analysis of reflex responses to pharmacological or mechanical manipulations of baroreceptors, and the analysis of spontaneously occurring changes in blood pressure and heart rate.

VASOACTIVE DRUGS

An increase in systemic arterial pressure increases the firing rate of baroreceptors which causes vagal excitation and sympathetic inhibition, thus decreasing heart rate; BRS can be quantified as the measure of the reflex bradycardia which follows the blood pressure rise induced by the injection of an alpha-adrenoreceptor stimulant (2).

In normal subjects 25-100 mcg of phenylephrine are flushed into a vein to increase systolic arterial pressure (SAP) by 15-40 mmHg. The dosage of phenylephrine and time of injection may vary widely according to the patients under evaluation. In patients after a recent myocardial infarction (3) phenylephrine has been injected over 30 seconds, and boluses of 150-350 mcg (2-4 mcg/Kg) have been safely administered. In patients with congestive heart

H.-H. Osterhues et al. (eds.),
Advances in Noninvasive Electrocardiographic Monitoring Techniques, 51–57.
© 2000 *Kluwer Academic Publishers. Printed in the Netherlands.*

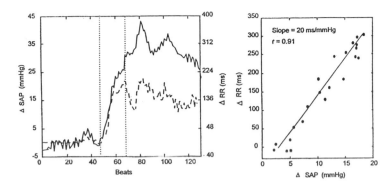

Figure 1. Example of a preserved BRS. On the left beat-to-beat changes in systolic arterial pressure (SAP) (dotted line) and in RR interval (continuous line) with respect to baseline values are reported. Analysis is limited to the first major increase in systolic arterial pressure with the attendant changes in RR interval (points included between dotted lines). These points are used for calculation of the regression line (on the right). The increase in SAP is greater than 20 mmHg and is accompanied by a consistent increase in RR interval. Accordingly the slope of the regression line is 20 ms/mmHg and represents a response primarily characterized by an increase in efferent vagus nerve activity to the sinus node.

failure (4) even higher doses (up to 10 mcg/kg) have been used to elicit baroreceptor responses.

Heart rate and blood pressure are recorded continuously because, given the rapidity of vagal responses, it is commonly assumed that, at normal resting heart rates each heart period value is mainly related on a cause-effect basis to the previous systolic pressure peak, and that this relation is linear. Prolongations of successive RR intervals with respect to baseline values (i.e. pre-injection) are therefore plotted as a function of preceding SAP changes and an analysis window is selected between the beginning and the end of the first significant (> 15 mmHg) increase in SAP. The slope of the regression line fitted to the selected points (expressed as msec/mmHg) - that is, the absolute increase in RR interval produced by a 1 mmHg rise in SAP - represents BRS. Pearson's correlation coefficient is used to test the goodness of the linear association between SAP and RR interval changes. When the correlation coefficient is higher than 0.7 - 0.8, and the pairs of data included in the analysis are greater than 10, a test of significance is not required since this correlation is obviously statistically significant. For lower values a test of significance is required to test the association between SAP and RR interval changes. However, when BRS values are near zero (- 0.5 ÷ + 0.5 ms/mmHg) - thus describing the absence of any response between pressure elevation and RR interval -, as it is commonly observed among patients with severe

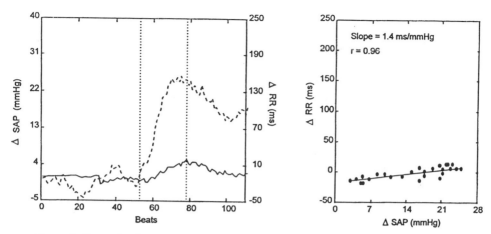

Figure 2. Example of a poor BRS. Detailed description as in Figure 1. The increase in SAP is accompanied by a modest increase in RR interval and the slope of the regression line is 1.4 ms/mmHg and represents a response characterized by weak vagal reflexes.

congestive heart failure, the correlation coefficient is obviously not significant (4).

Several injections are generally repeated at intervals of a few minutes and the corresponding slopes are averaged in order to reduce measurement variability between tests. The final slope is generally obtained by at least three slopes with the higher correlation coefficients. Estimates of BRS are very similar when SAP is measured directly from the radial or brachial artery or from a noninvasive pressure monitor (5)

In normal young subjects average BRS values of 14.8 ± 9.2 msec/mmHg (SD) (6) and 16.0 ± 1.8 msec/mmHg (SEM) (7) have been reported. When analyzing a test of BRS such a slope is generally interpreted as the result of the interplay between effective vagal reflexes and tonic sympathetic activity (FIGURE 1). Overall, BRS decreases whenever the autonomic balance shifts toward sympathetic dominance and increases whenever the autonomic balance shifts toward parasympathetic dominance. Significant impairment in the baroreflex control of heart rate is produced by pathological conditions including hypertension (6) and cardiac disease (1,3,4,7). The mean BRS was 7.2 ± 4.6 msec/mmHg (SD) and 3.9 ± 4.0 msec/mmHg (SD) in two large series of patients with a previous myocardial infarction (1) and with congestive heart failure (4) respectively. Accordingly a depressed BRS slope is interpreted as a reduced capability of vagal reflexes which may also be associated with the presence of elevated sympathetic activity (FIGURE 2).

NECK CHAMBER TECHNIQUE

The neck chamber is formed from a malleable lead collar by which controlled positive or negative pneumatic pressures are applied to the neck region. An increase in neck chamber pressure is sensed by the baroreceptors as a decrease in arterial pressure and thus it activates a double response which determines vagal withdrawal and sympathetic activation to the heart and the arterial vessels. Conversely, a decrease in neck chamber pressure results in reflex reduction of blood pressure and heart rate, which initially is mainly vagal.

Neck suction is presently the preferred stimulus of the two, as it is easier to use than pressure and is well tolerated by the subject. Neck suction is critically dependent on the rate of the stimulus and its duration. Different investigators have used quite different stimuli from less than 1 second to 5 or 10 seconds. The negative pressure is applied in separate steps and ranges in magnitude from -7 to - 40 mmHg. Each step is generally repeated three times and the steps are applied in random order. The maximal lengthening in RR interval observed over the three beats following the neck suction application generally represents the reflex response and the slope of the regression of RR interval over neck pressure is taken as the carotid baroreflex sensitivity. Given the fact that the "equivalent arterial pressure increase" following neck suction stimulation is unknown, the slopes obtained are not comparable with those obtained with phenylephrine injection (8).

A very interesting feature of the neck suction technique is the possibility of analyzing the dynamic behaviour of baroreceptors by the administration of a sinusoid suction at different frequencies within the spectrum of short-term blood pressure variability (0.02÷0.25 Hz). At each stimulating frequency the power of the corresponding spectral component of the RR signal is considered to be related to neck suction stimulation when the coherence value is > 0.5. A sinusoid stimulation of the carotid baroreceptors at a frequency > 0.2 can be followed only by vagal efferent activity while stimulation at 0.1 Hz can be followed normally by both vagal and sympathetic reflex activity. By this technique it has been found that carotid baroreceptors have an important role in the determination of the RR interval oscillations particularly in the low frequency band (around 0.1 Hz) (9) and that in heart transplant patients the occurrence of sympathetic reinnervation may be easily detected by the presence of a reflex oscillation at 0.1 Hz in response to baroreceptor stimulation at the same frequency (10).

ANALYSIS OF SPONTANEOUS BAROREFLEX SENSITIVITY

Spontaneous fluctuations in arterial pressure and RR interval may also provide information about cardiovascular control on the basis that naturally occurring small amplitude fluctuations of arterial pressure trigger changes of arterial baroreceptor firing, which in turn, trigger changes of vagal motoneurons firing. Both "time domain" and "frequency-domain" measurements have been proposed.

In time domain analysis, those sequences of three or more consecutive heart beats characterized by a progressive increase in SAP and a progressive lengthening in RR interval, or characterized by a progressive reduction in SAP and a progressive shortening in RR interval are identified and the slope of the regression line between changes in SAP and RR interval is computed (11). The threshold values for SAP and pulse interval changes are set at 1 mmHg and 6 milliseconds, respectively.

The underlying concept in the "frequency domain" approach is that each spontaneous oscillation in blood pressure elicits an oscillation of similar frequency in the RR interval by the effect of arterial baroreflex activity. Hence, the baroreflex gain can be obtained by dividing the amplitude of the RR oscillation by the amplitude of the corresponding oscillation of the blood pressure. The function that describes this gain at each oscillatory frequency is the modulus of the so-called transfer function between systolic pressure and RR interval.

Although several investigators, by studying normal subjects or hypertensive patients, have proposed that spectral estimations of baroreflex gain are reliable alternatives to the phenylephrine test (12,13), in patients with a previous myocardial infarction and different degrees of left ventricular dysfunction, the agreement between spectral measurements and phenylephrine in the estimation of baroreflex gain is weak because the difference can be as large as the BRS value being estimated (14,15).

GENERAL CONCLUSION

In summary several methods have been developed to measure the baroreflex control of heart rate and blood pressure. At this time only the phenylephrine-based baroreflex sensitivity has been demonstrated to carry prognostic information (1). The neck chamber technique should be regarded primarily as a tool for physiological studies. Although some correlation does exist between phenylephrine-based baroreflex sensitivity and measures derived from spectral analysis the two methods are not interchangeable for risk stratification. The prognostic implication of spontaneus variability need to be addressed.

REFERENCES

1. La Rovere MT, Bigger JT Jr, Marcus FI, Mortara A, Schwartz PJ for the ATRAMI Investigators: Baroreflex sensitivity and heart rate variability in prediction of total cardiac mortality after myocardial infarction. Lancet 351: 478-484, 1998
2. Smyth HS, Sleight P, Pickering GW: Reflex regulation of arterial pressure during sleep in man: a quantitative method for assessing baroreflex sensitivity. Circ Res 24: 109-121, 1969
3. La Rovere MT, Specchia G, Mortara A, Schwartz PJ: Baroreflex sensitivity, clinical correlates and cardiovascular mortality among patients with a first myocardial infarction. A prospective study. Circulation 1988; 78: 816-824
4. Mortara A, La Rovere MT, Pinna GD, Prpa A, Maestri R, Febo O, Pozzoli M, Opasich C, Cobelli F, Tavazzi L: Arterial baroreflex modulation of heart rate in chronic heart failure. Clinical and hemodynamic correlates and prognostic implications. Circulation 96: 3450-3458, 1997
5. Parati G, Casadei R, Groppelli A, Di Rienzo M, Mancia G: Comparison of finger and intra-arterial blood pressure monitoring at rest and during laboratory testing. Hypertension 13: 647-655, 1989
6. Bristow JD, Honour AJ, Pickering GW, Sleight P, Smyth HS: Diminished baroreflex sensitivity in high blood pressure. Circulation 1969; 39: 48-54
7. Eckberg DL, Drabinsky M, Braunwald E: Defective cardiac parasympathetic control in patients with heart disease. N Engl J Med 285: 877-883, 1971
8. Osculati G, Grassi G, Giannattasio C, Seravalle G, Valagussa F, Zanchetti A, Mancia G: Early alterations of the baroreceptor control of heart rate in patients with acute myocardial infarction. Circulation 81: 939-948, 1990
9. Sleight P, La Rovere MT, Mortara A, Maestri R, Leuzzi S, Bianchini B, Tavazzi L, Bernardi L: Physiology and physiopathology of heart rate and blood pressure variability in humans: is power spectral analysis largely an index of baroreflex gain? Clinical Science 1995; 88: 103-109
10. Bernardi L, Bianchini B, Spadacini G, Leuzzi S, Valle F, Marchesi E, Passino C, Calciati A, Vigano' M, Rinaldi M, Martinelli L, Finardi G, Sleight P: Demonstrable cardiac reinnervation after human heart transplantation by carotid baroreflex modulation of RR interval. Circulation 1995; 92: 2895-2903
11. Parati G, Di Rienzo M, Bertinieri G, Pomidossi G, Casadei R, Groppelli A, Pedotti A, Zanchetti A, Mancia G: Evaluation of the baroreceptor-heart rate reflex by 24-hour intra-arterial blood pressure monitoring in humans. Hypertension 12: 214-222, 1988
12. Robbe HWJ, Mulder LJM, Ruddel H, Langewitz WA, Veldman JBB, Mulder G: Assessment of baroreceptor reflex sensitivity by means of spectral analysis. Hypertension 10: 538-543, 1987

13. Pagani M, Somers V, Furlan R, Dell'Orto S, Conway J, Cerutti S, Sleight P, Malliani A: Changes in autonomic regulation induced by physical training in mild hypertension. Hypertension 12: 600-610, 1988

14. Maestri R, Pinna GD, Mortara A, La Rovere MT, Tavazzi L: Assessing baroreflex sensitivity in post-myocardial infarction patients: comparison of spectral and phenylephrine techniques. J Am Coll Cardiol 31: 344-351, 1998

15. Pitzalis MV, Mastropasqua F, Passantino A, Massari F, Ligurgo L, Forleo C, Balducci C, Lombardi F, Rizzon P: Comparison between noninvasive indices of baroreceptor sensitivity and the phenylephrine method in post-myocardial infarction patients. Circulation 97: 1362-1367, 1998

6. ROLE OF THE AUTONOMIC NERVOUS SYSTEM IN CARDIOVASCULAR DISEASES

RICHARD L. VERRIER

The activity of the autonomic nervous system exerts a pervasive influence on cardiovascular health. For many major forms of cardiovascular disease, evidence has been accrued to implicate neurogenic factors either as acute triggers or as longterm catalysts or both. Among the most prominent conditions with an underlying neural component exacerbating cardiovascular dysfunction are hypertension, heart failure, coronary artery disease, and arrhythmias (1). The underlying mechanisms are multifactorial and complex. There are both direct and intermediary factors responsible for the adverse influence of disturbed autonomic activity on cardiovascular health. These range from perturbations in hemodynamic function, particularly elevated arterial blood pressure, and direct effects of neurotransmitters on the myocardium and vascular endothelium.

The goals of this brief review are to summarize the current knowledge regarding sympathetic and parasympathetic neural infiuences on cardiac electrical stability and to discuss the evidence which implicates behavioral stress as a *bona fide* risk factor in cardiac events. We will focus primarily on propensity to arrhythmias, because of the relevance of ambulatory ECG monitoring to the audience and the fact that the basic principles have been elucidated by research on this topic.

SYMPATHETIC NERVE INFLUENCES

Sympathetic nerve activation has been extensively implicated in provoking life-threatening arrhythmias both in animals and humans (2,3). Stimulation of

H.-H. Osterhues et al. (eds.),
Advances in Noninvasive Electrocardiographic Monitoring Techniques, 59–68.
© 2000 *Kluwer Academic Publishers. Printed in the Netherlands.*

TABLE 1
DIRECT CARDIAC ELECTROPHYSIOLOGIC EFFECTS OF SYMPATHETIC NERVOUS SYSTEM STIMULATION

- Shifts pacemaker from sinus node to junctional region
- Alters P-wave morphology
- Abbreviates P-R interval
- Increases Purkinje fiber automaticity
- Increases early afterdepolarizations
- Prolongs QT-interval on body surface
- Increases TQ-depression and enhances reentry during acute myocardial ischemia
- Decreases ventricular fibrillation threshold
- Induces T-wave alternans in the long QT-syndrome and during acute myocardial ischemia

From Verrier RL, Kovach JA: Primary role of beta-adrenergic receptors in arrhythmogenesis during sympathetic nervous system activation. In Podrid PJ, Kowey PR (eds): Cardiac Arrhythmias: Mechanism, Diagnosis and Management. Baltimore, Williams & Wilkins, 1995.

central and peripheral adrenergic structures, infusion of catecholamines, and imposition of behavioral stress result in increased cardiac vulnerability in the normal and ischemic heart (4-8). These profibrillatory influences are substantially reduced by beta-adrenergic receptor blockade. Diverse supraventricular arrhythmias can also be precipitated by autonomic activation.

A striking surge in sympathetic nerve activity occurs within minutes of myocardial ischemia due to experimental left anterior descending coronary artery occlusion, as documented by both direct nerve recording measurements and more recently by complex demodulation of heart rate variability. This increase in sympathetic nerve activity is associated with a marked augmentation of vulnerability to ventricular fibrillation, as evidenced by the spontaneous occurrence of the arrhythmia, reduction in ventricular fibrillation threshold, and increased T-wave alternans magnitude (5,6). Upon reperfusion, a second peak in vulnerability ensues, probably due to washout of ischemic byproducts from the myocardium. Stellectomy blunts the surge in vulnerability to ventricular fibrillation during occlusion but augments its magnitude during reperfusion. These observations concur with the understanding that adrenergic factors are pivotal in arrhythmogenesis during ischemia and that stellectomy enhances reactive hyperemia during reperfusion resulting in greater release of profibrillatory ischemic byproducts.

The mechanisms whereby enhanced sympathetic nerve activity increases cardiac vulnerability in the normal and ischemic heart are complex (Table 1).

The major indirect effects include impaired oxygen supply-demand ratio due to increased cardiac metabolic activity and coronary vasoconstriction, particularly in vessels with injured endothelium and in the presence of altered preload and afterload. The direct profibrillatory influences on cardiac electrophysiologic function are attributable to derangements in impulse formation, conduction, or both. Increased levels of catecholamines activate beta-adrenergic receptors which consequently alter adenylate cyclase activity and intracellular calcium flux. These actions are probably mediated by the cyclic nucleotide and the protein kinase regulatory cascade, which can disrupt spatial heterogeneity of calcium transients and consequently increase dispersion of repolarization. The net influence is an increase in vulnerability to ventricular fibrillation. Conversely, stellectomy has proved to be antifibrillatory as the technique decreases cardiac sympathetic drive.

ANTIFIBRILLATORY INFLUENCES OF VAGUS NERVE ACTIVATION

Vagus nerve activation reduces the incidence of ischemia-induced spontaneous ventricular fibrillation. The extensive experimental studies demonstrate the cardioprotective effect of vagus nerve activation. These include vagus nerve stimulation, administration of vagomimetic agents, and vagotomy and have recently been reviewed (9). The main results can be summarized as follows. Vagotomy is profibrillatory during acute myocardial ischemia and reperfusion. In conscious animals, stress-induced decreases in cardiac electrical stability are markedly lowered when vagus nerve activity is blocked by atropine. Electrical stimulation of the vagus nerves decreases the incidence of fibrillation associated with exercise superimposed on acute ischemia in animals with a prior infarction.

The major component of the antifibrillatory action of the vagus nerve results from antagonism of the detrimental effects of sympathetic nerve activity (2). The molecular and cellular basis for this accentuated antagonism appears to be presynaptic inhibition of norepinephrine release and activation of muscarinic receptors, which inhibits second messenger formation by catecholamines (Fig. 1). Vagus nerve activity is not effective in preventing reperfusion-induced ventricular fibrillation during fixed rate pacing. However, during spontaneous rhythm, the rate-reducing effect of vagus nerve excitation decreases susceptibility to fibrillation by increasing diastolic perfusion time and reducing myocardial oxygen deficit, a process which lessens the amount of ischemic byproducts released.

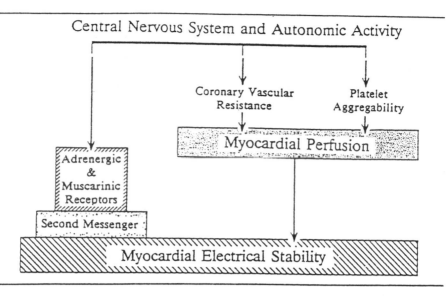

Figure 1. Summary of the mechanisms mediating the effects of the autonomic nervous system on ventricular electrical stability. Adapted from: Verrier RL. Central nervous system modulation of cardiac rhythm. In: Rosen MR, Palti Y, eds. Lethal Arrhythmias Resulting from Myocardial Ischemia and Infarction. Boston: Kluwer Academic Publishers, 1988;149-164.

In humans there is no direct evidence for an antiarrhythmic effect of vagus nerve activation at the ventricular level. However, inferential data suggest that some of the mechanisms described in experimental animals may operate in the clinical setting. Impairment of or a decrease in either vagal tone, as assessed by heart rate variability, or in reflex activation of the nerve, as assessed by baroreceptor sensitivity to phenylephrine infusion, are both associated with increased mortality and incidence of sudden death among post-myocardial infarction patients (10,11). The potential hazard of blocking tonic vagus nerve activity during the acute phase of myocardial ischemia is underscored in a case reported by Pantridge (12) in which atropine administration triggered ventricular fibrillation.

In summary, vagus nerve activation is capable of exerting significant beneficial effects on heart rhythm (Table 2). Vagus nerve stimulation can impart a potent antifibrillatory influence by presynaptic inhibition of norepinephrine release from adrenergic nerve endings and by direct muscarinic opposition of second messenger formation. Cardiac vagal tone also protects the heart against ischemia-induced susceptibility to ventricular fibrillation by reducing heart rate and the attendant cardiac metabolic demands. However, if

---

TABLE 2

BENEFICIAL EFFECTS OF ENHANCED VAGAL ACTIVITY ON VENTRICULAR ELECTRICAL STABILITY

Vagal tone exerts a rate-independent increase in myocardial electrical stability which reduces vulnerability to ventricular fibrillation during myocardial ischemia

Vagally induced reduction in heart rate plays an important role during both myocardial ischemia and reperfusion, because it increases diastolic perfusion time and reduces cardiac metabolic demand

Enhanced vagal activity has an additional antifibrillatory effect due to antagonism of adrenergic influences

The bases for sympathetic-parasympathetic interactions are:

• Inhibition of norepinephrine release from nerve endings

• Attenuation of response to catecholamines at receptor sites

Beneficial effects of vagal activity may be vitiated if profound bradycardia and hypotension ensue.

Myocardial infarction may alter autonomic influences by damaging neural fibers

---

Adapted from Verrier RL: Behavioral stress, myocardial ischemia, and arrhythmias. In Zipes DP, Jalife J (eds): Cardiac Electrophysiology: From Cell to Bedside. New York, WB Saunders, 1990.

---

the reduction in rate is excessive, the beneficial effects of vagus nerve activity may be offset by the development of hypotension and impaired coronary perfusion.

BEHAVIORAL STRESS AS A CARDIAC RISK FACTOR

There is increasing evidence of the role of behavioral stress in triggering major cardiovascular events, including myocardial ischemia and infarction, arrhythmias, and sudden cardiac death (Table 3). Cardiac events constitute the leading cause of death in men and women in the industrially developed world. In the United States alone, there are 1 million nonfatal infarctions and 250,000 sudden cardiac deaths annually. Descriptive studies indicate that emotional stress, particularly anger, fear, anxiety, bereavement, and depression, precedes both fatal and nonfatal myocardial infarction in approximately 14 to 18% of cases (3).

A recent report from the ONSET Study evaluated the role of anger as an acute precipitant of nonfatal infarction (7). Investigators interviewed 1623

TABLE 3

LETHAL PHYSIOLOGIC CHARACTERISTICS OF ACUTE BEHAVIORAL STRESS

Characteristics	Consequences
Rapid-onset sinus tachycardia	Impaired diastolic perfusion time leading to ischemia in stenosed coronary circulation
Acute hypertension	Increased cardiac metabolic demand
	Sheer stress and potential for coronary plaque rupture
Surge in catecholamines, particularly norepinephrine	Predisposition to coronary constriction especially in the presence of impaired endothelial function
	Heightezned platelet aggregability
	Increased cardiac electrical instability in the form of repolarization abnormalities, T-wave alternans and ventricular tachyarrhythmias
Abrupt offset of state with attendant imbalances between coronary hemodynamic and neurohumoral factors	Delayed myocardial ischemia due to an abrupt fall in coronary perfusion pressure in the presence of persistently elevated catecholamines
	This acute poststress state can be conducive to both myocardial infarction and arrhythmic death

From: Verrier RL, Mittleman MA. Life-threatening cardiovascular consequences of anger in patients with coronary heart disease. In: Deedwania PC, Tofler GH, eds. Triggers and Timing of Cardiac Events. Cardiology Clinics 1996;14:289-307.

patients with acute infarction an average of 4 days following onset of cardiac symptoms. In this study population, 2.4% of patients reported that they had been "very angry" during the two-hour period before myocardial infarction.

The most frequent triggers of anger were arguments with family members (25%), conflicts at work (22%), and legal problems (8%). When each patient's usual exposure during the prior year was used as the control information, the risk of myocardial infarction was found to be elevated only during the first two hours after an outburst of anger. When the control information on the usual frequency of anger was used, the relative risk of infarction onset in the 2-hour period immediately after "very angry" episodes was found to be 2.3 (95% confidence interval, 1.7-3.2). This result was similar to that obtained from control information based on exposure on the day before infarction (relative risk, 4.0; 95% confidence interval, 1.9-9.4). Finally, these results were consistent with analyses based on the anger subscale of the State-Trait Personality Inventory, which resulted in a relative risk of 1.9 (95% CI, 1.3-2.7). In this report, state anxiety was also found to be associated with a transient 1.6-fold (95% CI, 1.1-2.2) increase in risk of myocardial infarction onset. The cogent epidemiologic evidence implicating behavioral stress in cardiac risk has recently been reviewed (3).

IMPACT OF ANGERLIKE STATE ON CARDIAC ELECTRICAL PROPERTIES IN THE NORMAL AND ISCHEMIC HEART

Provocation of the angerlike state in the experimental laboratory has demonstrated that intense stress can result in substantial changes in cardiac vulnerability even in the normal heart (4). During the peak of the angerlike confrontation there was a 30-40% reduction in the threshold for inducing repetitive extrasystoles. This level of change was comparable to that produced by a shock-avoidance aversive conditioning paradigm. In the aversive setting, which produced a comparable degree of ventricular instability as did anger, the incidence of fibrillation during myocardial ischemia induced by acute coronary artery occlusion was more than three times greater than in a tranquil environment.

Recently, we determined that T-wave alternans, defined as a beat-to-beat fluctuation in T-wave magnitude, could be used to monitor anger-induced cardiac electrical instability during acute myocardial ischemia (3). This endpoint has proved to be a reliable indicator of susceptibility to ventricular fibrillation under diverse physiologic and pharmacologic interventions including acute myocardial ischemia and reperfusion, sympathetic nerve stimulation and denervation, vagus nerve activation and administration of various drugs including beta-blockers, calcium channel blockers, and nitroglycerin (13). Also, alternans magnitude is comparable to programmed electrophysiological testing in predicting arrhythmia-free survival (14). In the experimental paradigm, precordial lead V4 was recorded before and during a 3-minute period of LAD occlusion with and without provocation of the angerlike state in the canines. When anger was induced prior to ischemia. there was a substantial increase in the baseline level of T-wave alternans. This level was markedly enhanced when the arousal state was induced during coronary artery occlusion. As beta-adrenergic blockade with metoprolol markedly reduced the augmentation of T-wave alternans magnitude, it appears that the enhanced vulnerability was due to stimulation of these adrenergic receptors.

These observations carry important scientific and clinical implications. They indicate an important influence of anger on cardiac electrical properties in both the normal and ischemic heart, and that these effects are largely mediated by $beta_1$-adrenergic receptors. Clinically, the observations are significant as they suggest the potential vulnerability of patients with ischemic heart disease to anger-induced ventricular tachyarrhythmias. In addition, the findings suggested a potential noninvasive means for dynamically tracking the impact of arousal states on cardiac electrical stability.

CONCLUSIONS

The evidence reviewed underscores the pervasive impact which autonomic nervous system activity exerts on cardiovascular health. The potentially deleterious influence is manifest in many of the major forms of heart disease, including hypertension, heart failure, coronary artery disease, and susceptibility to life-threatening cardiac arrhythmias. In general, hyperadrenergic activity is deleterious and parasympathetic neural influences are cardioprotective as they antagonize the noxious actions of excessive release of catecholamines. Given the large body of evidence which has been accrued from the experimental laboratory and from human studies, behavioral stress should be regarded as a bona fide risk factor. As the actions of the autonomic nervous system are transitory but potent and are the consequence of the stresses of daily life, ambulatory monitoring of the ECG represents more than ever a valuable component of the clinical armamentarium for diagnosis and evaluation of efficacy of therapy. Particularly significant is the potential application of new ECG indexes of vulnerability to life-threatening arrhythmias (5,6,8) which can be tracked by dynamic signal processing techniques to detect transitory but potent influences of autonomic nervous system activity on cardiac vulnerability.

REFERENCES

1. Braunwald E, ed. Heart Disease: A Textbook of Cardiovascular Medicine, 5th edition. W.B. Saunders: Philadelphia, 1997.
2. Lown B, Verrier RL. Neural activity and ventricular fibrillation. N Engl J Med 1976;294: 1165-1170.
3. Verrier RL, Mittleman MA. Life-threatening cardiovascular consequences of anger in patients with coronary heart disease. In: Deedwania PC, Tofler GH, eds. Triggers and Timing of Cardiac Events. Cardiology Clinics 1996;14:289-307.
4. Verrier RL, Hagestad EL, Lown B. Delayed myocardial ischemia induced by anger. Circulation 1987;75:249-254.
5. Nearing BD, Huang AH, Verrier RL. Dynamic tracking of cardiac vulnerability by complex demodulation of the T-wave. Science 1991;252:437-440.
6. Nearing BD, Oesterle SN, Verrier RL. Quantification of ischaemia-induced vulnerability by precordial T-wave alternans analysis in dog and human. Cardiovasc Res 1994;28:1440-1449.
7. Mittleman MA, Maclure M, Sherwood JB, et al. Triggering of acute myocardial infarction onset by episodes of anger. Circulation 1995;92:1720-1725.
8. Verrier RL, Nearing BD, MacCallum G, Stone PH. T-wave alternans during ambulatory ischemia in patients with coronary heart disease. Annals of Nominvasive Electrocardiology 1996;1:113-120.
9. De Ferrari GM, Vanoli E, Schwartz PJ. Cardiac vagal activity, myocardial ischemia, and sudden death. In Zipes DP, Jalife J, eds: Cardiac Electrophysiology: From Cell to Bedside. New York, WB Saunders, 1995, pp. 422-434.
10. Kleiger RE, Miller JP, Bigger JT Jr, et al. The Multicenter Post-Infarction Research Group. Decreased heart rate variability and its association with increased mortality after acute myocardial infarction. Am J Cardiol 1987;59:256-262.
11. La Rovere MT, Bigger JT Jr, Marcus FI, Mortara A, Schwartz PJ. Baroreflex sensitivity and heart-rate variability in prediction of total cardiac mortality after myocardial infarction. ATRAMI (Autonomic Tone and Reflexes After Myocardial Infarction) Investigators. Lancet 1998;351:478-484.
12. Pantridge JF. Autonomic disturbance at the onset of acute myocardial infarction. In Schwartz PJ, Brown AM, Malliani A, Zanchetti A, eds. Neural Mechanisms in Cardiac Arrhythmias. New York, Raven Press, 1978.
13. Verrier RL. Physiology of electrical alternans. Cardiac Electrophysiology Review 1997;3 :383-388.
14. Rosenbaum DS, Jackson LE, Smith JM, et al. Electrical alternans and vulnerability to ventricular arrhythmia. N Engl J Med 1994;330:235-241.
15. Verrier RL. Central nervous system modulation of cardiac rhythm. In Rosen MR, Palti Y, eds. Lethal Arrhythmias Resulting from Myocardial Ischemia and Infarction. Boston, Kluwer Academic Publishers, 1988.
16. Verrier RL, Kovach JA. Primary role of beta-adrenergic receptors in arrhythmogenesis during sympathetic nervous system activation. In Podrid PJ, Kowey PR, eds. Cardiac

Arrhythmias: Mechanism, Diagnosis and Management. Baltimore, Williams & Wilkins, 1995.

17. Verrier RL. Behavioral stress, myocardial ischemia, and arrhythmias. In Zipes DP, Jalife J, eds. Cardiac Electrophysiology: From Cell to Bedside. New York, WB Saunders, 1990.

7. THERAPEUTICAL OPTIONS TO INFLUENCE THE AUTONOMIC NERVOUS SYSTEM

EMILIO VANOLI, PAOLO VALENTINI
AND ROBERTO PEDRETTI

SUMMARY

The evidence of the predictive value of autonomic markers has generated a growing interest for interventions able to influence autonomic control of heart rate. The efficacy of β-blockers is well established and recent data document the effectiveness of this intervention even in patients with congestive heart failure. It has to be noted that efficacy of ß-blockers is associated with and, at least in part, due to heart rate reduction. As an alternative to antiadrenergic intervention, the hypothesis exists that an increase in cardiac vagal activity, as detected by an increase in Heart Rate Variability (HRV) or baroreflex sensitivity (BRS), may be beneficial in the ischemic heart. Supportive of this approach is the evidence that ventricular fibrillation during acute myocardial ischemia may be largely prevented by electrical stimulation of the right cervical vagus or by pharmacological stimulation of cholinergic receptors with oxotremorine. However, there is an inherent danger in the so far unwarranted assumption that modification of HRV or BRS translates directly in cardiac protection. It should be remembered that the target is the improvement in cardiac electrical stability and that BRS or HRV are just markers of autonomic activity. Low dose scopolamine increases HRV in patients with a prior myocardial infarction (MI). This observation has lead to study of the effect of vagal modulation by low dose scopolamine on arrhythmic risk after MI. We tested low dose scopolamine in a clinically relevant experimental preparation

H.-H. Osterhues et al. (eds.),
Advances in Noninvasive Electrocardiographic Monitoring Techniques, 69–86.
© 2000 *Kluwer Academic Publishers. Printed in the Netherlands.*

for sudden death in which other vagomimetic interventions are effective and found that this intervention does indeed increase cardiac vagal markers but has minimal antifibrillatory effects. This is at variance from exercise training that, in the same experimental model, had a marked effect on both baroreflex sensitivity and HRV and at the same time provided strong protection from ischemic ventricular fibrillation. Thus, based on the current knowledge it seems appropriate to call for caution before attributing excessive importance to changes in "markers" of vagal activity in the absence of clear-cut evidence for a causal relation with an antifibrillatory effect.

Key Words: Vagal activity, ventricular fibrillation, myocardial infarction

INTRODUCTION

Experimental and clinical evidence have established and described the existence of a tight relation between autonomic nervous system, acute myocardial ischemia and occurrence of lethal cardiac arrhythmias (1-5). Specifically, dominance of sympathetic or vagal reflexes during acute myocardial ischemia markedly increases or decreases, respectively, the risk for developing lethal arrhythmias and sudden death.

This information has lead to the successful use of autonomic markers, like baroreflex sensitivity (BRS) and heart rate variability (HRV) for risk stratification after myocardial infarction. The hypothesis that the analysis of autonomic function could have been helpful in arrhythmia risk detection was initially suggested in an experimental preparation of sudden death in conscious dogs with a healed myocardial infarction. In this model a depressed BRS identified a large proportion of dogs at high risk of developing sudden death at the time of a new ischemic episode. Subsequently, the clinical relevance of this information was proposed by some pilot studies (8,9) and recently confirmed by the multi-center prospective international study ATRAMI (Autonomic Tone and Reflexes After Myocardial Infarction). In 1284 post-myocardial infarction patients ATRAMI has shown that both BRS and HRV have a strong and independent predictive value for cardiac and arrhythmic mortality (10).

The concept of manipulating autonomic nervous system after myocardial infarction is widely accepted and has resulted in the effective use of β-blockers after myocardial infarction. Nowadays, two opposite trends seems to influence the use of these interventions. On one side, β-blockers are frequently not adequately or properly used (11). On the other hand, the evidence of the predictive value of autonomic markers has generated a growing interest for new interventions able to influence autonomic control of heart rate and, specifically, the vagal component. The though underlying this interest is that an increase in cardiac vagal activity, as detected by an increase in HRV or BRS, may be beneficial in the ischemic heart. As matter of fact, the concept that interventions augmenting vagal activity might be protective against lethal ischemic arrhythmias is supported by numerous experimental data (12). Among them, the evidence that ventricular fibrillation during acute myocardial ischemia may be largely prevented by electrical stimulation of the right cervical vagus (13) or by pharmacological stimulation of cholinergic receptors with oxotremorine (14,15). There is, however, an inherent danger in the so far unwarranted assumption that modification of HRV or BRS translates directly in cardiac protection. This may and may not be the case. It should be remembered that the true target is the improvement in cardiac electrical stability and that BRS or HRV are just markers of autonomic activity.

Hereafter experimental and clinical data concerning the influences of pharmacological and non pharmacological interventions able to modulate autonomic markers and ventricular electrical stability will be discussed.

THE PREDICTIVE VALUE OF AUTONOMIC MARKERS

Autonomic markers and risk for ventricular fibrillation

Several information on the mechanisms involved in the genesis of sudden cardiac death had been obtained in an experimental model in which ventricular fibrillation could be reproducibly induced by clinically relevant stimuli (6). This conscious animal preparation, already described in several circumstances, combines three elements highly relevant to the genesis of malignant arrhythmias in man: a healed myocardial infarction, acute myocardial ischemia, and physiologically elevated sympathetic activity. In brief, 30 days after an anterior wall myocardial infarction, chronically instrumented dogs perform a submaximal exercise stress test. When heart rate reaches approximately 210-220 b/min, a 2-minute occlusion of the circumflex coronary artery is performed by means of a pneumatic occluder previously positioned around the vessel. After 1 minute exercise stops while the occlusion continues for another minute. This "exercise and ischemia test" triggers ventricular fibrillation in almost 50% of the animals. The outcome of the test is highly reproducible over time in the same animal and allows to the clear separation of two groups: 1) animals that develop ventricular fibrillation and are classified "susceptible" to sudden death; 2) dogs that survive and are defined "resistant". A critical difference between the two groups of dogs was that "resistant" dogs very often had marked reduction in heart rate during acute myocardial

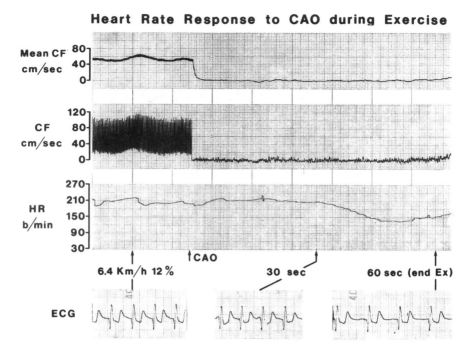

Figure 1. Heart rate response to acute myocardial ischemia in a dog resistant to ventricular fibrillation. From top to bottom, mean and actual coronary flow (CF), the tachogram and the electrocardiogram (ECG) before and at 30 and 60 seconds of acute ischemia. Within 30 seconds of ischemia a marked bradycardia occurs despite the ongoing exercise and the animal is protected from lethal events. Atropine completely prevents the reflex heart rate reduction during ischemia.

ischemia despite the ongoing exercise while susceptible dogs had an opposite response, i.e. an increase in heart rate (6). The reflex heart rate increase during ischemia could have been readily explained by the combination of the baroreflex response to the decline in arterial blood pressure and of the excitatory cardio-cardiac sympathetic reflex (16). However resistant and susceptible dogs have similar blood pressure during ischemia the unexpected heart rate reduction induced by myocardial ischemia in the resistant dogs was clearly dependent on a vagal reflex, as it could be prevented by atropine (Figure 1).

This evidence triggered the idea of measuring vagal reflexes by analysing BRS, specifically looking to the vagally mediated reflex bradycardia consequent to blood pressure rise. By using the Sleight's method (18), BRS was expressed by the slope of the regression line correlating consecutive R-R intervals with the increasing values of systolic blood pressure due to the bolus

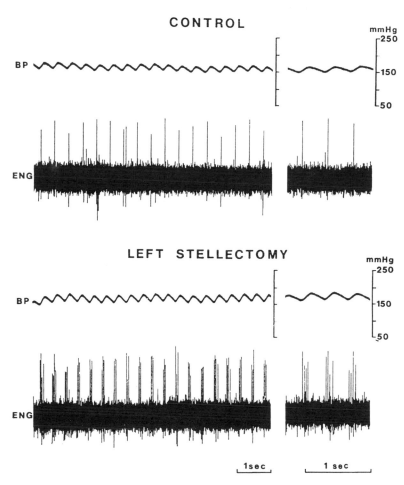

Figure 2. Tracings showing the activity of a single cardiac vagal efferent fiber, at the same blood pressure level before and after (bottom panel) left stellectomy. The fiber shows a pulse-synchronous activity that is clearly increased after left stellectomy.

injection of phenylephrine. The main finding of this study was that in 86 dogs resistant to sudden death BRS was significantly lower than in 106 dogs at high risk for ventricular fibrillation (17.7 ± 6.0 vs. 9.1 ± 6.5 ms/mm p<0.001). The link between altered autonomic control of heart rate and risk for lethal arrhythmias was further described by the use of HRV (19,20). The predictive value of this marker has been extensively described (21).

Mechanisms of autonomic imbalance after myocardial infarction

The comprehension of the potential factors involved in autonomic imbalance after MI is critical for the use of autonomic markers for post-MI risk stratification and for the interpretation of the effects of autonomic interventions. Such mechanisms are not yet fully understood, but neural reflexes of cardiac origin are likely involved. Among the various possibilities (4), cardio-cardiac sympatho-vagal reflexes (16) may play an important role. The changes in the geometry of a beating heart secondary to the presence of a necrotic and noncontracting segment may quite conceivably increase beyond normal the firing of sympathetic afferent fibers by mechanical distortion of their sensory endings. Such a sympathetic excitation affects and impairs the baroreceptor reflex, i.e. interferes with the physiological increase in the activity of vagal fibers directed to the sinus node (22,23). This hypothesis is supported by experimental evidence obtained by recording vagal efferent activity prior to and after removal of the left sided afferent and efferent cardiac sympathetic fibers by left stellectomy in anesthetized cats (22) (Figure 2). In 16 anesthetized cats removal of the left stellate ganglion increased resting level of vagal activity from 1.2 ± 0.2 to 2.1 ± 0.3 imp/sec, ($+ 75\%$, $p<0.01$). In the same cats, vagal activity during similar blood pressure rises induced by phenylephrine was also higher after left stellectomy (4.7 ± 0.7 vs. 2.2 ± 0.4 imp/sec, $p<0.001$), with an increment of 134 ± 24 vs. $86 \pm 18\%$, ($p<0.05$) versus the resting level. These data support the hypothesis that the depression in vagal control of heart rate observed often after MI may depend largely on an increase in afferent sympathetic traffic of cardiac origin.

MODULATION OF AUTONOMIC CONTROL OF HEART RATE

Non Pharmacological interventions: Exercise training

A physiologic way to achieve an increase in vagal control of heart rate is represented by exercise training. It is a common knowledge that exercise training produces a lower resting and exercising heart rate (24). This typical response has been interpreted as the consequence of a combined effect of exercise training on both limbs of the autonomic nervous system.

The exercise training-induced changes in cardiac vagal activity are the results of several significant modifications on the heart and on the autonomic nervous system (25). Surprisingly, there is very little information on the effects of exercise training on autonomic markers. An increase in heart rate variability and baroreflex sensitivity after exercise training has been described in normal

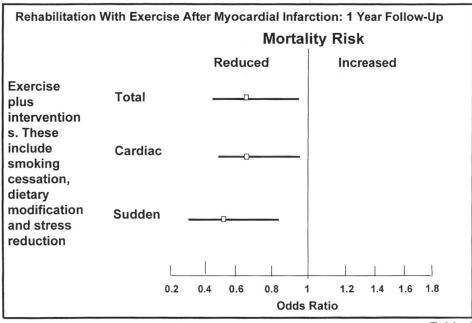

and in mild hypertensive subjects (26). A critical aspect of exercise training is its health benefit, and specifically the potential positive impact on cardiovascular mortality (table 1, 27-29).

The availability of the experimental model in conscious dogs where occurrence or prevention of lethal arrhythmias primarily depends upon autonomic reflexes allowed us to investigate the relation between autonomic modifications induced by exercise training and risk for sudden cardiac death. In a first study (30), we observed that 6 weeks of exercise training significantly increased the depressed baroreflex sensitivity of 8 dogs with a healed myocardial infarction susceptible to ventricular fibrillation (from 5.4 + 1.2 to 13.2 + 4 msec/mmHg). At the same time, another group of susceptible dogs was kept for six weeks in cage rest and did not show any autonomic change. The main finding of the study was that, concomitant with the increase in BRS, all 8 trained dogs became resistant to lethal arrhythmias during the exercise and ischemia test while all but one cage-rested dogs had no change in BRS and had recurrence of ventricular fibrillation. The one dog that behaved differently in this latter group had an increase in its BRS and became resistant to sudden cardiac death. The advantage of this experimental preparation is that, at variance from clinical trials, by definition no changes in lifestyle other than exercise training occurred in the subjects under study. In this controlled environment this was the first documentation that training could be an independent factor able to concomitantly modify a marker of cardiac vagal activity and to reduce risk for ventricular fibrillation.

Our initial observation in conscious dogs was interpreted as potentially dependent upon an increased cardiac performance in hearts damaged by the anterior wall myocardial infarction. We recently extended the initial observation to dogs without myocardial infarction to test whether exercise training prior to an ischemic event could be of benefit at the time of its occurrence (31). Seven healthy dogs that developed ventricular fibrillation during a control exercise and ischemia test were exposed to six weeks of exercise training. After this treatment, the low to high frequency ratio in the spectral analysis of heart rate variability was decreased by 52%, BRS increased by 69% from 16±8 to 27±14 msec/mmHg and the electrical threshold for ventricular repetitive responses was increased by 44%, from 32±6 to 46±4 mA. At the same time, none of the dogs developed again ventricular fibrillation during a second exercise and ischemia test. A likely mechanism involved in this antifibrillatory effect involves the fact that exercise training increases metabolic efficiency during ischemia (indeed, exercise training seems to be able to specifically act at various site and on various mechanisms involved in genesis of ischemia-dependent ventricular tachyarrhythmias). However, the fact that repetitive extrasystole threshold was also significantly increased after training strongly support the hypothesis that this intervention, by modulating autonomic balance, significantly improves the electrical stability of the ventricles.

Thus, exercise training appears to be very effective in increasing vagal control of heart rate. This results in an improvement of cardiac electrical stability and, ultimately, in a reduced risk for arrhythmic events in the ischemic heart as the consequence of several concomitant actions on ventricular performance, metabolic activity, cardiac reflexes.

Pharmacological interventions:

Beta-adrenergic receptors blockers

The effectiveness of ß-blocker therapy after myocardial infarction has been extensively documented and this therapy is a primary choice in high risk patients, specifically with ischemic heart disease. Despite this established evidence very little information exists about the influence of beta-blockers on autonomic markers. Few clinical reports have indicated that ß-blockers can positively affect heart rate variability (32). Recent data suggest that carvedilol may increase baroreflex sensitivity in patients with congestive heart failure

(33). On the other hand, the analysis of the interaction between bisoprolol, a selective ß1-receptors blocker, heart rate and survival in heart failure patients has shown interesting data (34). The CIBIS II study documented, for the first time prospectively, that ß-blocker therapy, in this case using bisoprolol, reduces mortality in heart failure patients (35). Bisoprolol significantly reduced heart rate and its variability in a subgroup of patients from the first CIBIS study (36,37) . In this study, heart rate reduction over time was a strong predictor of survival. However, patients receiving bisoprolol were at lower risk than those on placebo whatever their heart rate change was over time while in the placebo group the risk of dying decreased only when heart rate decreased. This analysis documents that the interaction between antiadrenergic interventions heart rate and survival is complex but also underscore the fact that analysis of heart rate provide information on the efficacy of ß-blocker therapy in heart failure.

Low dose of muscarinic receptors blocking agents

Low dose of muscarinic receptors blockers may produce a paradoxical increase in vagal efferent activity. Atropine is known to induce bradycardia (as a "paradoxical" vagomimetic effect) at low doses and the expected heart rate increase (as the typical antimuscarinic effect) at higher doses (38). For atropine the effect at low dose has been recognized since the beginning of the century (39), but the precise mechanisms has not yet been fully clarified.

In 1993 four different studies from independent groups reported similar findings using transdermal administration of scopolamine (40-43). The main finding common to the four studies was that in patients with a healed myocardial infarction low dose scopolamine were able to significantly increase various measures of HRV both in time and frequency domain. The conclusion derived from the HRV results were also strengthened by the study of BRS performed in three of these four studies. BRS was increased by scopolamine by an extent ranging from 42 to 98%.

In one of these studies (42) the influences of transdermal scopolamine on cardiac electrical properties were also evaluated. Effective refractory periods of right atrium, atrioventricular node, and right ventricle were assessed before and after scopolamine in 20 patients with a recent MI. After wearing one patch of transdermal scopolamine for 24 hours, right atrium refractory period decreased from 242 ± 44 to 223 ± 41 msec ($p<0.01$), atrioventricular node refractory period increased from 320 ± 65 to 357 ± 77 msec ($p<0.05$) and right ventricle refractory period increased from 224 ± 14 to 235 ± 16 msec ($p<0.001$)

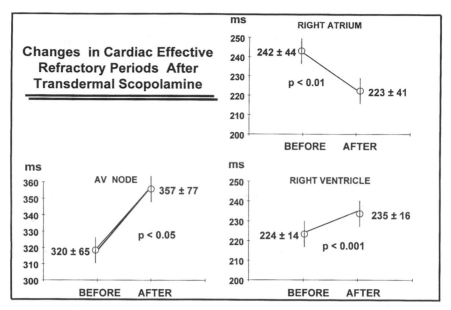

Figure 3. Effect of low dose scopolamine on refractoriness in the right atrium and ventricle and on the atrioventricular node (av node). The increase in cardiac vagal activity after scopolamine results in an increased refractoriness of the av node and of the right ventricle and in reduced refractoriness at the atrial level.

More recently attention has been devoted to pirenzepine, an antimuscarinic agent widely used for peptic ulcer therapy, that, at variance from scopolamine, does not have central action, and, more importantly can be used orally for long time with minimal side effects.

In a single-blind placebo-controlled crossover trial (44) 20 patients underwent evaluation of short-term RR-variability and BRS 19 ± 6 days after the infarction. Analysis was performed in control condition and during placebo, oral pirenzepine and transdermal scopolamine administration. In an initial dose-response study 5 of 8 post-MI patients showed a significant increase in BRS and were considered responders to pirenzepine. BRS was reassessed after 2 days of therapy for each oral dose tested. If a BRS increase > 4 ms / mm Hg occurred, the patient was considered responder to pirenzepine and that dose was defined effective. All responder patients underwent treatment with a higher dose to assess the possibility of a further increase of vagal activity. In all responder patients administration of a pirenzepine dose higher than the effective one did not induce a further increase in baroreceptor reflex sensitivity value.

Compared with placebo pirenzepine, at the dose of 25 mg BID, significantly increased all time and frequency domain measures of RR-variability, and augmented BRS by 60% (10.37 ± 6.82 vs. 6.47 ± 3.22 msec/mmHg, p = 0.0025). Pirenzepine showed a vagomimetic effect that was comparable with that observed with scopolamine, but with a markedly lower incidence of adverse effects. Oral pirenzepine may have a potential therapeutic application for long term treatment of post-MI patients.

Overall, these data combined with the experimental evidence of the antifibrillatory effect of vagal stimulation fostered the idea that low dose antimuscarinivc agents might be an effective tool to improve autonomic balance after MI. However, confirmatory data are necessary to prove that such a change in autonomic markers would indeed result in a significant increase in the electrical stability of the ischemic heart.

Experimental evidence: the effect of scopolamine on autonomic markers and on ventricular fibrillation.

In order to investigate whether a relation exists between changes in markers of cardiac vagal activity and changes in cardiac electrical stability an experimental study was designed with the specific goal to verify if an intervention known for its ability to increase HRV and BRS would, at the same time, be effective in reducing the incidence of ischemia-induced ventricular fibrillation in the clinically relevant animal preparation (6). The effects of low dose scopolamine i.v. on HRV and cardiac electrical stability were studied in dogs with a prior MI that had or had not ventricular fibrillation during an exercise and ischemia test (45).

Prior to scopolamine, susceptible animals had an average StD of the mean R-R interval lower than that of the resistant ones (136+30 vs. 224+ 33 msec, -65%, p< 0.01). This difference was progressively reduced by increasing doses of scopolamine and, at 1 and 3 µg/kg, the values among the two groups became similar: 223±35 vs. 322±31 msec (NS). At higher dose, 10 µg/kg, StD decreased. The coefficient of variance (i.e. the StD of RR interval corrected for heart rate) showed the same pattern observed for the StD. Prior to scopolamine, it was lower by 45% in the susceptible dogs when compared with the resistant (203±40 vs. 294±33, P <0.01). This difference was reduced to 2% after administration of 3 µg/kg of scopolamine (198±23 vs. 224±43; NS).

Thus, the effect of scopolamine in autonomic markers in this experimental study parallelled the clinical findings observed in the 4 studies in post-MI patients. Additionally, 3.0 µg/kg of scopolamine reduced heart rate at rest and during the lower levels of exercise and ischemia test. However, the chronotropic effect of scopolamine disappeared at higher levels of exercise. During the exercise and ischemia test just prior to the occlusion of the circumflex coronary artery heart rate was 227+8 b/min in the control test and

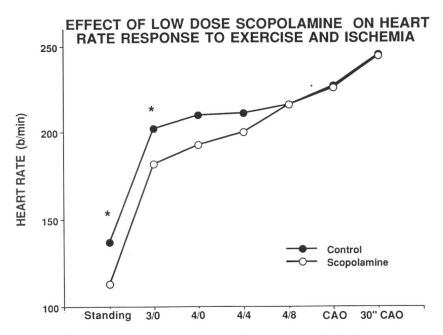

Figure 4. Heart rate response to exercise and acute myocardial ischemia in control conditions and after scopolamine.

226±7 b/min with scopolamine. The reflex response to acute myocardial ischemia was also, in this setting, unaffected by scopolamine. Heart rate at 30 seconds of ischemia was 245±15 b/min in the control tests and 244±15 b/min with scopolamine (Figure 4).

The critical finding of the study was that scopolamine had minimal antifibrillatory effect. Ventricular fibrillation was indeed prevented in only 1 (14%) of the 7 susceptible dogs in which it was tested (Figure 5).

Mechanisms of action of low dose muscarinic receptors blockers and possible explanation of the observed failure
Low dose atropine increases neural activity directly recorded in the vagus (46). Acetylcholine mediates the effects of inhibitory fibers projecting from the ventrolateral respiratory reticular formation on the vagal motoneurons (47). Specifically, during inspiration acetylcholine released from these fibers causes an hyperpolarization of vagal motoneurons and, consequently, a reduction in their firing rate. Atropine, by blocking these inhibitory mechanisms may increase the vagal motoneurons activity. This hypothesis is supported by the fact that iontophoretic administration of atropine in the area of the nucleus ambiguous increases the firing of vagal-cardiac motoneurons (47). In addition

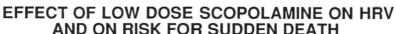

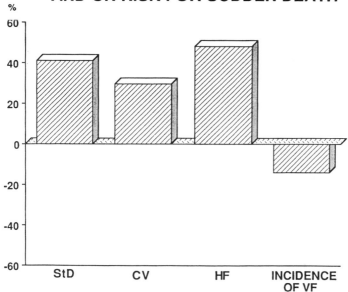

Figure 5. Effect of low dose scopolamine on different measures of heart rate variability and on risk for ventricular fibrillation during the exercise and ischemia test. Std=standard deviation of RR intervals; CV=coefficient of variance; HF= power in the high frequency band of spectral analysis of heart rate variability.

to central actions, peripheral mechanisms, notably blockade of the presynaptic muscarinic modulation of acetylcholine release (48), may contribute to the effect of low dose scopolamine on HRV. This is suggested by the evidence that pirenzepine, that does not seem to have central actions, increases HRV.

The chronotropic effects of scopolamine progressively decreased with exercise and were largely lost at the highest workload of the submaximal test. The reflex response to acute myocardial ischemia was also unaffected by scopolamine. Overall, the vagal antagonism of the detrimental electrophysiologic effects of adrenergic activation was absent when mostly needed. Based on these findings, the failure of scopolamine in preventing ventricular fibrillation is no longer surprising, particularly in a preparation in which sympathetic reflexes are major contributors to the occurrence of lethal arrhythmias (49).

Clinical Implications
The clinical implications of the present data are that low dose of muscarinic receptors blockers have a positive effect on autonomic markers but seems to be

of little effect in reducing risk for lethal events in the acutely ischemic heart specifically at a time when sympathetic activity is elevated. This is quite at variance with what has been observed with exercise training, that by affecting several aspects of the cardiovascular system and regulation significantly increases autonomic markers and also provides a striking protection from VF.

On the other hand the potential importance of a chronic (as with exercise training) versus an acute (as with scopolamine) modulation of the autonomic activity should not be underestimated. In this prospective the use of pirenzepine, a muscarinic antagonists that, as just described, increases autonomic markers and can be used chronically may open the prospective of a long term treatment. The possibility of a chronic modulation of cardiac vagal activity in high risk post-MI patients deserves attention. This aspect should be carefully taken in consideration in view of the evidence that scopolamine exerts beneficial effects on HRV also in patients with left ventricular dysfunction and heart failure (50). Specifically, in 21 patients with moderate to severe heart failure scopolamine increased the standard deviation of RR-variability by 45%, without markedly influencing heart rate (-5%). Chronic heart failure is associated with a marked vagal withdrawal and with a very high risk of cardiac and arrhythmic mortality strongly related to the level of sympathetic activation (51). Scopolamine or pirenzepine might open the way to the development of new interventions able to modulate autonomic imbalance in heart failure without affecting left ventricular function or causing significant bradycardia as it may occur with ß-blockers. If maintained over time, vagal stimulation may then favorably influence the risk for lethal events.

CONCLUSIONS

The rationale for the attempts to increase autonomic markers in post-MI patients rests on the multiple evidence that the risk for cardiac mortality and sudden death is higher among individuals with signs of decreased vagal activity. Beta-blockers, so far, represent one of the most effective treatment after MI and likely in congestive heart failure. ACE inhibitors, that are also effective in reducing mortality after MI, probably exert an useful action on sympathovagal balance (52).

A major limitation to the use of autonomic markers to predict efficacy is represented by the fact that the degree of increase in vagal activity that may produce antifibrillatory effects is still unknown. Exercise training acts on several aspects of cardiovascular regulation and function , shifts the autonomic balance toward a vagal dominance and significantly increases cardiac electrical stability. On the other hand, low dose of muscarinic antagonists, while positively affecting autonomic markers, seem to have little effect on cardiac electrical stability specifically in condition of elevated sympathetic activity. A possible explanation of this failure stands on the fact that acute administrations of these compounds looses efficacy when mostly needed, i.e. in condition of elevated sympathetic activity. The possibility that chronic treatment with low dose muscarinic antagonists may result beneficial deserves further investigation. However, based on the current knowledge it seems appropriate to call for caution before attributing excessive importance to changes in "markers" of vagal activity in the absence of clear-cut evidence for a causal relation with an antifibrillatory effect.

REFERENCES

1. Lown B, Verrier RL: Neural activity and ventricular fibrillation. (1976) New England J Medicine 294, 21:1165-1170.

2. Corr PB, Yamada KA, Witkowski FX: Mechanisms controlling cardiac autonomic function and their relation to arrhythmogenesis (1986). In: The heart and cardiovascular system. Vol. II (Fozzard HA, Haber F., Jennings RB, Katz AM, Morgan HE, Eds.) Raven Press, New York, pp 1343-1403.

3. Schwartz PJ, Priori SG: Sympathetic nervous system and cardiac arrhythmias. In: Cardiac electrophysiology (1990). From cell to bedside (Zipes DP, Jalife J, Eds) WB Saunders Co, Philadelphia, pp 330-343.

4. Schwartz PJ, La Rovere MT, Vanoli E (1982). Autonomic nervous system and sudden cardiac death. Circulation 85(suppl I):I-77-91.

5. Vanoli E and Schwartz PJ (1990) Sympathetic-parasympathetic interaction and sudden death. Basic Res in Cardiol 85(Suppl 1):305-321.

6. Schwartz PJ, Billman GE, Stone HL (1984). Autonomic mechanisms in ventricular fibrillation induced by myocardial ischemia during exercise in dogs with a healed myocardial infarction. An experimental preparation for sudden cardiac death. Circulation 69:780-790.

7. Schwartz PJ, Vanoli E, Stramba-Badiale M, De Ferrari GM, Billman GE, Foreman RD (1988). Autonomic mechanisms and sudden death. New insights from the analysis of baroreceptor reflexes in conscious dogs with an without a myocardial infarction. Circulation 78: 969-979.

8. La Rovere MT, Specchia G, Mortara A, Schwartz PJ (1988) Baroreflex sensitivity, clinical correlates and cardiovascular mortality among patients with a first myocardial infarction. A prospective study. Circulation 78:816-824.

9. Farrell TG, Paul V, Cripps TR, et al. (1991)Baroreflex sensitivity and electrophysiological correlates in patients after acute myocardial infarction. Circulation 83:945-952.

10. La Rovere MT, Bigger JT, Jr, Marcus FI, Mortara A, Schwartz PJ. Baroreflex sensitivity and heart rate variability in prediction of total cardiac mortality after myocardial infarction. The Lancet 1998; 351:478-484

11. Viskin S, Barron HV (1996). Beta blockers prevent cardiac death following a myocardial infarction: so why are so many infarct survivors discharged without beta blockers? Am J Cardiolpgy 79: 821-822

12. De Ferrari GM, Vanoli E, Schwartz PJ (1995). Cardiac vagal activity, myocardial ischemia and sudden death. In: CARDIAC ELECTROPHYSIOLOGY. FROM CELL TO BEDSIDE. II EDITION Zipes DP and Jalife J (Eds.) WB Saunders Co., Philadelphia, pp. 422-434.

13. Vanoli E, De Ferrari GM, Stramba-Badiale M, Hull SS Jr, Foreman RD and Schwartz PJ (1991). Vagal stimulation and prevention of sudden death in conscious dogs with a healed myocardial infarction. Circ Res 68:1471-1481.

14. De Ferrari GM, Vanoli E, Curcuruto P, Tommasini G, Schwartz PJ (1992). Prevention of life-threatening arrhythmias by pharmacologic stimulation of the muscarinic receptors with oxotremorine. Am Heart J 124:883-890.

15. De Ferrari GM, Salvati P, Grossoni M, Ukmar G, Vaga L, Patrono C, Schwartz PJ (1993). Pharmacologic modulation of the autonomic nervous system in the prevention of sudden cardiac death. A study with propranolol, methacholine and oxotremorine in conscious dogs with a healed myocardial infarction. J Am Coll Cardiol 21:283-290.

16. Malliani A, Schwartz PJ, Zanchetti A (1969) A sympathetic reflex elicited by experimental coronary occlusion. Am J Physiol 217:703-709.

17. De Ferrari GM, Vanoli E, Stramba-Badiale M, Hull SS Jr, Foreman RD, Schwartz PJ (1991). Vagal reflexes and survival during acute myocardial ischemia in conscious dogs with healed myocardial infarction. Am J Physiol 261:H63-H69.

18. Smyth HS, Sleight P, Pickering GW (1969). Reflex regulation of arterial pressure during sleep in man. Circ Res 24:109-121.

19. Hull SS, Evans AR, Vanoli E, Adamson PB, Stramba-Badiale M, Albert DE, Foreman RD, Schwartz PJ (1990). Heart rate variability before and after myocardial infarction in conscious dogs at high and low risk of sudden death. J Am Coll Cardiol 16:978-985.

20. Vanoli E, Adamson PB, Cerati D, Hull SS: Heart rate variability and risk stratification post-myocardial infarction (1995). In.: HEART RATE VARIABILITY M Malik and AJ Camm (Eds.) Futura publishing, Armonk NY, pp 347-361.

21. Task Force of the European Society of Cardiology and the North American Society of Pacing and Electrophysiology (Bigger JT Jr, Breithardt G, Camm AJ, Cerutti S, Cohen RJ, Coumel P, Fallen EL, Kennedy HL, Kleiger RE, Lombardi F, Malik M, Malliani A, Moss AJ, Rottman JN, Schmidt G, Schwartz PJ, Singer DH): Heart rate variability (1996). Standards of measurement, physiological interpretation, and clinical use. Circulation 93:1043-1065, and Eur Heart J 17:354-381.

22. Cerati D, Schwartz PJ (1991). Single cardiac vagal fiber activity, acute myocardial ischemia, and risk for sudden death. Circ Res 69:1389-1401.

23. Gnecchi Ruscone T, Lombardi F, Malfatto G, Malliani A (1987). Attenuation of baroreceptive mechanisms by cardiovascular sympathetic afferent fibers. Am J Physiol 253:H787-H791

24. Scheuer J, Tipton CM (1977). Cardiovascular adaptations to physical training.   Ann Rev Physiol 39:221-251.

25. Stone HL (1977). Cardiac function and exercise training in conscious dogs. J Appl Physiol 42:824-832

26. Pagani M, Somers V, Furlan R, Dell'Orto S, Conway J, Baselli G, Cerutti S, Sleight P (1988) Changes in autonomic regulation induced by physical training in mild hypertension. Hypertension 12:600-610.
27. Ekelunnd GL, Haskell WL, Johnson JL, Whaley FS, Criqui MH, Sheps DS (1988) Physical fitness as a predictor of cardiovascular mortality in asymptomatic North American men: the Lipid Research Clinics Mortality Follow-up Study. N Engl J Med 319:1379-1384.
28. Sandvik L, Erikssen J, Thaulow E, Erikssen G, Mundal R, Rodahl K (1993) Physical fitness as a predictor of cardiovascular mortality among healthy,middle-aged norwegian men. N Engl J Med 328:533-537.
29. O'Connor GT, Buring JE, Yusuf S, Goldhaber SZ, Olmstead M, Paffenbarger RS Jr, Hennekens CH (1989) An overview of randomized trials of rehabilitation with exercise after myocardial infarction. Circulation 80:234-244.
30. Billman GE, Schwartz PJ, Stone HL (1984) The effects of daily exercise on susceptibility to sudden cardiac death. Circulation 69, 6:1182-1189.
31. Hull SS Jr, Vanoli E, Adamson PB, Verrier RL, Foreman RD, Schwartz PJ (1994) Exercise training confers anticipatory protection from sudden death during acute myocardial ischemia. Circulation 89:548-552.
32. Sandrone G, Mortara A, Torzillo D, et al. (1994). Effects of β-blockers (atenolol or metoprolol) on heart rate variability after acute myocardial infarction. Am J Cardiol 74: 340-345
33. Mortara A, La Rovere MT, Capomolla S, Febo O, Riccardi G, Pozzoli M, Opasich C, Tavazzi L (1997). In chronic heart failure β-blockade therapy is associated with restoration of arterial baroreflex gain. Circulation 96; Suppl I:644
34. Lechat P, Escolano S, Golmard JL, Lardoux H, Witchitz S, Henneman JA, Maisch B, Hetzel M, Jaillon P, Boissel JP, Mallet A, on behalf of the CIBIS Investigators (1997). Prognostic value of Bisoprolol-induced hemodynamic effects in heart failure during the cardiac insuffuciency Bisoprolol study (CIBIS) Circulation 96: 2197-2205.
35. CIBIS II Investigators and committees (1999). The cardiac insufficiency bisoprolol study II (CIBIS ii): A randomized trial. The Lancet 353:9-13.
36. Pousset F, Copie X, Lechat P, Jaillon P, Boissel JP, Hetzel M, Fillette F, Remme W, Guize L, Le Heuzey JY (1996). Effects of bisoprolol on heart rate variability in heart failure. Am J Cardiol 77: 612-617.
37. CIBIS Investigators and Committees (1994). A randomized trial of β-blockade in heart failure: the Cardiac Insufficiency BIsoprolol Study (CIBIS). Circulation 90: 1765-1773
38. Wellstein A, Pitschner HF (1988). Complex dose-response curves of atropine in man explained by different functions of M1- and M2-cholinoceptors. Naunyn-Schmiedeberg's Arch Pharmacol 338: 19-27.
39. Wilson FN (1915): The production of atrioventricular rhythm in man after the administration of atropine . Arch Intern Med, 16:989-1007
40. Casadei B, Pipilis A, Sessa F, Conway J, Sleight P (1993). Low doses of scopolamine increases cardiac vagal tone in the acute phase of myocardial infarction. Circulation 88:353-357.

41. De Ferrari GM, Mantica M, Vanoli E, Hull SS Jr, Schwartz PJ (1993). Scopolamine increases vagal tone and vagal reflexes in patients after myocardial infarction. J Am Coll Cardiol 22:1327-1334.
42. Pedretti R, Colombo E, Sarzi Braga S, Carù B (1993). Influence of transdermal scopolamine on cardiac sympathovagal interaction after acute myocardial infarction. Am J Cardiol 72:384-392.
43. Vybiral T, Glaeser DH, Morris G, Hess KR, Yang K, Francis M, Pratt CM (1993). Effects of low doses scopolamine on heart rate variability in acute myocardial infarction. J Am Coll Cardiol 22:1320-1326
44. Pedretti RFE, Colombo E, Sarzi Braga S, Ballardini L, Carù B (1995). Effects of oral pirenzepine on heart rate variability and baroreceptor reflex sensitivity after acute myocardial infarction. J Am Coll Cardiol 25:915-921.
45. Hull SS Jr, Vanoli E, Adamson PB, De Ferrari GM, Foreman RD, Schwartz PJ (1995). Do increases in markers of vagal activity imply protection from sudden death? The case of scopolamine. Circulation 91:2516-2519.
46. Katona PG, Lipson D, Dauchot PJ (1977) Opposing central and peripheral effects of atropine on parasympathetic cardiac control Am J Physiol 232:H146-H151.
47. McCloskey DI: Cardiorespiratory integration (1994). In: VAGAL CONTROL OF THE HEART: EXPERIMENTAL BASIS AND CLINICAL IMPLICATIONS Levy MN and Schwartz PJ (eds.). Futura Publishing Co, Armonk, NY, pp 481-508.
48. Wetzel GT, Brown JH (1985): Presynaptic modulation of acetylcholine release from cardiac parasympathetic neurons. Am J Physiol 248:H33-H39
49. Schwartz PJ, De Ferrari GM (1995). Interventioons changing heart rate variability after acute myocardial infarction. In: Malik M, Camm AJ (eds) Heart rate varibility. Futura Publishing Company Inc, Armonk, NY pp 407-420.
50. La Rovere MT, Mortara A, Pantaleo P, Maestri R, Cobelli F, Tavazzi L (1994). Scopolamine improves autonomic balance in advanced congestive heart failure Circulation 90: 838-843.
51. Gheorghiade M, Bonow RO (1998). Chronic heart failure in the United States. A manifestation of coronary artery disease. Circulation 97: 282-289.
52. Bonaduce D, Petretta M, Morgano G, et al (1992). Effects of converting enzyme inhibition on baroreflex sensitivity in patients with myocardial infarction. J Am Coll Cardiol 20: 587-93.

CHAPTER TWO: ECG ASPECTS INVESTIGATED BY DIFFERENT METHODS

SECTION ONE: P-WAVE AND QRS

8. THE SIGNAL AVERAGED P-WAVE

ROHAN PERERA AND JONATHAN S. STEINBERG

ABSTRACT

The role of impaired conduction in the atrium as a pre-requisite for atrial fibrillation (AF) is undisputed. This tendency was identifiable only by changes in the standard ECG or indirect methods such as echocardiography until the development of P-wave signal averaged ECG (SAECG). The process of 'signal averaging' produces a magnified and crisper signal better suited for detailed analysis. The study of the P-wave in particular requires specific modifications in technology and refinements that have further enhanced the reliability of this method. The two clinical entities where the P-wave SAECG has been most tested has been to predict a propensity for developing AF in patients undergoing cardiac surgery and in patients with histories of paroxysmal AF.

In both scenarios, the collective results indicate a validation of the P-wave SAECG as a valuable screening test. **Conclusion:** The P-wave SAECG has been shown to serve as a non-invasive indicator of a tendency to develop AF. At present this utility has been demonstrated best in patients undergoing cardiac surgery and in patients with histories of paroxysmal AF but with the continuing interest its clinical use will likely expand.

INTRODUCTION

In atrial fibrillation (AF), the role of a substrate of depressed intra-atrial conduction contributing to multiple re-entrant circuits has been convincingly

H.-H. Osterhues et al. (eds.),
Advances in Noninvasive Electrocardiographic Monitoring Techniques, 89–97.

proven by invasive and experimental mapping studies. Delay and inhomogeniety of atrial conduction could give rise to high-frequency low-amplitude signals and prolong the duration of the P-wave on the ECG. Recent studies have indeed shown good correlation between the duration of the signal averaged P-wave on the surface ECG and the likelyhood of developing AF (1), a predictive accuracy superior to standard ECG and echocardiographic criteria (2,3).

Signal averaging of the surface ECG involves amplification and filtering of electrical signals to display the low amplitude components (which could relate to abnormal myocardial conduction) while simultaneously eliminating any confounding noise. Limited initially to the QRS-complex and ventricular arrhythmias, this technique has found a special and robust role in the study of atrial arrhythmias as well.

METHODOLOGY

Acquisition

The key to recording the signal-averaged ECG lies in acquisition of a tracing with minimal artifact and noise contamination. Recordings should preferably be done in an area of low ambient noise interference, away from the usual hospital environment. The patient should be as motionless as possible and the skin well prepared for electrode contact. Three orthogonal bipolar leads are commonly used: lead X at the 4th intercostal space and mid-axillary line on the left (+) and right (-) sides, lead Y at the mid-clavicular line inferior to clavicle (+) and to the left of the umbilicus (-) and lead Z at 4th intercostal space at left sternal border (+) and similar posterior position to the left of the vertebral column (-). Signals from each lead are amplified and digitally recorded at a rate of 1000-2000 samples/sec and 12-16 bit resolution.

A signal for detection of the P-wave and 'window' alignment is required and this is referred to as the 'trigger' or fiducial point. The triggering mechanism can be "single" (P-wave or R-wave only) or "double" with the R-wave triggering first and subsequently the smaller P-wave (4-6). Ideally manual positioning of the P-wave correlation window should be possible in addition to automatic pre-configuration. The R-wave fiducial point for P-wave signal averaging must be located to the extreme right of the correlation window to expose the P-wave and PR-segment for analysis. Software modification is necessary to use a chosen sinus P-wave as template. In our laboratory, the window width is set between 100 to 150 ms and within that window we look for 95 to 99% correlation coefficient before accepting any P-wave signals into the average. Recording continues until the noise in the TP-segment is as low as 0.3 µV root mean square (RMS), a process which typically requires 200-500 beats and can take 15 to 20 minutes.

When a digitization pattern is established, acquisition can begin in the following stages: a) Template designation: As the sinus P-wave may vary in the same patient resulting in two or three recurring forms one needs to ensure averaging is applied to the predominant P-wave morphology. Hence the importance of additional manual control over the P-wave selection. b) P-wave alignment: Every incoming beat is subject to a cross correlation function and any ectopic beats or beats with excessive PR-interval variation should be rejected. The correlation window can be pre-set aiming for a 95-99% match (a cross correlation coefficient of 0.95-0.99). c) Calculation of the residual noise value: usually done in a 'quiet' portion of the ECG (e.g., TP-segment) where a window is placed to measure the noise following completion of the average. d) Termination: To indicate the signal averaging end, a point can be preset by using a predetermined number of beats when the noise level is expected to be sufficiently low or preferably to a low noise value such as 0.3µV.

Processing

Filtering is necessary to emphasize the main waveform of interest and limit low frequency contaminants. Filtering techniques previously used in P-wave SAECG are unidirectional, bidirectional, finite impulse response, least squares fit and spectral filters. Comparison among the above mentioned filter types carried out in our laboratory (7) indicate that total P-wave vector duration after filtering with the least-squares-fit filter to be superior to the others in correlating with the occurrence of AF (Table 1).

We have also studied various bandpass filtering frequencies applied to the least-squares-fit filter (Table 2) and shown that a bandpass filtering frequency of 29-250 Hz produced the strongest association with AF with an odds ratio of 26 (95% CI, 7-45).

APPLICATIONS

AF Prediction

The P-wave SAECG has been used to predict AF in a variety of settings. It has been studied in patients with paroxysmal AF, lone AF, AF recurrence after DC cardioversion and AF following coronary artery bypass surgery (CABG).

Table 1. Signal Averaged P-wave Duration by Filter Type in Patients Vs Controls

Filter Type	Group I(AF) (n=15) (ms)	Group II (controls) (n=15) (ms)	p	Odds Ratio
Unidirectional	150±17	136±16	.04	2.3
Bidirectional	150±17	136±16	.04	2.3
Finite impulse response	122±25	110±16	NS	1.0
Least-squares-fit	159±14	137±12	.005	26
Spectral	143±19	122±23	.02	5.5

Adapted from: Ehlert FA, Steinberg JS. J. Electrocardiol. 28;Suppl., 33-38, 1995 (With permission W.B. Saunders).

Table 2. Signal-averaged P-wave Duration by Patient Group and Filtering Frequency Using Least-squares-fit Filter Type

Filter Frequency	Group I(AF) (n=15) (ms)	Group II(controls) (n=15) (ms)	p	Odds Ratio
14-250 Hz (ww*=200ms)	132±24	108±15	.01	3
29-250 Hz (ww*=100ms)	159±14	137±12	.005	26
60-250 Hz (ww*=50ms)	138±14	128±15	NS	4

*Window width

Adapted from: Ehlert FA, Steinberg JS. J. Electrocardiol. 28; Suppl., 33-38, 1995 (With permission W.B. Saunders).

Table 3. Prediction of Atrial Fibrillation After Cardiac Surgery.

Study	No of patients	Criteria	Sensitivity %	Specificity %
Steinberg et al. (3)	130	P-wave duration > 140 msec	77	55
Klein et al. (10)	45	P-wave duration > 155 msec	69	79
Frost et al (9)	189	P-wave duration RMS voltage	Filtered P-wave duration and RMS voltage did not differ.	
Zaman et al. (11)	105	P-wave duration > 155msec	86	45
Stafford et al. (2)	201	P-wave duration >141 ms	73	48

P-Wave SAECG Use in Patients Undergoing Cardiac Surgery

Over a third of patients more than 70 years of age having bypass surgery are prone to post-surgical AF (8). Several investigators have examined P-wave SAECG in the role of a screening test for post operative AF (Table 3). Steinberg and colleagues reported the first prospective study of this kind (3), wherein they performed pre-operative P-wave SAECG on 130 consecutive patients undergoing open heart sugery. Patients were required to be in sinus rhythm with no history of AF and not using class I or III antiarrhythmic drugs. Thirty-three patients (25%) developed de novo AF lasting at least 30 minutes and their P-wave duration by SAECG was significantly longer (152 ± 18 vs 139 ± 17 ms, respectively; P<0.0001) than that of patients who remained in sinus rhythm.

Furthermore, a logistic regression model was constructed including ejection fraction, left ventricular hypertrophy by electrocardiogram, P-wave duration in standard lead II and P-wave duration on SAECG. Only the P-wave duration on SAECG proved to be an independent predictor of AF. A later study from the same authors (9) looked at a larger number of patients (n=272) and identified several factors such as older age, lower ejection fraction, valve surgery, preoperative use of digoxin and prolonged P-wave duration on SAECG as all associated with an increased incidence of post-operative AF.

Multivariate analysis showed that only P-wave duration on SAECG >140ms (odds ratio 3.1, 95% CI1.37-6.82, p<0.01) and LVEF<40% (odds ratio 2.8, 95% CI 1.32-5.82, p<0.01) independently predicted post-operative AF. Dissenting results were obtained by Frost et al. (10), albeit in a study which considered AF to have occurred only if it was clinically significant thus excluding all occurrences of asymptomatic AF, a phenomenon not uncommon in post-cardiac surgical patients. Following on Steinberg's initial efforts, three separate studies (2,11,12) have also asserted the predictive value of P-wave SA ECG for forecasting AF in patients after cardiac surgery and one of them has shown an incremental effect on specificity if P-wave SAECG is combined with postoperative serum magnesium level (12).

P-Wave SAECG in Paroxysmal AF

Several investigators have examined the P-wave duration on SAECG in patients who suffer bouts of paroxysmal AF. Guidera and Steinberg (1) studied a group of patients with a history of paroxysmal AF and compared them with age- and disease-matched controls who had no history of AF. A filtered vector composite of the three orthogonal leads was found to be significantly longer in the patient group than in the controls (162 ± 15 vs 140 ± 12 ms, p<0.01). A P-wave duration of ≥ 155ms using a filtered vector composite was associated with a sensitivity and specificity of 80% and 93%, respectively, and a positive predictive value of 92%, for separating patients with a history of AF from those without AF. Similar results were obtained by frequency as well as time domain analysis by others (5,13).

Recently Abe and co-workers followed 122 consecutive patients with PAF after P-wave SAECG recording and echocardiography at study entry. They defined the abnormality in P-wave SAECG as a duration of ≥ 145 ms and root-mean-square voltage for the last 30 ms (LP30) < 3.0μV. Of the 122, 23 had abnormal P-wave SAECG recordings and these constituted the study patients, the remainder serving as controls. During a mean follow-up of 26±12 months, 43% of those with the abnormality (compared with 4% of controls) developed AF lasting for at least 6 months (14). The sensitivity, specificity and predictive accuracy for the P-wave duration and the LP 30 to predict AF were 86%, 71% and 80% and 79%, 71% and 72%, respectively. When these two measures were combined the sensitivity, specificity and predictive accuracy were 71%, 91%, and 89% respectively. Of the echocardiographic criteria, left atrial dimensions were significantly higher (40.5± 5.1 against 36.4± 5.2 mm, p<.05) in the group with P-wave SAECG abnormality while there was no difference in left ventricular dimensions in the two groups.

Other applications of P-wave SAECG:

Attempts have been made to use P-wave SAECG in the study of sinus node disease (15,16), and also to identify a propensity to developing AF in patients with mitral valve prolapse, hypertrophic cardiomyopathy and the Wolf-Parkinson-White syndrome (17-19).

There is also some early work to identify the risk of AF in other conditions such as hyperthyroidism, chronic pulmonary disease, hypertension and myocardial infarction.

PITFALLS IN P-WAVE SAECG:

Some potential difficulties with this technique may need to be addressed in the future.

In electrocardiograms with short PR intervals it might be difficult to separate the end of the P and the beginning of the QRS. The use of a composite vector might result in loss of data from individual orthogonal leads. It is also possible that Purkinje conduction is incorporated into the P-wave. P-wave SAECG might vary with autonomic tone (20), and hemodynamic alterations such as volume overload or the use of nitrates (21). Finally there is a need for universal normal values for P-wave duration and other measurements, and possibly age, height and gender specific adjustments.

CONCLUSION

The weight of evidence supports the role of the signal-averaged P-wave as a predictor of AF and for use as a noninvasive measure of atrial activation for clinical and research objectives. It has been tested against the standard surface ECG and found to be superior, and the predictive qualities and indications will doubtlessly improve with refinements in the methodology.

REFERENCES

1. Guidera SA and Steinberg JS. The signal averaged P-wave duration: a rapid and non-invasive marker of atrial fibrillation. J Am Coll Cardiol 1993; 21:1645-51.
2. Stafford PJ, Kolvekar S, Cooper J et al. Signal averaged P-wave compared with standard electrocardiography or echocardiography for prediction of atrial fibrillaion after coronary bypass grafting. Heart 77: 417-422,1997.

3. Steinberg JS, Zelenkofske S, Wong SC et al. Value of the P-wave signal averaged ECG for predicting atrial fibrillaion after cardiac surgery. Circulation 88: 2618-2622, 1993.
4. Engel TR, Vallone N and Windle J. Signal averaged electrocardiogram in patients with atrial fibrillation or flutter. Am Heart J 115: 592-597, 1988.
5. Fukunami M, Yamada T, Ohmori M et al. Detection of patients at risk for paroxysmal atrial fibrillaion during sinus rhyrhm by P-wave triggered signal averaged electrocardiogram. Circulation 83: 162-169, 1991.
6. Chan EKY. Early potential analysis (EPA) version 1.10 software add-on for the LP-Pac Q™, user's manual. Austin, TX, Arrhythmia Research Technology, Inc., 1995, pp 7-18 and pp 23-26.
7. Steinberg JS, Kornstein D. Comparison of techniques for analysis of the P-wave signal averaged ECG (abstract) Circulation 88: I-311, 1993.
8. Lauer MS, Eagle KA, Buckley MJ et al. Atrial fibrillaion following coronary artery bypass surgery. Prog Cardiovasc Dis. 31: 367-378, 1989.
9. Hutchinson LA and Steinberg JS. A prospective study of atrial fibrillation after cardiac surgery:Multivariate risk analysis using P-wave signal-averaged ECG and clinical variables. Annals of Noninvasive Elec. 1:133-140,1996.
10. Frost L, Lund B, Pilegaard H et al. Re-evaluation of the role of P-wave duration and morphology as predictors of atrial fibrillation and flutter after coronary artery bypass surgery. Eur Heart J 17:1065-1071, 1996.
11. Klein M, Evans SJL, Blumberg S et al. Use of P-wave triggered, P-wave signal-averaged electrocardiogram to predict atrial fibrillation after coronary artery bypass surgery. Am Heart J.129:895-901, 1995.
12. Zaman AG, Alamgir F, Richens T et al. The role of signal averaged P-wave duration and serum magnesium as a combined predictor of atrial fibrillation after elective coronary artery bypass surgery.Heart 77: 527-531, 1997.
13. Yamada T, Fukunami M, Ohmori M et al. Characteristics of frequency content of atrial signal-averaged electrocardiograms during sinus rhythm in patients with paroxysmal atrial fibrillation.J Am Coll Cardiol 19:559-563, 1992.
14. Abe Y, Fukunami M, Yamada T et al. Prediction of transition to chronic atrial fibrillation in patients with paroxysmal atrial fibrillation by signal averaged electrocardiography: A Prospective Study. Circulation 96;2612-2616, 1997.
15. Yamada T, Fukunami M, Kumagai K et al. Detection of patients with sick sinus syndrome by use of low amplitude potentials early in filtered P-wave. J Am Coll Cardiol 28 (3): 738-744, 1996.
16. Keane D, Stafford P, Baker S et al. Signal-averaged electrocardiography of the sinus and paced P-wave in sinus node disease. Pacing Clin Electrophysiol. 18(7):1346-53, 1995.
17. Banasiak W, Pajak I, Ponikowski P et al. P-wave signal-averaged electrocardiograms in patients with. idiopathic mitral valve prolapse syndrome and supraventricular arrhythmias. Int J Cardiol 50(2):175- 80,1995.
18. Cecchi F, Montereggi A, Olivotto I et al. Risk for atrial fibrillation in patients with hypertrophic cardiomyopathy assessed by signal averaged P-wave duration. Heart 78(1):44-9,1997.

19. Maia IG, Cruz Filho FE, Fagundes ML et al. Signal-averaged P-wave in patients with Wolf-Parkinson-White syndrome after successful radiofrequency catheter ablation. J Am Coll Cardiol 26(5)·1310- 4,1995

20. Cheema AN, Ahmed MW, Kadish AH et al. Effects of autonomic stimulation and blockade on signal averaged P-wave duration. J Am Coll Cardiol 26; 497-502, 1995.

21. Vainer J, Cheriex EC, van der Steld B, et al. Effect of acute volume change on P-wave characteristics:correlation with echocardiographic findings in healthy men. J Cardiovasc Electrophysiol 5:999-1005,1994.

9. WENCKEBACH PATTERN OF VENTRICULAR LATE POTENTIALS

P. STEINBIGLER, R. HABERL, A. SPIEGL, G. JILGE AND
G. STEINBECK

ABSTRACT

Ventricular late potentials are considered a marker of an arrhythmogenic substrate especially in patients with a history of myocardial infarction. The classic way of late potential analysis, the vector analysis in the time domain, the so called Simson method, is useful in the post-infarction risk stratification with its great ability to predict a very low risk when the results are normal. However, the positive prediction is only poor, especially of ventricular fibrillation and sudden cardiac death rather than the prediction of sustained, slow, monomorphic and reproducibly inducible ventricular tachycardia [1].

Up to now recording of late potentials from the body surface, signals in the range of microvolts, requires the application of signal averaging techniques in order to improve the signal-to-noise ratio [2]. However, the primary shortcoming of these methods is that they do not allow the recognition of dynamic variations that may occur on a beat-by-beat basis.

Invasive registrations have shown that in ischemic regions of a postinfarction heart, the origin of late potentials, activation patterns sometimes varied with successive sinus beats. In certain areas 2:1 or Wenckebach like conduction patterns were observed. In canine models it has been demonstrated that the presence of these conduction sequences represent the possibility of initiating a reentrant rhythm rather than the presence of a conduction delay following the regular 1:1 pattern [3].

H.-H. Osterhues et al. (eds.),
Advances in Noninvasive Electrocardiographic Monitoring Techniques, 99–107.
© 2000 *Kluwer Academic Publishers. Printed in the Netherlands.*

Since these dynamics are not amenable to signal-averaging techniques but theoretically can be represented on the body surface in a beat-to-beat fashion, methods for single-beat late potential analysis both in the time and the frequency domain have been developed.

BEAT-TO-BEAT LATE POTENTIAL VARIABILITY IN HIGH-RESOLUTION RECORDINGS IN THE TIME DOMAIN

Many investigators introduced either technical equipment or digital approaches in order to improve the signal-to-noise ratio and were indeed able to show, that late potential analysis on a beat-to-beat basis is possible. However, only a few descriptions or quantifications of distinct patterns of late potential variations are available.

Using a combination of a variety of techniques to improve the signal-to-noise ratio such as volume conductor electrodes in an electrically quiet room and spatial signal averaging of a multichannel lead system with a high-resolution electrocardiogram beat-to-beat variations observed in intracardiac registrations were recognized at the body surface [4, 5]. Within a small study population of 21 patients after myocardial infarction, in whom 12 had malignant ventricular arrhythmias late potentials were described in 15 patients. They varied in amplitude between 2 and 25 µV, in extension into the ST-segment between 20 to 190ms after the end of QRS and moreover in 6 patients in configuration and in timing in successive sinus beats, probably reflecting a Wenckebach-type conduction pattern [4]. Employing similar equipment, in a larger patient group consisting of 44 patients, the dynamicity of late potentials was demonstrated [5]. In 11 of 27 patients with late potentials, late potentials occurred only intermittently. In those 22 patients with ventricular ectopic beats in only one patient was a Wenckebach-like periodocity reported, whereas a single ectopic potential prior to the ectopic beat was seen in 13/22 patients named as "focal" type of late potential occurrence. In another study of 27 patients with coronary artery disease in those 17 patients with ventricular late potentials the duration of the terminal signal below 44µV (TDS) showed more variability compared to patients without late potentials [5]. In the same study also a greater variability of TDS was evident in those 9 patients with sustained ventricular tachycardia than in 18 patients without ventricular arrhythmias. Moreover, successful therapy with Sotalol significantly reduced the late potential variability.

However, the validation of abnormal signals in single-beat late potential analysis in the time domain is difficult and automatic determination of late potential variability may be useful to avoid observer variability [6].

BEAT-TO-BEAT LATE POTENTIAL VARIABILITY IN HIGH-RESOLUTION RECORDINGS IN THE FREQUENCY DOMAIN USING SPECTRAL PATTERN RECOGNITION ALGORITHM (SPRA)

Frequency analysis of multiple segments (=Spectrotemporal Mapping with fast Fourier transform) of the high-resolution electrocardiogram proved to enable a powerful signal-to-noise discrimination capable of single-beat anaysis [7]. By this method late potentials are characterized by a typical spectral pattern after signal averaging (figure 1, upper left side). However, further refinement to allow description and quantification of beat-to-beat variations within spectral maps of single beats is needed (figure 1, lower right panel).

We therefore developed the method of Spectral Pattern Recognition Algorithm (SPRA) which is based mathematically on the two-dimensional correlation function [8]. Using the typical spectral representation of late potentials in spectral maps (figure 1, upper right panel) as a two-dimensional template, two-dimensional correlation looks for similarity within the spectral map step by step while the template is shifted in spatial and temporal direction over the spectral map. Thereby at identity the correlation factor amounts to one and at no similarity at all it amounts to zero. Multiplication of the spectral map with all correlation factors leads to an enormous enhancement of the signal of interest within the spectral maps of single beats (figure 1, lower left panel). Thereby late potentials become clearly visible and measurement of amplitude and time extention into the ST-segment is possible. The determination of a Late Potential Index (LPI) enables user-indepentent evaluation.

In a recently published study [8] high resolution surface electrocardiograms of 385 patients after myocardial infarction (85 with documented sustained ventricular tachycardia, 100 with fast, polymorphic ventricular tachycardia (>270 cycles/min) or primary ventricular fibrillation, 200 without ventricular arrhythmias) and 45 healthy volunteers were investigated. Spectrotemporal Pattern Recognition Algorithm detected late potentials in single beats in 89% of patients with ventricular tachycardia, in 79% of patients with ventricular fibrillation, in only 22% of patients without ventricular arrhythmias and in 4% of normals. Beat-to-beat variability was quantified by standard deviation of the mean localization of the late potential with respect to the end of QRS and standard deviation of the mean frequency content of the late potential measured within a period of 5 minutes. Interestingly, beat-to-beat variability of late potentials with respect to frequency content and extension into the ST-segment was markedly higher in patients with a history of primary ventricular fibrillation compared to those with a history of sustained ventricular tachycardia (53 ± 15 vs. 15 ± 12Hz and 35 ± 10 vs. 13 ± 11ms). Visual inspection after SPRA identified alternating, i.e. 2:1, possibly 'focal patterns', and

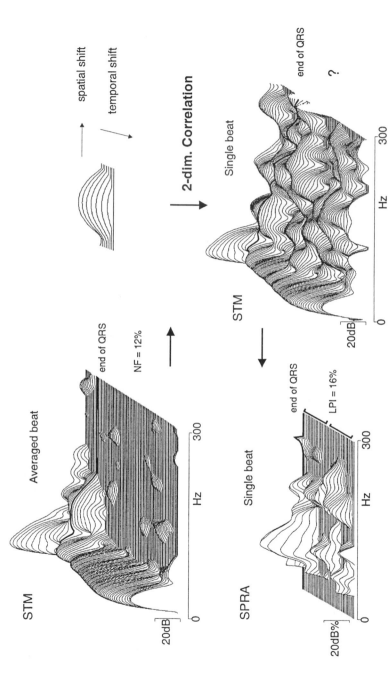

Figure 1. Principle of Spectrotemporal Pattern Recognition Algorithm (SPRA). Late potentials show a characteristic spectral pattern in the Spectrotemporal Mapping (STM) by fast Fourier transform of an averaged beat with pathologic Normality Factor (NF) (upper left panel). This pattern (upper right panel) serves as a template and is shifted in both spatial and temporal direction over the Spectrotemporal Mapping of a single beat of the same patient (lower right panel). At each step a correlation factor between 0 and 1 is calculated by two-dimensional correlation and multiplied with the spectrotemporal map. This results in the map of SPRA of the single beat clearly demonstrating the late potentials (lower left panel). The Late Potential Index (LPI) is pathologic.

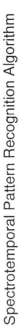
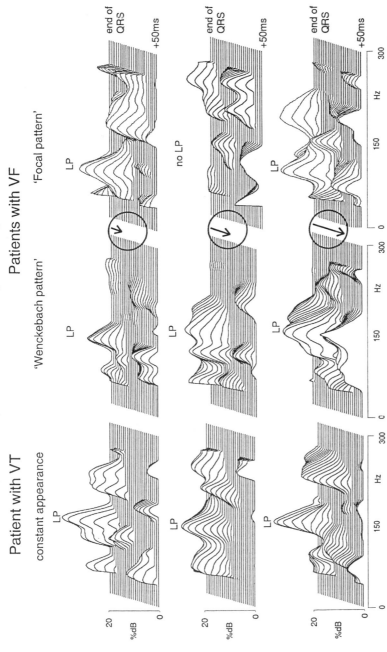

Figure 2. Beat-to-beat variability of late potentials identified by SPRA. In a patient with sustained, ventricular tachycardia (<270/min) late potentials are constant whereas in patients after ventricular fibrillation (mid and right panels) late potentials demonstrate 'Wenckebach patterns' with variable extension into the ST-segment or a focal pattern, i.e. late potentials appearing with constant spectral representation but not in every beat.

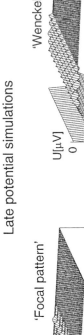

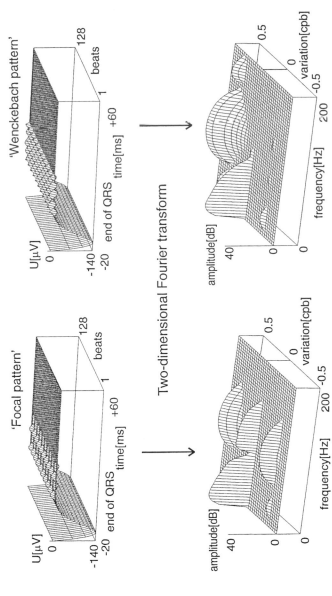

Figure 3. Quantification of beat-to-beat late potential variability using the two-dimensional Fourier transform. Test signal reflecting the end of QRS with simulated 'late potentials' appearing in every third beat representing a 'focal' pattern of late potential variability (upper left panel) or with variable extension into the ST-segment representing the 'Wenckebach pattern' (upper right panel). The power spectrum of two-dimensional Fourier transform gives the frequency content in the X-axis, the magnitude in the Y-axis and the periodicity of the frequency content in cycles per beat (cpb) in the Z-axis. Thereby 'focal' patterns can be identified as symmetric (lower left panel) and 'Wenckebach patterns' as asymmetric (lower right panel). Only frequency contents without periodicity at 0 cpb are detectable with one-dimensional Fourier transform.

variable appearance, possibly 'Wenckebach patterns', of late potentials in patients with a history of ventricular fibrillation, whereas constant appearance characterized patients after sustained, slow and monomorphic ventricular tachycardia (figure 2).

QUANTIFICATION OF BEAT-TO-BEAT LATE POTENTIAL VARIABILITY IN HIGH-RESOLUTION RECORDINGS USING SINGLE BEAT SPECTRAL VARIANCE (SBSV)

Two-dimensional fast Fourier transform is able to quantify beat-to-beat variabilities within the high resolution surface electrocardiogram [9]. Based on this algorithm we developed the method of Single-Beat Spectral Variance (SBSV) in order to receive a user-independent information about the periodicity of microvolt signals at the terminal QRS-complex [10]. In figure 3 the principle is shown. A test signal (panel A) contains 128 consecutive beats with late potentials in the range of microvolts at the end of the QRS-complex appearing only in every third beat or with alternating extension into the ST-segment in every third beat (panel B). The power spectra of two-dimensional fast Fourier transform give the magnitude in the Y-axis, the frequency content of 'late potentials' in the X-axis and the periodicity of 'late potentials' from beat to beat in the Z-axis. Here, the periodicity was 0.33 cycles per beat. Additionally, the symmetry of the power spectra reveals information about the alternating or variable pattern of the periodicity. These facts were summarized in a complex index function. Thus, a pathologic index function includes both constant late potentials, still detectable after signal averaging and variable late potentials not detectable by common methods.

In a retrospective study [10] 80 post-infarction patients were investigated, 20 patients had a history of documented, sustained, monomorphic slow (<230/min) ventricular tachycardia (group 1), 20 patients were resuscitated from ventricular fibrillation (group 2), 40 patients had no ventricular arrhythmias (group 3). Additionally 10 healthy voluteers were included. Conventional late potential analysis after signal averaging revealed late potentials in 60% of group 1, in 15% of group 2, in 20% of group 2 and in 20% of normals. SBSV showed a pathologic result in 80% of group 1, in 65% of group 2, in 7% of group 3, but not in normals. Time varying late potentials not detectable after signal averaging could be identified in 12% of group 1, in 50% of group 2 but not in group 3. In 50% of patients of group 2 'Wenckebach patterns' were present.

CLINICAL APPLICATION

The new methods of Spectrotemporal pattern recognition algorithm and Single Beat Spectral Variance offer the possibility analyzing high-resolution electrocardiograms even in a normal hospital environment and the user-indepedent quantification of beat-to-beat variabilities of ventricular late potentials as they are known from invasive registrations. They promise a more precise investigation of functional changes seen during transient conditions such as acute ischaemia, heart rate accelerations or transitory decreased heart rate variability. Especially in patients prone to fast, polymorphic ventricular tachycardia or ventricular fibrillation retrospective and preliminary prospective studies show, that analysis of beat-to-beat variability of late potentials might be useful in post-infarction risk stratification. Since the predictive accuracy of late potential analysis during sinus rhythm at rest is still low, these functional late potential analyses might offer a more accurate risk stratification of post-infarction patients in the future. A preliminary prospective study already showed a higher predictive value of late potential analysis by considering late potential functionality and periodic appearance especially in digital Holter electrocardiograms compared to conventional methods of late potential analysis [11].

REFERENCES

1. Breithardt G, Borggrefe M, Fetsch T, Böcker D, Mäkijärvi M, Reinhardt L (1995) Prognosis and risk stratification after myocardial infarction. Eur Heart J 16 (Suppl. G), 10-19.
2. Breithardt G, Cain E, El-Sherif N, Flowers NC, Hombach V, Janse M, Simson MB, Steinbeck G (1991) Standards for analysis of ventricular late potentials using high-resolution or signal-averaged electrocardiography. J Am Coll Cardiol 17: 999-1006.
3. El-Sherif N (1993) Electrophysiologic basis of ventricular late potentials. Prog Cardiovasc Dis, Vol. 35 (6), 417-427.
4. El-Sherif N, Mehra R, Restivo M (1992). Beat-to-beat recording of a high-resolution electrocardiogram: technical and clinical aspects. in: El-Sherif, Turitto G (eds) High resolution electrocardiography, Futura Publishing Inc., pp 189-210.
5. Hombach V, Höher M, Kochs M, Eggeling T, Weismüller P, Wiecha J (1993) Clinical significance of high resolution electrocardiography - sinus node, His bundle and ventricular late potentials. in: JA Gomes. Signal-averaged electrocardiography- Concepts, methods and applications. Kluwer Academic Publishers, pp. 267-295.
6. Zimmermann M, Adamec R, Richez J (1992) Detection of ventricular late potentials on a beat-to-beat basis: Methodological aspects and clinical application. in: El-Sherif, Turitto G (eds) High resolution electrocardiography, Futura Publishing Inc., pp 259-276.

7. Haberl R, Hengstenberg E, Pulter R, Steinbeck G (1986) Frequenzanalyse des Einzelschlag-Elektrokardiogrammes zur Diagnostik von Kammertachykardien. Z Kardiol 75: 659-65.

8. Steinbigler P, Haberl R, Jilge G, Steinbeck G (1998) Single-beat-analysis of ventricular late potentials in the surface-electrocardiogram using the Spectrotemporal Pattern Recognition Algorithm in patients with coronary artery disease. Eur Heart J 19: 435-446.

9. Spiegl A, Haberl R, Steinbigler P, Manz C, Schmücking I, Knez A, Steinbeck G (1998) Analysis of Beat-to-beat variability of frequency contents in the electrocardiogram using two-dimensional Fourier transforms. IEEE 45 (2): 235-241.

10. Steinbigler P, Haberl R, Spiegl A, Manz C, Schmücking I, Steinbeck G (1995) Single-Beat-Spectral-Variance - A new method to differentiate time varying and constant late potentials for improved post-infarction risk stratification. Circulation 92 (8): I-144 (0680-abstract).

11. Steinbigler P, Haberl R, Vogel J, Spiegl A, Schmücking I, Nespithal K, Brüggemann T, Andresen D, Steinbeck G (1996) Functional late potential analysis in Holter-electrocardiographic recordings improves post-infarction risk stratification (1996) Eur Heart J Vol. 17, Suppl., p 124: 747 (abstract).

10. DETECTION OF QRS-VARIABILITY

MARTIN HÖHER, SIEGFRIED BAUER AND HANS A. KESTLER

The standard approach for micro-potential analysis from the high-resolution electrocardiogram is signal-averaging and time-domain analysis of ventricular late potentials (VLP) [1]. VLP's indicate local depolarization abnormalities and have been successfully applied as a non-invasive marker of an increased risk for malignant ventricular arrhythmias. However, due to the preceding signal-averaging process, VLP analysis is restricted to the detection of static micro-potentials. The presence of such static VLP's can be interpreted as a marker of a local depolarization delay indicating the existence of a potentially arrhythmogenic substrate. Since standard time-domain analysis of VLP according to Simson [2] is restricted to the detection of pathological signals at the end of the QRS, more sophisticated frequency domain and time-frequency techniques have been developed to detect VLP's inside the QRS.

Variant micropotentials in contrast to static VLP's are known from the early days of high-resolution electrocardiography [3,4] and have been supposed to be more closely tied to the pathogenesis of spontaneous occurring arrhythmias. In these initial studies, variant micro-potentials were defined as singular, variant low amplitude potentials visually identified from non-averaged high-resolution ECG recordings. Variant potentials were found in 9-32% of recordings from patients with different types of arrhythmias and had a higher sensitivity in terms of the detection of patients with malignant arrhythmias or sudden death during follow-up [5]. Due to the successful standardization of the Simson technique, micropotential analysis has concentrated on the signal-averaged ECG.

Looking for an automatic analysis of QRS-micropotential variability, variant signals can be identified by several features:

H.-H. Osterhues et al. (eds.),
Advances in Noninvasive Electrocardiographic Monitoring Techniques, 109–119.

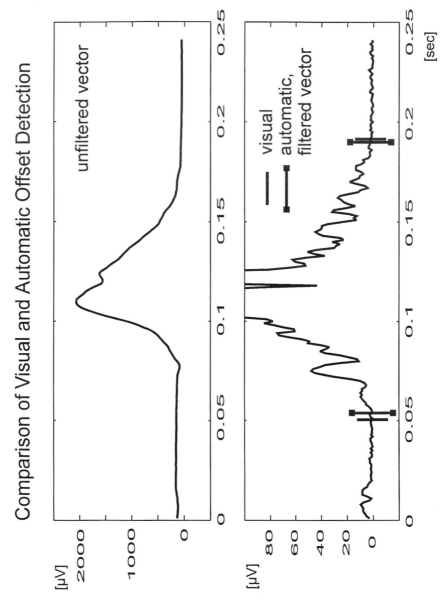

Figure 1. Correspondence of visual and automatic QRS-onset and QRS-offset determination from the high-pass filtered vector magnitude (bottom). For comparison the unfiltered QRS is shown in the upper panel.

- Amplitude variability (Y-axis)
- Duration variability (time axis)
- Spectral variability (variability of Fourier or high-order spectra)
- Time-Frequency variability (wavelets, Wigner-Ville distribution)
- Identification of individual signal patterns (pattern recognition, neural networks)

BEAT-TO-BEAT VARIABILITY OF QRS DURATION

In a previous visually-evaluated analysis of the non-averaged high-resolution ECG we showed an significantly increased beat-to-beat variability of QRS duration and of terminal signal duration in patients with malignant arrhythmias [6]. Based on these data our group concentrated on the development of an automatic analysis of QRS variability to study this parameter in larger patient groups and from longer ECG recordings.

ECG recording

High-resolution ECG's of 30 min duration were recorded from bipolar, orthogonal X,Y,Z leads. The skin was carefully prepared and recordings were done in Faraday cage. Sampling rate was 1000 Hz, A/D resolution was 16 bit, and a bandpass filter of 0.05-350 Hz used (anti-aliasing).

The ECG's were recorded with the Predictor hardware (Corasonix Inc, Oklahoma, USA). QRS triggering, reviewing of the ECG, and arrhythmia detection was done on a high-resolution ECG analysis platform developed by our group [7].

QRS variability calculation

Each lead was filtered with a 40 Hz bidirectional, 4-pole Butterworth high-pass filter and the filtered vector magnitude was calculated:

$$V_f = \sqrt{X_f^2 + Y_f^2 + Z_f^2}$$

QRS-onset and QRS-offset were measured for each individual beat. In each beat pre-QRS and post-QRS local noise was determined as the minimum standard deviation within a 40 ms noise window shifted through the ST or TP-segment. A rough initial QRS-endpoint estimate was calculated at mean ± 3 standard deviations of noise. Afterwards it was fine-tuned by an algorithm maximizing the ratio between the standard deviations of two consecutive windows shifted outwards of the QRS, during stepwise reduction of the window lengths. For comparison, visual evaluation of QRS-onset and QRS-offset of the high-pass filtered signal was performed (Figure 1).

Variability of the duration of the total QRS (QDV), the initial portion of the QRS (IDV) and of the terminal portion of the QRS (TDV) were calculated as the standard deviation of the time-series of all normal-to-normal QRS sequences. Noisy beats with a noise level above 10 µV in the high-pass filtered vector were excluded.

Study groups

We compared a group of cardiac patients with ventricular tachycardia (VT) and a group of healthy subjects. The VT group consisted of 31 patients with inducible, monomorphic, sustained VT. Out of them 28 had a documented episode of spontaneous, sustained VT or ventricular fibrillation. The underlying heart disease was coronary artery disease (n=23), dilative cardiomyopathy (n=5), arrhythmogenic right ventricular disease (n=2) or valve disease (n=1). All patients with coronary artery disease had a previous myocardial infarction. Intraventricular conduction abnormalities were present in 6/31 patients. 23/31 patients were VLP positive in the signal-averaged ECG.

The group of normals consisted of 10 healthy young volunteers and 13 patients without organic heart disease. The healthy volunteers had a normal resting ECG, a normal echocardiography, no history of cardiac symptoms and a negative coronary risk profile. The patient group without organic heart disease consisted of patients in whom a suspected cardiac disease had been excluded by a complete cardiac diagnostic program including left and right heart catheterization.

Increased QRS variability in VT patients

Similar to our previous data [6], visual inspection of the high-pass filtered vector showed a higher beat-to-beat variability in VT patients as compared to normals (Figure 3). In addition to the increased variability in time of QRS-onset and QRS-offset, there was an increased signal variability inside the QRS. Automatic analysis revealed a significantly higher beat-to-beat variability of the duration of the terminal QRS and of the total QRS in VT patients as compared to the group of healthy subjects (TDV: 7.49 ± 3.10 ms versus 4.60 ± 1.82 ms, p=0.0002; QDV: 9.01 ± 3.03 ms versus 6.68 ± 2.23 ms, p=0.003) (Figure

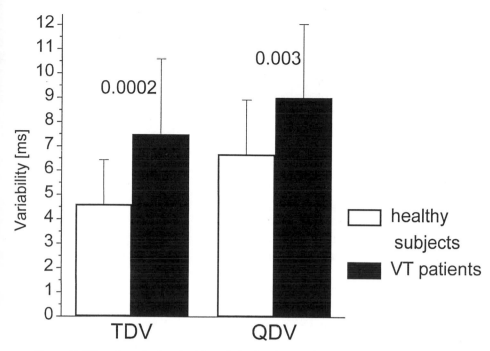

Figure 2. VT patients had a significantly higher beat-to-beat variability of the terminal QRS (TDV) and the total QRS (QDV) duration as compared to healthy subjects.

2). The variability of the initial portion of the QRS did not differ between both groups.

Since the non-averaged high-resolution ECG is associated with a higher noise level as compared to the conventional signal-averaged ECG, detailed statistical analyses were performed to detect any potential interference between noise and beat-to-beat variability. The mean noise level of the filtered vector magnitude (mean amplitude of a 50 ms noise window starting 20 ms after QRS-offset) was 2.4 ± 0.6 µV, the mean beat-to-beat variation of noise (standard deviation of the time-series of noise values from consecutive beats) was 0.8 ± 0.3 µV. There was no correlation between QRS duration variability and mean noise level or beat-to-beat variation of noise. Likewise, noise did not differ between the study groups of subjects with and without inducible VT.

Mean QRS-duration was also significantly longer in VT-patients (150.4 ± 21.9 ms) as compared to the group of healthy subjects (122.8 ± 9.2 ms). To study the relation between QRS-variability and mean QRS-duration, we calculated variation coefficients of the initial and the terminal portions of the QRS. Variation coefficients were 3.3% in the initial and 6.9% in terminal portion of the QRS (p<0.0001), indicating that QRS variability is not simply a

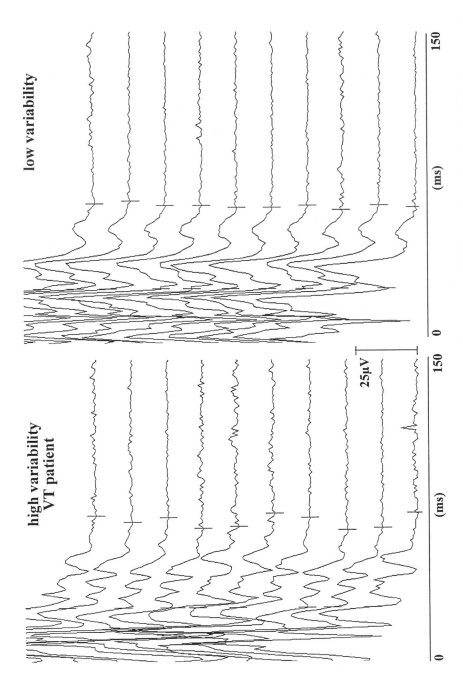

Figure 3. Variant micropotentials and high beat-to-beat variability of the terminal QRS in a patient with inducible VT (left) compared to a patient without malignant arrhythmias (right).

function of QRS-duration but dependent on variant signals in the terminal QRS.

To compare QDV with alternative parameters of variability, time-domain heart rate variability was calculated using the standard deviation of consecutive RR intervals. In accordance with other studies, VT patients had a significantly lower heart-rate variability (37 ± 21 ms) as compared to healthy subjects (69 ± 20 ms; $p<0.001$). Yet there was no significant correlation between heart-rate variability and QRS-duration variability within both patient groups.

QRS VARIABILITY ASSESSMENT BY NEURAL NETWORKS

In addition to the above described automatic analysis of QRS-duration variability we investigated neural networks as an alternative way to detect QRS-onset and QRS-offset less dependent on noise. In contrast to conventional algorithmic approaches comparing the signal of interest with some measure of surrounding noise, neural networks perform a pattern analysis and estimate QRS-offset by 'experience' from learning.

Principle of neural network analysis

The signal processing of neural networks resembles the functioning of neurons within the central nervous system. The basic idea is to solve problems by adaptive learning instead of a fixed algorithm. Information processing of a neural network is highly parallel in contrast to the sequential processing of algorithmic approaches.

In the biological neural network each neuron of the network represents a simple microprocessing unit, which receives a set of incoming information from other neurons through its dendrites. If the sum of the incoming excitation is strong enough, the neuron is activated and transfers its activation via the axon and connecting synapses to the next line of neurons. The information processing at the synapses and in the neuron form the basic memory mechanisms of the brain. In an artificial (computerized) neural network the unit analogous to the biological neuron is called a processing element consisting from multiple inputs, a summation and a transfer function. The incoming information of all inputs is combined by a weighted summation process resulting in the internal activation level of the processing element. This activation is then translated into the output of the element by a non-linear transfer function, resembling the threshold mechanism of a biological neuron.

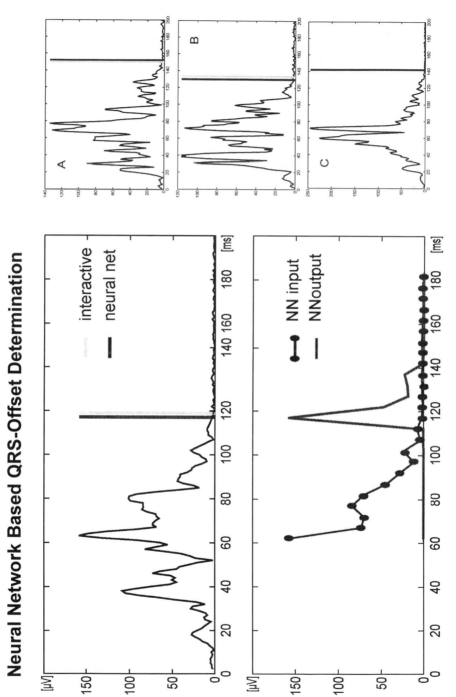

Figure 4. QRS-offset estimation by a backpropagation neural network (see text).

The output of a single processing element connects to the input paths of the next layer of processing elements. The weighting factor of each connection corresponds to the synaptic strength of the biological model. Within a computerized neural network the processing elements are typically organized in layers with full or partial connections between consecutive layers.

QRS-offset recognition by a backpropagation neural network

The interesting feature of such an artificial neural network is its learning ability. In general "learning" of an artificial neural network means its adaptation to a given problem by changing its internal parameters, e.g. the weights of the input function or the numbers of neurons. Different types of learning schemes are known. For QRS-offset recognition we used a backpropagation network which was trained by supervised learning; the output of the network is compared to the desired response to a given input, which must be provided by a knowledgeable teacher.

For training of the network we used 1040 randomly selected high-pass filtered QRS from our high-resolution ECG database [7], in which QRS-onset and QRS-offset had been visually marked. Data were down-sampled to 200 Hz and a backpropagation network with 40 inputs, one hidden layer containing 30 elements, and one output layer with 40 elements. The network was trained to predict the QRS-offset by a "1 out of n" coding. The output element with the highest output was chosen as QRS-offset of the network. Training of the network was very slow and required almost three days of computing time on a UNIX workstation (HP9000/700 C100). Afterwards the network was tested with a different set of 1040 QRS-complexes. Figure 4 shows four examples of the neural network offset estimation in very different QRS-morphologies. In 67% of the QRS-complexes the difference between the neural net and interactive, visual assessment was ±1 data point, and in 92% of the QRS it was ±2 data points.

DISCUSSION

In this study we evaluated a statistical approach to analyze variant micropotentials by measuring the beat-to-beat variability of QRS-duration. This concept differs from previous studies which were aimed to identify singular, variant ventricular late potentials [3,8,9]. The concept of measuring the standard deviation of QRS-duration does not depend on a yes/no decision for each individual potential but provides a global parameter of variability and seems to be less sensitive to noise.

Based on our earlier, visually-evaluated data [6] the aim of this study was to develop an automatic algorithm for QRS-variability analysis. Our data showed a significantly higher beat-to-beat variability of the high-pass filtered QRS duration in patients with spontaneous or inducible ventricular tachycardia as compared to healthy subjects or patients without organic heart disease. Furthermore there was a significantly higher variation coefficient within the terminal portion of the QRS as compared to the initial portion. Both findings indicate the presence of variant micropotentials as the pathophysiological base of QRS-variability. Since such micropotentials are induced by local depolarization delays, they are more likely to occur within the rear part of the QRS.

QRS-variability seems to be independent from heart-rate variability. Based on the concept of variant micropotentials we conclude, that QRS-variability is a marker of intrinsic cardiac variation complementing heart-rate variability, which reflects more the external neural control mechanisms.

The described algorithm allows to apply QRS-variability analysis to a larger set of ECG-data in order to evaluate the clinical relevance of this non-invasive risk marker.

However, there are certain limitations. Comparing the signal with local noise is sensitive to intermittent noise and additional criteria have to be developed to exclude noise-dependent variability from the analysis. The neural network estimation of QRS-offset is very promising and seems to resemble much more the visual type of inspection [10]. Although de-noising seems to be useful, the optimal filter type for continuous high-resolution ECG recordings has to be defined [11,12].

To assess the clinical value of QRS-variability we are currently analyzing the ECG's from our high-resolution ECG database [5]. This database includes ECG recordings from 1052 patients (6 min: n=782; 30 min: n=270). The patient distribution is: 766 coronary artery disease, 31 dilative cardiomyopathy, 54 other cardiac diseases, 201 without organic heart disease (45 with arrhythmias). From these, 690 had a myocardial infarction and 150 had an episode of VT or VF. A one- and two-years follow-up including cardiac death, myocardial infarction and arrhythmic events, currently conducted, will allow us to asses the prognostic relevance of QRS-variability.

REFERENCES

1. G. Breithardt, M.E. Cain, N. El Sherif, N. Flowers, V. Hombach, M. Janse, M.B. Simson, and G. Steinbeck, Standards for analysis of ventricular late potentials using high resolution or signal-averaged electrocardiography. *Eur.Heart J*, vol. 12, pp. 473-480, 1991.

2. M.B. Simson, Use of signals in the terminal QRS-complex to identify patients with ventricular tachycardia after myocardial infarction. *Circulation*, vol. 64, pp. 235-242, 1981.

3. V. Hombach, U. Kebbel, H.W. Höpp, U. Winter, and H. Hirche, Noninvasive beat-by-beat registration of ventricular late potentials using high resolution electrocardiography. *Int.J Cardiol.*, vol. 6, pp. 167-183, 1984.

4. N. El Sherif, J.A.C. Gomes, M. Restivo, and R. Mehra, Late potentials and arrhythmogenesis. *Pace.*, vol. 8, pp. 440-462, 1985.

5. V. Hombach, M. Hoeher, M. Kochs, T. Eggeling, P. Weismueller, and J. Wiecha. Clinical significance of high resolution electrocardiography - sinus node, His bundle and ventricular late potentials. In: *Signal averaged electrocardiography*, ed. J.A. Gomes. Dordrecht, The Netherlands: Kluwer Academic Publishers, 1993.pp. 267-295.

6. M. Hoeher, J. Axmann, T. Eggeling, M. Kochs, P. Weismuller, and V. Hombach, Beat-to-beat variability of ventricular late potentials in the unaveraged high resolution electrocardiogram - Effects of antiarrhythmic drugs. *Eur.Heart J*, vol. 14 (Suppl. E), pp. 33-39, 1993.

7. D.E. Ritscher, E. Ernst, H.G. Kammrath, V. Hombach, and M. Hoeher, High-Resolution ECG Analysis Platform with Enhanced Resolution. *IEEE Computers in Cardiology*, vol. 24, pp. 291-294, 1997.

8. N. El Sherif, M. Restivo, W. Craelius, R. Henkin, G. Kelen, J.M. Fontaine, S.N. Ursell, and G. Turitto. High resolution electrocardiography. Basic and clinical aspects. In: *Electrocardiography and cardiac drug therapy*, eds. V. Hombach, H.H. Hilger, and H.L. Kennedy. Dordrecht, Netherlands: Kluwer Academic Press, 1989.pp. 172-203.

9. M. Zimmermann, R. Adamec, P. Simonin, and J. Richez, Beat-to-beat detection of ventricular late potentials with high- resolution electrocardiography. *Am Heart J*, vol. 121, pp. 576-585, 1991.

10. M. Hoeher, H.A. Kestler, G. Palm, and V. Hombach, Intra QRS-variability of high-resolution ECG beat-to-beat recordings classified by neural networks. *Eur.Heart J*, vol. 18 (Abstr Suppl), pp. 308, 1997.

11. H.A. Kestler, M. Hoeher, F. Schwenker, and V. Hombach, Filtering Beat-to-Beat Recordings of the High Resolution Electrocardiogram. *IEEE Computers in Cardiology*, vol. 23, pp. 461-464, 1996.

12. H.A. Kestler, M. Haschka, W. Kratz, F. Schwenker, G. Palm, V. Hombach, and M. Hoeher, De-noising of high-resolution ECG signals by combining the discrete wavelet transform with the Wiener filter *IEEE Computers in Cardiology*, vol.25, pp.233-236, 1998.

CHAPTER TWO: ECG ASPECTS INVESTIGATED BY DIFFERENT METHODS

SECTION TWO: QT-VARIABILITY/QT-DISPERSION

11. QT-DISPERSION: ROLE IN CLINICAL DECISION MAKING

THOMAS KLINGENHEBEN, MARKUS ZABEL AND
STEFAN H. HOHNLOSER

ABSTRACT

For almost fifty years, the QT interval has been known to vary significantly between the individual 12 leads of the surface ECG [1]. A potential clinical application of this interlead difference was proposed in 1990 by Day, McComb and Campbell [2]. They suggested that this interlead QT difference may provide a measure of repolarization inhomogenity which they called "QT-dispersion". The method subsequently gained popularity as a new marker of ventricular arrhythmogenity and the association between QT-dispersion (QTD) and antiarrhythmic therapy [3,4] or the efficacy of antiadrenergic therapy in patients in which the congenital long QT syndrome was examined [5]. Subsequently, the potential role of QTD for risk stratification was examined in patients prone to sudden arrhythmogenic death such as patients after myocardial infarction [6,7] or with congestive heart failure [8,9].

In this review, important clinical data available on QTD are summarized and its role for risk stratification in clinical practice is discussed.

H.-H. Osterhues et al. (eds.),
Advances in Noninvasive Electrocardiographic Monitoring Techniques, 123–130.
© 2000 Kluwer Academic Publishers. Printed in the Netherlands.

INITIAL STUDIES ON DISPERSION OF VENTRICULAR REPOLARIZATION

The first data on dispersion of repolarization came from various experimental models [10,11]. Kuo et al., for example, performed simultaneous recordings of multiple monophasic action potentials from the epicardium of the isolated canine heart. They could induce dispersion of repolarization by regional hypothermia, resulting in susceptibility to malignant ventricular tachyarrhythmias due to reentry [11]. Mirvis et al. were the first to evaluate spatial variation of the QT interval in normal volunteers and patients with acute myocardial infarction by means of precordial mapping [12]; they found higher values for the maximal difference in QT interval in the patient group compared to normal individuals. These findings were subsequently confirmed using the 12 lead ECG [13]. A link between the early experimental data on dispersion of repolarization and the clinical finding of QTD in the surface ECG was provided by Zabel et al. [14]. Using an isolated rabbit heart model, they validated different parameters of dispersion of repolarization (such as QT, JT-dispersion, T-wave area, and the "T-peak-to-end" [TPE] interval) by demonstrating a relevant correlation of these variables with the dispersion of action potential duration (see Tab.1).

Tabel 1. Correlation between dispersion of action potential duration (ADP_{90}) and different ECG variables of dispersion [14]

Markers from the surface ECG	**Dispersion of ADP_{90}**	
	Correlation coefficient	*p-value*
QTD (ms)	0.61	< 0.001
JTD (ms)	0.64	< 0.001
Area under T-wave (ms x mV)	0.79	< 0.0001
T-peak-to-end-interval (ms)	0.81	< 0.0001

QT-DISPERSION AND THE CONGENITAL LONG-QT SYNDROME

In their first study on QTD, Day and Campbell found a significant correlation between this parameter and the risk of subsequent ventricular tachyarrhythmias in patients with the congenital long-QT syndrome (LQTS) [2]. These findings were extended by a study by Priori et al in 1994 [5]. In twenty-eight patients with LQTS, QTD measures were obtained before institution of therapy and during treatment (ß-blocker /left cardiac sympathetic denervation) and were compared to those of a control group [5]. Two parameters of dispersion were assessed, QTD/QT_cD and the "relative QTD/QT_cD" (=standard deviation of

QT/QT average x 100). Whereas QTD averaged 46+ 18 ms in controls, it was significantly higher in the LQTS patients (133 ± 21 ms; p<0.05). In LQTS patients responding to betablockers, QTD decreased significantly to 75 ± 38 ms whereas it remained unchanged in betablocker-resistant patients (137 ± 52 ms; p<0.05). After left cardiac sympathetic denervation, the latter patients had a QTD of 78± 45 ms, thus comparable to the betablocker responders [5]. The authors concluded that QTD may be an effective tool for assessment of arrhythmic rsik and guidance of therapy in LQTS patients.

EFFECT OF ANTIARRHYTHMIC DRUGS ON QTD

Proarrhythmia induced by antiarrhythmic drugs - predominantly by class I and III drugs - usually takes the form of torsade de pointes tachycardia [15]. As to the electrophysiologic mechanism of this polymorphic tachycardia, inhomogeneity of ventricular repolarization and the genesis of early afterdepolarizations are considered the most relevant factors [15]. Thus, it seems useful to assess QTD to identify drug-induced inhomogenity of prolonged ventricular repolarization [16,17]. Hii and coworkers evaluated the 12 lead ECGs from 38 patients who were treated with class Ia drugs and subsequently received chronic amiodarone therapy [4]. Nine of these patients had torsade de pointes with class Ia drugs. In these patients, QTD was significantly increased as compared to baseline (101+37 vs 44+12 ms; p=0.002) and returned to normal values (49+26 ms) with amiodarone although both drugs prolonged the QT interval to a comparable extent. In the remaining 29 patients, there was no difference in QTD on either treatment (50+6 ms with class Ia vs 69+7 ms with amiodarone) [4]. Whether the beta-blocking actions of amiodarone are responsible for its low incidence to cause torsades by counterbalancing its class III properties or whether the drug causes a more homogenous than inhomogenous prolongation of ventricular repolarization, remains to be elucidated.

QT-DISPERSION - A MARKER FOR RISK STRATIFICATION IN STRUCTURAL HEART DISEASE ?

Although prophylactic antiarrhythmic therapy with the implantable defibrillator can be realized today [18], its widespread use is hampered by the low predictive power of different methods to identify patients with survived myocardial infarction (MI) or congestive heart failure at risk for subsequent arrhythmic death. Therefore, several studies were performed using QTD as a marker of risk in these patient populations [6,7,19-23]. Most of these studies are, however, retrospective or were conducted as case-control trials. For example, Perkiömäki et al measured QTD and heart rate variability (HRV) in 30 survivors of ventricular fibrillation (VF) with previous MI and inducible unstable ventricular tachyarrhythmia, in 30 patients with a previous MI and inducible stable monomorphic ventricular tachycardia (VT), and in 30 post MI control patients without a history of ventricular arrhythmias [7]. They found prolonged QTD in both arrhythmia groups but not in the control group, whereas HRV was reduced in the VF survivor group only and they concluded that increased QTD was associated with vulnerability to VF and VT [7]. In a retrospective analysis from the LIMIT-2 trial, Glancy et al. found that QTD assessed early (3 days) after acute MI did not predict mortality during long term follow-up. However, if ECGs at 4 weeks after MI were analyzed, a lack of decrease in QTD was associated with mortality [6]. In this and other studies, a selection bias with respect to overrepresentation of patients with recurrent myocardial ischemia needs to be discussed [7,23]. In a recent report from the "Rotterdam Study" QT_cD was found to predict cardiac mortality in older men and women irrespective of an underlying cardiac disease [24].

Tab. 2. Different ECG parameters of dispersion compared between alive and deceased patients (pts) and patients with vs without arrhythmic event [19]

Dispersion parameter	Survivors	Deceased pts	p-value	Pts without arrhythmic event	Pts with arrhythmic event	p-value
	(N=259)	*(N=21)*		*(N=261)*	*(N=19)*	
QTD (ms)	65±29	61±22	NS	65±29	58±20	NS
JTD (ms)	64±29	58±23	NS	64±29	56±18	NS
T area (ms x mV)	31±14	34±17	NS	31±14	37±17	NS
TPE interval (ms)	96±20	100±20	NS	95±20	101±22	NS

The first prospectively designed study in patients after acute MI assessing the predictive value of QTD as well as other ECG markers of repolarization was recently reported by our group [19]. In 280 consecutive infarct survivors none of the dispersion variables - measured with a newly developed digital ECG analysis program - were of predictive value neither for all-cause mortality or arrhythmic events (see Tab.2). Of note, the extensive use of beta-blockers and revascularization procedures in this study minimizes the potential influence of ischemia on QTD. In contrast to QTD, variables such as left ventricular ejection fraction, HRV, or the mean 24-hour heart rate proved to be of potential use for risk stratification in these patients [19].

Similarly to these findings in postinfarction patients, conflicting results concerning the predictive value of QTD were reported in patients with congestive heart failure. Whereas some investigators found QTD to be a useful risk stratifier [8,22], others did not [9,25]. A variety of methodological difficulties underlying determination of QTD may account for these contradictory findings from different centers [26,27].

METHODOLOGICAL CONSIDERATIONS OF QT-DISPERSION MEASUREMENT

The lack of methodological standardization of assessment of QTD makes comparison of many of the above mentioned studies difficult. Although sophisticated computerized methods were recently developed to accurately measure QT intervals [28], there are problems remaining unsolved of which one is the determination of the end of the T-wave, and the relevance of U-waves for measuring repolarization duration [26]. In addition, a wide range of inter- and intraobserver reproducibility of QTD measurements has been reported [26,29]. No standards are defined concerning the selection of leads to be measured, or the optimal paper speed of the ECG tracings. Finally, the usefulness of rate correction needs to be discussed as recent data suggest that dispersion of myocardial repolarization is independent of heart rate [30].

PRESENT CLINICAL ROLE OF QT-DISPERSION AND IMPLICATIONS FOR FUTURE RESEARCH

At present, measuring QTD can be considered useful in patients with the congenital or the acquired form of LQTS with respect to guide therapy in these patients and, in particular, to identify those prone to developing proarrhythmic side-effects on treatment with drugs that prolong the QT interval. With respect to using QTD as a tool for risk stratification for instance following myocardial infarction, the results from the currently available studies are contradictory. Technical problems of QTD measurement as the lack of digitizing techniques in the earlier studies may be the key to these differences [27]. Thus, more sophisticated techniques of measuring dispersion of repolarization from the surface ECG need to be developed and subsequently analyzed with regard to their prognostic value. New concepts of assessing repolarization abnormalities such as T-wave alternans [31,32] and T-wave complexity [33] have been introduced and need to be validated in prospective controlled trials.

REFERENCES

1. Lepeschkin E, Surawicz B. The measurement of the QT interval of the electro-cardiogram. Circulation 1952;6:378-388
2. Day CP, McComb JM, Campbell RWF.QT-dispersion: an indication of arrhythmia risk in patients with long QT intervals. Br Heart J 1990;63:342-344
3. Day CP, McComb JM, Matthews J, Campbell RWF. Reduction in QT-dispersion by sotalol following myocardial infarction. Eur Heart J 1991;12:423-427
4. Hii JTY, Wyse DG, Gillis AM, Duff HJ, Solylo MA, Mitchell LB. Precordial QT-interval dispersion as a marker of torsade de pointes:disparate effects of class Ia antiarrhythmic drugs and amiodarone. Circulation 1992;86:1376-1382
5. Priori SG, Napolitano C, Diehl L, Schwartz PJ. Dispersion of the QT interval: a marker of therapeutic efficacy in the idiopathic long QT syndrome. Circulation 1994; 89:1681-1689
6. Glancy JM, Garratt CJ, Woods KL, de Bono DP. QT-dispersion and mortality after myocardial infarction. Lancet 1995;345:945-948
7. Perkiömäki JS, Huikuri HV, Koistinen JM, Mäkikalliio T, Castellanos A, Myerburg RJ. Heart rate variability and dispersion of QT interval in patients with vulnerability to ventricular tachycardia and ventricular fibrillation after previous myocardial infarction. J Am Coll Cardiol 1997;30:1331-1338
8. Barr CS, Naas A, Freeman M, Lang CC, Struthers AD. QT-dispersion and sudden unexpected death in chronic heart failure. Lancet 1994;343:327-329
9. Fei L, Goldman JH, Prasad K, Keelin PJ, Reardon K, Camm AJ, McKenna WJ. QT-dispersion and RR variations on 12-lead ECGs in patients with congestive heart failure secondary to idiopathic dilated cardiomyopathy. Eur Heart J 1996;17:258-263
10. Han J, Moe GK. Nonuniform recovery of excitability in ventricular muscle. Circ Res 964;14:44
11. Kuo CS, Munakata K, Reddy CP, Surawicz B. Characteristics and possible mechanism of ventricular arrhythmia dependent on the dispersion of action potential durations. Circulation 1983;67:1356-1367
12. Mirvis DM. Spatial variation of QT intervals in normal persons and patients with acute myocardial infarction. J Am Coll Cardiol 1985;3:625-631
13. Cowan JC, Yusoff K, Moore M, Amos PA, Gold AE, Bourke JP, Tansuphaswadikul S, Campbell RWF. Importance of lead selection in QT interval measurement. Am J Cardiol 1988;61:83-87
14. Zabel M, Portnoy S, Franz MR. Electrocardiographic indexes of dispersion of ventricular repolarization: an isolated heart validation study. J Am Coll Cardiol 1995; 25:746-752
15. Haverkamp W, Shenasa M, Borggrefe M, Breithardt G. Torsade de pointes. In Zipes DP, Jalife J (eds). Cardiac Electrophysiology. WB Saunders, Philadelphia,1994, pp. 885-899

16. van de Loo A, Klingenheben T, Hohnloser SH. Amiodarone therapy after previous sotalol-induced torsade de pointes: analysis of QT-dispersion to predict proarrhythmia. J Cardiovasc Pharmacol Therapeut 1996;1(I):75-78

17. Mattioni TA, Heutlin TA, Sarmiento JJ, Parker M, Lesch M, Kehoe RF. Amiodarone in patients with previous drug-mediated torsade de pointes: Long-term safety and efficacy. Ann Int Med 1989;111:574-580

18. Moss AJ, Hall WJ, Cannom DS, Daubert JP, Higgins SL, Klein H, Levine JH, Saksena S, Waldo AL, Wilber D, Brown MW, Heo M. Improved survival with an implanted defibrillator in patients with coronary disease at high risk for ventricular arrhythmias. N Engl J Med 1996;335:1933-1940

19. Zabel M, Klingenheben T, Franz MR, Hohnloser SH. Assessment of QT-dispersion for prediction of mortality or arrhythmic events after myocardial infarction: results of a prospective long-term follow-up study. Circulation 1998;97:2543-2550

20. Higham PD, Furniss SS, Campbell RWF. QT-dispersion and components of the QT interval in ischemia and infarction. Br Heart J 1995;73:32-36

21. Trusz-Gluza M, Wozniak-Skowerska I, Giec L, Szydlo K. Dispersion of the QT interval as a predictor of cardiac death in patients with coronary heart disease. PACE 1996;19:1900-1904

22. Pinsky DJ, Sciacca RR, Steinberg JS. QT-dispersion as a marker of risk in patients awaiting heart transplantation. J Am Coll Cardiol 1997;29:1576-1584

23. Zareba W, Moss AJ, le Cessie S. Dispersion of ventricular repolarization and arrhythmic cardiac death in coronary artery disease. Am J Cardiol 1994;74:550-553

24. de Bruyne MC, Hoes AW, Kors JA, Hofman A, van Bemmel JH, Grobbee DE. QTc disperion predicts cardiac mortality in the elderly: The Rotterdam Study. Circulation 1998;97:467-472

25. Zabel M, Ney G, Fisher SR, Singh SN, Fletcher RD, Franz MR. QRS width in the 12 lead surface ECG but not variables of QT-dispersion predict mortality in the CHF stat trial. PACE 1996;19:589 (abstract)

26. Statters DJ, Malik M, Ward DE, Camm AJ. QT-dispersion: problems of methodology and clinical significance. J Cardiovasc Electrophys 1994;5:672-685

27. Coumel P, Maison-Blanche P, Badilini F. Dispersion of ventricular repolarization. Reality? Illusion? Significance? Circulation 1998;97:2491-2493

28. Zabel M, Portnoy S, Fletcher RD, Franz MR. A program for digitizing of ECG tracings on paper and accurate interactive measurement of QT intervals and ECG parameters of ventricular repolarization. J Am Coll Cardiol 1995;25:374A (abstract)

29. van de Loo A, Arendts W, Hohnloser SH. Variability of QT-dispersion measurements in the surface electrocardiogram in patients with acute myocardial infarction and in normal subjects. Am J Cardiol 1994;74:1113-1118

30. Zabel M, Franz MR, Klingenheben T, Auth B, Mansion B, Hohnloser SH. Rate-dependence of the QT interval and of QT-dispersion: comparison of atrial pacing and exercise testing. Circulation 1997;86(suppl.I):324 (abstract)

31. Rosenbaum DS, Jackson LE, Smith JM, Garan H, Ruskin JN, Cohen RJ. Electrical alternans and vulnerability to arrhythmias. N Engl J Med 1994;330:235-241

32. Hohnloser SH, Klingenheben T, Zabel M, Li YG, Albrecht P, Cohen RJ. T-wave alternans during exercise and atrial pacing in humans. J Cardiovasc Electrophysiol 1997;8:987-993

33. Priori SG, Mortara DW, Napolitano C, Diehl L, Paganini V, Cantù F, Cantù G, Schwartz PJ. Evaluation of the spatial aspects of T-wave complexity in the long QT syndrome. Circulation 1997;96:3006-3012

12. DYNAMIC QT-INTERVAL ANALYSIS

J.M.NEILSON

BACKGROUND

For almost eighty years interest has continued in the relationship between the heart rate and the duration of electrical systole, more usually expressed as the QT/RR relationship. In 1920 Fridericia (1) concluded that the relationship could best be described by a cube root formula and, within weeks, Bazett (2) independently suggested that a square root formula $QT = k \sqrt{RR}$ fitted his data and that of several other workers. By 1947 this had become accepted as "Bazett's Law" (3) and was in widespread use for estimating from the QT and RR-intervals observed at a particular time, the value of "QTc," the QT-interval "corrected" to a standard RR-interval of one second so allowing comparison of QT-intervals between individuals or the change in QT-interval over time in a single individual.

Since then numerous empirical formulae have been advocated claiming to improve on the Bazett formula which nevertheless remains in almost universal clinical use.

Controversy continues as to which is the best empirical formula, and whether the Bazett QTc is useful in risk stratification. (4-8)

DYNAMIC QT/RR ANALYSIS

Recent advances in electronic and computer technology (9,10) have made it possible to track the RR-interval and the corresponding QT-interval

H.-H. Osterhues et al. (eds.),
Advances in Noninvasive Electrocardiographic Monitoring Techniques, 131–141.
© 2000 *Kluwer Academic Publishers. Printed in the Netherlands.*

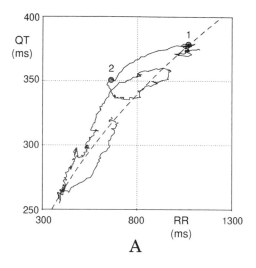

A

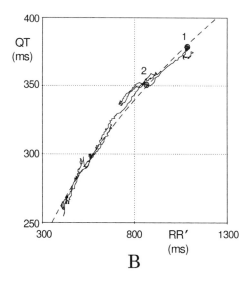

B

*Figure 1. **A**: A plot tracing continuously the dynamic relationship between QT and RR during a twenty minute ecg record superimposed on the curve representing the underlying steady state QT/RR characteristic.*
***B**: The plot of the same sequence after compensation for the QT lag by introducing a lag into the RR signal adjusted to mimic the QT lag and superimposed on the QT/RR characteristic derived from it.*

continuously in time. In our own laboratory at Edinburgh University we have developed a high speed RR and QT Analyser which can track these intervals on a beat by beat basis continuously throughout 24 hour ambulant tape recordings of the ecg and this technique is widely available [Reynolds Medical Limited, Hertford, England]

Using the continuous RR(t) and QT(t) signals from the Analyser it was instructive to plot one against the other as a QT/RR plot to reveal dynamically the characteristic curve of the QT/RR relationship.

This plot follows the consecutive (RR,QT) points, joining them to form a continuous trace. (Figure 1 A) The figure shows the plot of an episode lasting about 20 minutes and includes brief shortening of RR (points 1-2), then recovery almost to the original RR-interval, followed by a further tachycardia and partial recovery. It is clear from the looped nature of this plot that the relationship between the QT and RR-intervals is a complex one depending strongly on the time course of the RR-changes. In particular, the dynamic course of QT and RR follows a continuously changing path and not any of the widely reported characteristic curves (laws) which evidently do not apply in the dynamic situation.

These complex plots result from the well known fact that there exists a time lag in the response of the QT-interval to each change in RR-interval.

Watching the dynamic plot on an oscilloscope screen during a 24 hour record shows that from time to time the RR-interval remains relatively unchanging for long enough (several minutes) for the QT-interval to "catch up" and settle to the value corresponding to this steady RR-interval. At these times, and only at these times, the (RR,QT) point lies on the underlying steady state QT/RR characteristic curve and this is the basis of the steady state method (11) for studying the relationship. Unfortunately this elegant approach is limited by the facts that, firstly, there may be relatively few occasions in the entire record at which the RR-interval remains steady for long enough for an accurate estimate of the QT-interval to be obtained. Secondly, these occasions are not of the observer's choosing and may not arise at times when the RR-intervals are conveniently spaced so as to outline the steady state characteristic curve. Thirdly, the underlying steady state characteristic may change between observations at these steady state points so that they may not all relate to the same QT/RR characteristic.

QT LAG COMPENSATION

It became clear that if the effects of the lagging QT response to RR changes could be compensated for, the changes in the resulting QT and RR values

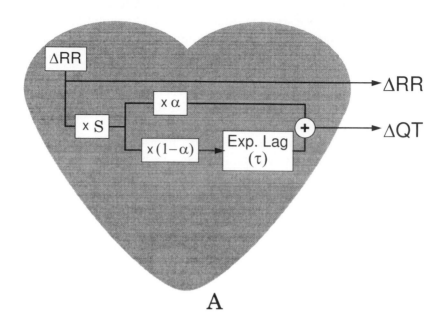

A

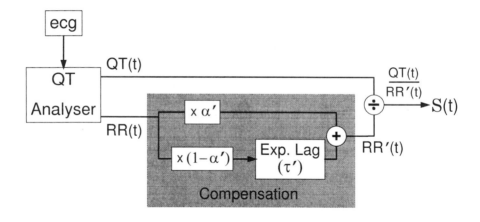

B

*Figure 2. **A** : The experimentally developed model of the QT lag showing how changes in QT respond to the changes in RR as a function of the fraction α and a time
constant τ. **B**: The RR'(t) signal is derived from the output RR(t) of the basic QT
analyser modified by operating on it by a lag network in which α' and τ' are adjusted to remove QT lag loops from the QT/RR' plot when α'= α and τ' = τ. The quo-
tient of QT(t) and RR'(t) then yields S(t) the slope of the QT/RR Characteristic.*

would be synchronised in time and the plots of these modified values would traverse the true underlying steady state characteristic curve. This might be achieved if the nature of the lag function could be adequately modelled and used either to de-convolute the lagging QT(t) signal so removing the effects of the lag, or alternatively to manipulate the RR(t) signal to impose on it a lag matching that of the natural QT signal.

After experimental investigation of several possible models using many tape recorded ecg's from our extensive database of twenty-four hour ecg's of healthy individuals and patients with a range of cardiac and non-cardiac disease, a model of the functional relationship within the heart between the changing RR-interval and the resulting change in the QT-interval emerged. This is illustrated diagramatically in Figure 2A.

For a given change in RR. the resulting QT change is related in the first place by the sensitivity of QT to change in RR. That is by the slope, S, of the QT/RR relationship, so that for very slow changes the ultimate (steady state) change in QT resulting from a sustained change in RR would be given by $\Delta QT = S.\Delta RR$.

For "dynamic" changes in heart rate taking place over periods shorter than several minutes, the change in QT comprises a 'direct', undelayed fraction $\alpha.(S.\Delta RR)$, and the remainder, a fraction $(1-\alpha).(S.\Delta RR)$, which has suffered a single pole lag with a time constant of τ seconds.

In Laplace Transform notation the lag function is thus:-

$$\Delta QT(s) = \{\alpha + (1-\alpha) / (1+s\tau) \}.S.\Delta RR(s)..............(1)$$

This model was refined by imposing just such a lag function electronically on the RR(t) signal emerging from the analyser as shown in Figure 2B and adjusting its constants α' and τ' to generate a modified signal, RR'(t), which lagged behind RR(t) in the same manner as QT(t).

When the model is correctly adjusted so that $\alpha'= \alpha$, and $\tau'= \tau$ the dynamic QT/RR' plot monitored on a digital storage oscilloscope loses its loops and traces and retraces along approximately a single curve which is the underlying steady state QT/RR characteristic.

As each record is examined the plot is observed at several places throughout the recording and, remarkably, it has been found that, for normal individuals, and across the range of diseases so far reviewed, the optimum value for α remained relatively constant in the range 0.2-0.4, (for 40 normal subjects, Mean $\pm$ SD = 0.29 $\pm$ 0.04) while τ was unchanging at approximately 60 seconds.

The compensated plot corresponding to the episode seen in Figure 1A is shown in Figure 1B.

From points on this trace the equation best fitting this curve was calculated as QT(ms)=369 [RR(ms) /1000] $^{0.372}$ and this calculated curve is shown as the dotted trace superimposed onto the compensated plot.

This same calculated curve has been superimposed onto the original dynamic QT/RR trace in Figure 1A to illustrate how far instantaneous values of (RR,QT) deviate from the underlying steady state characteristic.

In particular if samples of ecg had been taken at the times corresponding to points 1 and 2 in Figure 1A, an estimate of the slope of the steady state characteristic calculated from the co-ordinates at these points would deviate very significantly from that of the true underlying curve. Indeed the range of estimates of slope taken using points at arbitrary times along the dynamic curve is extremely wide.

Conversely, the slope of the steady state characteristic around the point being described at any time can be obtained free of the error due to the QT lag by dividing the change in QT by the corresponding change in RR' on the compensated curve of Figure 2B. This slope will depend on which part of the steady state characteristic is being described at the relevant time, and may also vary if , at some other time, the operating point moves onto another curve altogether in response to some physiological or pathological change.

CONTINUOUS ANALYSIS OF THE QT/RR RELATIONSHIP.

To explore further the behaviour of the steady state QT/RR relationship during twenty-four hour tape recorded ecg's and during various manoeuvres a hardware/software Analyser has been constructed and used in an initial assessment of the relationship in normal and diseased individuals.

This apparatus uses the QT(t) and RR(t) signals from the basic QT-interval analyser and further processes them to derive the compensated RR'(t) signal.

The QT(t) and RR'(t) signals are then cross-correlated within a selectable time window, of duration variable from one to a few minutes, which is swept continuously through the (usually twenty-four hour) ecg recording. A continuous estimate of the cross-correlation coefficient is thus generated and used automatically to gate the output of the system so that use is made of the processed results only during times when the cross-correlation coefficient r is greater than 0.8.

The slope S(t) of the QT/RR' characteristic is meanwhile continuously estimated as the linear regression coefficient within the window and used to define further the underlying characteristic.

It is assumed that the steady state characteristic can be modelled adequately by a curve of the general form:-

$$QT = QTo \ (RR'/RRo)^{J} \ ....(2)$$

where QTo is the standard QT-interval which would apply at RRo, a chosen reference RR-interval, and J is an exponent which determines the actual shape of the curve. If the Bazett assumption was correct J would equal 0.5 always, and 0.33 if Fridericia's cube root relationship held.

For equations of this general form there is only one member of this family of curves which passes through a given point (RR', QT) and has a slope S at that point and it can be shown that for this curve the exponent J is given by :-

$$J = S. \ (RR' \ / \ QT \ )...........................(3)$$

It follows therefore that, in a dynamic situation when RR'(t), QT(t), and S(t) all vary with time, then J is also time varying and J(t) describes the varying shape of the underlying QT/RR characteristic.

When a reference RR-interval (RRo) is selected, then a continuous estimate can be made of QTo(t) the intercept of the varying characteristic curve with the ordinate at RRo using:-

$$QTo(t) = QT(t) \ (\ RR(t) \ / \ RRo)^{-J}..........(4)$$

The apparatus is thus programmed to generate continuous outputs of RR(t), QT(t), S(t), J(t) and QTo(t) which are plotted as time trends, usually throughout the twenty-four hours.

RESULTS

Figure 3 shows typical time trend graphs of the output of the analyser during high speed analysis of twenty-four hour ecg tapes from a representative normal subject and a sick patient.

Small gaps in the traces mark points in the record where the correlation coefficient r between RR(t) and QT(t) fell below 0.8 so that the output of the machine was temporarily inhibited.

Figure 3A shows the twenty four hour time course of the RR and QT-intervals from the ambulatory ecg record of a healthy young student together with the time course of J(t) and $QT_{1000}(t)$ [i.e. QTo(t), the minute by minute corrected QT-interval using a reference RRo of 1000ms.] It is noticeable that despite relatively large variation of RR during the recording the corrected

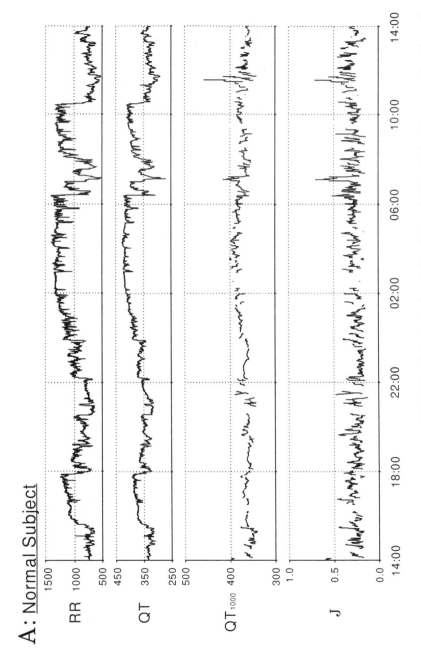

Figure 3. The twenty-four hour time course of RR, QT and the derived variables J (t) and $QT_{1000}(t)$ for (A) a young healthy male and (B) a patient with cardiomyopathy.

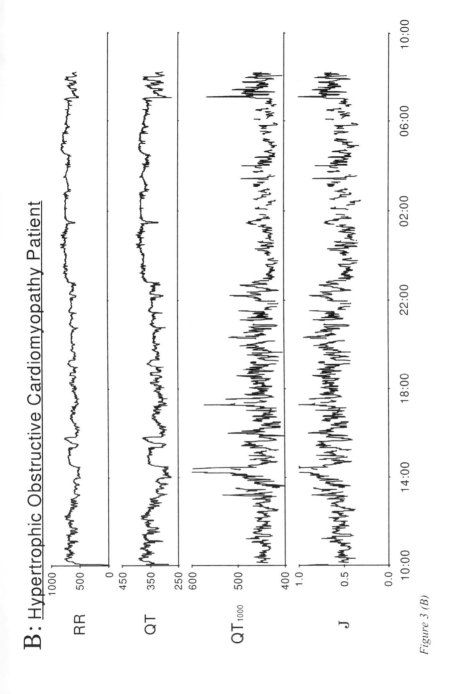

Figure 3 (B)

value of QT varies much less than the Bazett corrected QTc would have done with this much RR variation.

It can also be seen that J varies throughout the day and has a mean value of around 0.25 (half the Bazett value and slightly below the value of 0.33 favoured by Fridericia.) A few peaks reach briefly up to the Bazett level of 0.5

Figure 3B in contrast shows the picture obtained from a patient with significant heart disease.

There is generally less variation in RR through the day yet relatively more QT variation. This gave rise to an increased value of the slope of the QT/RR characteristic. The slope also showed more variation with time. Hence (Equation 3) there is a markedly higher mean value for J, the exponent governing the shape of the QT/RR characteristic.

In this case the mean value of J is seen to hover around 0.6 or 0.7 during the day only falling to 0.5 during the night but its variability is impressive, swinging from around 0.4 to around unity.

Corresponding to the dramatic variability of the shape of entire characteristic, QTo is seen to vary extensively, especially during waking hours, and has an average value of around 450ms with several peaks exceeding 500ms.

CONCLUSIONS

It has been shown that an electronic model of the natural QT lag can be constructed and adjusted using real ecg signals to compensate for the lag and allow continuous monitoring of the underlying QT/RR relationship. The technique has been extended to allow continuous estimation of the complete characteristic and hence changes in its shape and in particular to track the time course of QTo the "rate corrected" QT at any selected reference value of RR.

Observation of the 24 hour ecg's of numerous normal and sick subjects has illuminated the long standing controversy regarding the 'rate correction' of the QT-interval showing that none of the proposed formulae are right all of the time, and all are right some of the time, because the QT/RR relationship changes continuously throughout the day as J varies across a range of values from 0.2 to around unity.

It is expected that the technique will give fresh impetus to studies of the factors affecting the QT-interval, of drug effects in relation to arrhythmogenesis and therapy, and perhaps in risk stratification in disease.

REFERENCES

1. Fridericia L.S. Die Systolendauer im Elektrokardiogramm bei normalen Menschen und bei Herzkranken. Act. Med. Scand. 1920; 53 : 469-

2. Bazett H.C. An analysis of the time relations of electrocardiograms.

3. Taran L.M. & Szilagy N. The duration of electrical systole (QT) in acute rheumatic carditis in children. Am. Heart J. 1947; 33 : 14-26.

4. Franz, M.R. Time for yet another QT correction algorithm? Bazett and beyond. Editorial J.Am.Col.Cardiol. 1994; 23

5. Ward, D.E. Prolongation of the QT-interval as an indicator of risk of a cardiac event. Eur. Heart J.1988; 9 (Supplement G) : 139-44

6. Moss, A.J. Measurement of the QT-interval and the risk associated with QTc-interval prolongation: A review. Am.Heart. J. '93; 72 :23B - 25B.

7. Tomaselli, G. F. et al. Sudden cardiac death in heart failure. The role of abnormal repolarisation. Circulation. 1994; 90 ;2534-39

8. Fei et al. Is there an abnormal QT-interval in sudden cardiac death survivors with a "normal" QTc ? Am.Heart J. 1994; 128(1) : 73-76

9. Pisani et al. Performance evaluation of algorithms for QT-interval measurements in ambulatory ecg recording. In Computers in Cardiology. Los Alamitos IEEE Computer Society Press 1985 : 459-62

10. Laguna et al. New algorithm for QT-interval analysis in 24 hour Holter ecg Medical and Biological Engng & Comput. '90; 28 ; 67-73.

11. Maison-Blanche P. et al. QT-interval, heart rate and ventricular arrhythmias. In Moss, A.J. & Stern, S. Eds. Non-invasive electrocardiology: Clinical aspects of Holter monitoring. W.B. Saunders & Company Ltd. 1996 ; 383-404

13. QT-VARIABILITY: CLINICAL RESULTS AND PROGNOSTIC SIGNIFICANCE

HANS-H. OSTERHUES

QT-VARIABILITY: CLINICAL RESULTS AND PROGNOSTIC
SIGNIFICANCE

Terms such as *QT-Variability* or *Dynamic QT-Analysis* are usually used in different contexts. This raises the necessity to exactly define them for the purposes of this paper. At onset of the research there were a lot of studies publishing results from discontinuous measurement of the QT-interval for example by manual or automatic analysation of hourly strips from Holter registrations. Nowadays it is possible to perform a continuous "dynamic" QT-interval measurement in order to correlate the QT values with the RR values. At present, there are different devices used. Some perform a real beat-to-beat analysis, other systems use averaged QT values over different time windows, e.g. 30 seconds. All systems may calculate rate normalized QT-analysis, the so-called QTc value. This paper will focus on results of studies in which a continuous measurement of the QT-interval was used.

This real dynamic QT-analysis is very interesting with regard to the content of information. Just to mention the possible correlation with simultaneous measurements of the autonomic nervous system to judge its influence on re-polarisation. This may offer an insight into the physiology and pathophysiology of repolarisation. Furthermore this method may help us to control therapies, e.g. anti-arrhythmic therapy with influence on repolarisation. On the other hand, there are still a lot of problems, in particular technical problems in performing continuous QT-interval analysis. The basic signal for QT-analysis

H.-H. Osterhues et al. (eds.),
Advances in Noninvasive Electrocardiographic Monitoring Techniques, 143–153.
© 2000 *Kluwer Academic Publishers. Printed in the Netherlands.*

derived from Holter recordings is not always suitable for continuous measurement of the QT-interval. Problems such as baseline noise, insufficient quality of T-waves or changing T-waves might occur. Regarding the fact that there is an ongoing discussion about the correct measurement of T-waves (real end of T-wave, U-wave-problem) these open questions are also apparent for automatic QT-interval measurements from long-term recordings.

Another point is the question of the optimal correction formula to judge the relation of QT and heart rate. At present, the formula most frequently used is still the *Bazett* formula [1]. Nevertheless, there is an active discussion in particular on this formula, because of its inaccuracy, especially in high and low heart rates [2]. Consequently numerous new formulas for heart rate adjustment based on different mathematical models have been published [3,4]. The question is, which algorithm is optimal to correct the QT and RR ratio with regard to all frequency ranges. Despite the presentations of newer formulas with better fit than the Bazett formula there is still no agreement and no generally accepted formula.

INITIAL CLINICAL STUDIES ON CONTINUOUS "DYNAMIC" QT MEASUREMENT

First attempts for an automatic measurement of ventricular repolarisation duration were published by *Arthur Moss'* group in 1989 [5]. The computer algorithm of this group which carried out a beat-to-beat analysis of the time intervals between the peaks of the R and T-waves (RTm) was later used for the analysis of Holter ECGs. In combination with the simultaneous measurement of the RR-intervals an evaluation of the dynamic relation between repolarisation and cycle length was possible [6].

Another group which early described the clinical relevance of assessing QT dynamicity in Holter recordings was the group of *Paul Coumel*. This group also developed an original computer algorithm for the dynamic QT-interval measurement and linearly correlated the QT and RR values over a time period of 24 hours. The method used was independent from correction formulas. To judge the influence of heart rate and autonomic nervous system on repolarisation changes the group appropriately selected the QRST-complexes according to their environment. Coumel stated that not only the last RR cycle but the mean heart rate over the preceding minutes and the circadian influences must be controlled to differentiate the role of the short- and long-term influences. The study showed that the QT-interval is shorter, and the slope of the QT/RR regression line is steeper at daytime compared to nighttimes. Aging lengthens the QT-interval and reduces the day-to-night differences of QT duration and dynamicity but is gender independent. The investigations of several patients with different heart diseases, left ventricular hypertrophy or heart failure showed an alteration of QT dynamicity [7].

HEALTHY VOLUNTEERS

In 1996 *J. Molnar* and colleagues published their data of dynamic QT-interval measurement in healthy volunteers [8]. The Holter recordings of 21 healthy subjects (11 men, 10 women; mean age 57, range 36 to 76 y) were divided into 288 5-minutes segments. Average RR-interval, the QT-interval, the rate corrected QTc-interval according to the Framingham algorithm and the maximal QTc-interval was measured from these segments. The authors showed that the maximal QT-interval over 24-hours in normal subjects is longer than once thought: 511 ±16 ms in women and 479 ±12 ms in men (p=0.05). Furthermore the group confirmed the differences of the QT and QTc-interval in women and men: mean QT in women 404 ±26 ms, in men 410 ±13 ms (p=0.05) and mean QTc in women 457 ±10 ms, in men 434 ±12 ms (p=0.0001). The QT and QTc-intervals were longer during sleeping time and the QT-variability reached a peak shortly after awakening. This may reflect increased autonomic instability during early wakening hours.

Looking at our own data we had similar results. Our study included 57 healthy volunteers (28 men, 29 women, mean age 44 years, range 20 – 78 y). With regard to the female and male difference of the QTc-interval we could confirm these differences. But in our study the mean QTc-intervals were shorter than in Molnar`s study. Table 1 shows the results of our study (unpublished data).

Furthermore we correlated the QT and QTc-interval with the age of healthy persons. Despite the fact that there were increasing values of the QT and QTc duration depending on the age there was no clear correlation between these variables (Table 2 and Figure 1 and 2).

The results of these two studies focusing healthy persons show that there is still a need of larger studies to establish the normal values ranges of QT and QTc values in women and men.

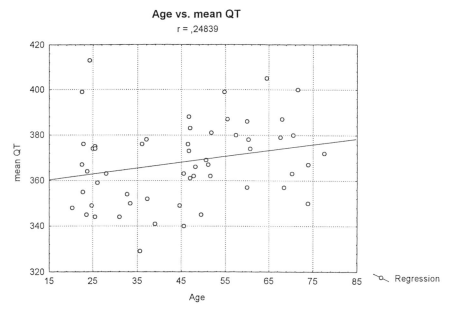

Figure 1. Corrrelation of age vs. mean QT interval of 57 healthy volunteers

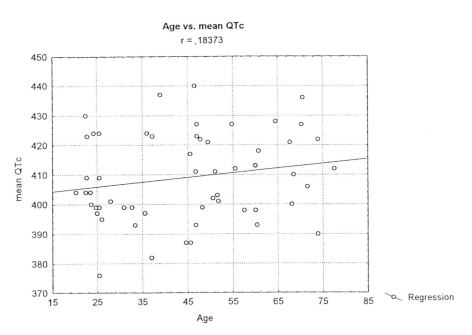

Figure 2. Corrrelation of age vs. mean QTc-interval of 57 healthy volunteers

Table 1. Results of 57 healthy volunteers (unpublished data); HR= heart rate

	All healthy volunteers (n=57)	Female (n=28)	Male (n=29)
Mean QT (ms)	367 ±18	368 ±18	367 ±17
Mean QTc * (ms)	409 ±15	417 ±12	401 ±13
HR min (beats/min)	43	45	41
HR max (beats/min)	136	140	130

* Bazett correction formula

Table 2. Results of 57 healthy volunteers according to different age classes

Normals:	**< 40 years (n=25)**	**40-60 years (n=18)**	**60 years (n=14)**
Mean QT (ms)	363 ±19	370 ±16	375 ±16
Mean QTc * (ms)	407 ±16	410 ±15	412 ±14

* Bazett correction formula

PATIENTS WITH LONG QT SYNDROME

It is not surprising that the first patients´ data of continuous QT measurement were performed in patients with long QT syndrome. The clinical course of these patients made obvious the connection of a QT-interval prolongation with rhythm disturbances. *M. Merri* and colleagues published one of the first investigations looking at these patients [6]. With regard to the better signal, the group analysed the R-wave peak and the maximum amplitude of the T-wave (RTm). Former investigations showed a close correlation between the QT-interval and the RT-interval [5]. The Holter recordings of 16 patients with congenital long QT syndrome were compared to 11 normal volunteers. The authors found a significant difference between these groups regarding the relation between ventricular repolarisation duration and cycle length during 24-hour recordings. Mean regression RTm/RR lines showed a significantly larger slope in the long QT patients compared to normal controls. The patients had an exaggerated delay in repolarisation at long RR cylce lengths. This kind

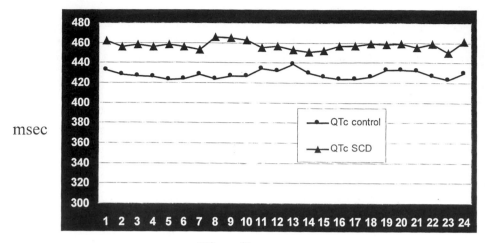

Time / hour

Figure 3.

of calculation expressed as the slope of the regression line represents one possible methodology for the judgement of the QT/RR -information.

In a study published by *T. Emori* and co-workers the results were confirmed in a group of 11 patients with long QT syndrome in comparison to 10 healthy controls[9].

PATIENTS WITH VENTRICULAR ARRHYTHMIAS WITH AND WITHOUT PREVIOUS MYOCARDIAL INFARCTIONS

E. Homs and *Antonio Bayes de Luna* compared patients with life threatening arrhythmias such as sustained ventricular tachycardia or out of hospital cardiac arrest (group 1, n=14), and patients without malignant arrhythmias (group 2, n=28). All patients had had a myocardial infarction. The comparison of the QTc values of the two groups showed significant differences for the time period of 24 hours: mean QTc-interval in group one 425 ±20 ms and in group two 405 ±17 ms (p=0.01).

Furthermore they could show that a significant proportion of patients of the group with life threatening arrhythmias exhibited more peaks of corrected QTc-intervals longer than 500 ms.

Homs recorded a circadian rhythm of peaks of QTc-intervals longer than 550 ms with a significantly higher incidence from 11 pm to 11 am. The authors concluded that a QTc-interval longer than 500 ms may be a cut-off point with poor prognostic impact [10].

A population with ventricular fibrillation but without heart disease was investigated by *R. Tavernier* and co-workers [11]. The study focussed on the QT-interval and its adaptation to heart rate in 6 patients compared to 21 normal persons. Both groups were not different with regard to mean heart rate, standard deviation of RR-intervals or RMSSD heart rate variability parameter and mean QT end.

Tavernier plotted the QT end against the corresponding average RR value to determine the slope of this regression. He documented significant differences between normals and ventricular fibrillation patients with a significantly lower slope of the fibrillation patients.

Results of our group confirmed the significant differences of the QTc-interval in patients with malignant ventricular tachycardias and sudden cardiac death compared to healthy controls. Figure 3 shows the QT-interval of a healthy control person from our investigation in comparison to a patient who died suddenly.

Patients in the chronic phase post myocardial infarctions were investigated by *T. Walter* and colleagues [12]. 42 patients without ventricular tachyarrythmias (VT) were compared with 24 patients with ventricular tachyarrhythmias. A control group consisted of 14 healthy volunteers. There were significant differences in QT dynamics of the patients with VT versus those without VT: mean QTc with VT: 431 ±39ms vs 406 ±11ms without VT ($p < 0.001$). Comparison of patients groups with healthy controls showed no significant difference in patients without VT versus controls but significant differences to patients with VT. This underlines the hypothesis of an altered repolarisation in post MI patients. The degree of these changes might be of prognostic value. However, a small study published by *M. Stopp* and colleagues focusing on the same patients population could not confirm these results [13].

Another starting point for dynamic QT-interval analysis has been published by *T. Brüggemann* and co-workers in the Annals of Noninvasive Electrocardiology [14]. In this retrospective analysis a continuous QT-interval measurement was carried out in patients after myocardial infarction. Additionally to the measurement of the QT-interval and corrected QTc-interval, Brüggemann performed an analysis of the so called "duration of late repolarization". This was defined as the duration of the down sloping part of the T-wave, which means the QT end minus the QT peak, RR corrected. This marker showed a significant difference between the patients with cardiac death after myocardial infarction in comparison to post MI patients without death during follow up. Significant differences of QT and QTc-intervals could not be detected between groups. Therefore the authors concluded that standard QT measurements have no predictive value in post MI patients.

In this beginning area of dynamic QT-interval measurement the most studies focused on QT-variability of patients post MI with and without arrhythmias. But there are already a few studies reporting from other heart diseases.

PATIENTS WITH CARDIOMYOPATHY

Ronald Berger and co-workers studied patients with dilated cardiomyopathy (DCM). They investigated the beat-to-beat QT-interval variability [15]. The authors compared 83 patients with cardiomyopathy: 54 with non-ischemic causes and 29 with idiopathic dilated cardiomyopathy with a control group consisting of 60 healthy volunteers. This study did not use Holter recordings as basis but 256 sec records of the surface ECG. The estimation of the beginning and the end of the QT-interval was manually selected by an operator. From this view it is only a short-term variation study of the QT-interval.

Comparisons showed significant differences of the mean heart rate and the mean QT-interval between patients and healthy controls. Further analysis included the calculation of a QT-variability index (QTVI) as the logarithm of the ratio of normalized QT variance to heart rate variance. DCM patients had greater QT variance than control subjects ($p<0.0001$) despite reduced heart rate variance. Coherence between heart rate and QT-interval fluctuations at physiological frequencies was lower in DCM patients compared to control subjects. The authors concluded that DCM is associated with beat-to-beat fluctuations in QT-interval which are larger than normal and uncoupled from variations in heart rate. This may lead to temporal lability in ventricular repolarisation.

PATIENTS WITH LEFT VENTRICULAR HYPERTROPHY

A study published by *J.P. Singh* and co-workers investigated patients with left ventricular hypertrophy and compared them with controls [16]. A computerized Holter system was developed to study the QT-interval reponse to changes in the RR-interval. The adaptive response of the QT-interval was measured as the ratio of the slope from 10% to 90% of the QT change relative to the RR-interval change (dQT/dRR_{10-90}). The investigators were able to show that the adaptive response of the QT-interval was increased in the left ventricular hypertrophy group compared to the control group during both acceleration and deceleration phases. This documents a rapid and exaggerated response of the QT-interval to changes in the RR-interval. The authors concluded that there are alterate repolarisation dynamics in patients with left ventricular hypertrophy which may make them vulnerable to serious ventricular arrhythmias.

CONTROL OF PHARMACOLOGICAL THERAPY

Several antiarrhythmic drugs lead to a prolongation of the cardiac repolarisation phase. Representative drugs with these effects are class III anti-arrhythmics such as Amiodarone and Sotalol. A link between pro-arrhythmic effects of these drugs and alterations of repolarisation phase may be possible. It is therefore of interest to study the short and long-term effects of these drugs on the QT-interval and circadian patterns of the heart rate.

M. Antimisiaris published the data of heart rate and QTc-interval measurements of three groups of patients who received Amiodarone over different time courses: 10 patients at baseline of drug administration, 11 patients treated for 3 to 6 months with Amiodarone and 13 patients treated longer than 1 year. Amiodarone reduced heart rate which reached steady state at 3 to 6 months. The corrected QT-interval (QTc) increased as a function of treatment duration. The circadian rhythm of QTc was abolished in patients with long term administration (> 1 year). A power spectral anaysis showed a tendency for Amiodarone to reduce both RR-variability and QT-interval variability. From these results, the authors concluded an inhibition of autonomic control of the heart by this drug. Pro-arrhythmic effects and a possible correlation with QT-interval alterations were not part of this investigation [17].

CONCLUSION

From these few studies it is not possible to give clear statements and to draw real conclusions. The data presented are limited due to the small number of patients and existing methodological problems of this method. Some results are antithetic to others and there is not enough data to judge the conflicting results.

Summarizing the available studies of normal volunteers, it is obvious that circadian QTc variations are a physiological phenomenon. These variations are not only influenced by heart rate but also occur independently. From these first studies it seems to be true that QTc peaks longer than 500 ms are rare in healthy persons. But we have to consider that there might be gender-specific differences.

The studies in patients show that the fluctuations of the QT-intervals un-coupled from variations of heart rate may reflect lability of repolarisation. This was shown for patients with ischemic and non-ischemic cardiomyopathy. The adaptive reponse of the QT-interval to heart rate changes seems to be of interest.

Furthermore, the available results could show that the slope of the regression lines of QT to RR is different in patients with cardiac diseases compared to healthy controls. This was found in post-MI patients with ventricular tachycardias, sudden cardiac death patients and iⁿ patients with long QT syndrome.

Nevertheless, the question of the prognostic value of this method cannot be answered at present time.

We are just at the beginning of this interesting field of measurement of dynamic QT-variability as an expression of repolarisation behaviour. Nevertheless, we do need larger prospective trials, especially for the judgement of the prognostic value of this method. Future studies should focus on different aspects such as comparison of different patient groups and controls or try to confirm cut-off points of the QT and QTc-interval. We have to investigate the meaning of RR-independent QT fluctuations and last but not least try to illuminate the interaction of different systems such as the autonomic nervous system and the repolarisation behaviour.

ACKNOWLEDGMENT
I thank Dagmar Schemminger for technical assistance

REFERENCES:

1. Bazett H: An analysis of time relation of electrocardiogram. Heart 1920;7:353-370
2. Ahnve S: Correction of the QT-interval for heart rate: review of different formulas and the use of Bazett´s formulas in myocardial infarction. Am.Heart J. 1985;109:568-574
3. Karjalainen J, Viitasalo M, Manttari M, Manninen V: Relation between QT-intervals and heart rates from 40 to 120 beats/min in rest electrocardiograms of men and a simple method to adjust QT-interval values. J.Am.Coll.Cardiol. 1994;23:1547-1553
4. Sagie A, Larson M, Goldberg R, Bengston J, Levy D: An improved method for adjusting the QT-interval for heart rate (the Framingham Heart Study). Am.J.Cardiol. 1992;70:797-801
5. Merri M, Benhorin J, Alberti M, Locati E, Moss AJ: Electrocardiographic quantitation of ventricular repolarization. Circulation 1989;80:1301-1308
6. Merri M, Moss AJ, Benhorin J, Locati EH, Alberti M, Badilini F: Relation between ventricular repolarization duration and cardiac cycle length during 24-hour Holter recordings. Findings in normal patients and patients with long QT syndrome. Circulation 1992;85:1816-1821
7. Coumel P, Fayn J, Maison BP, Rubel P: Clinical relevance of assessing QT dynamicity in Holter recordings. J.Electrocardiol. 1994;27 Suppl:62-66

8. Molnar J, Weiss JS, Rosenthal JE: The missing second: what is the correct unit for the Bazett corrected QT-interval? Am.J.Cardiol. 1995;75:537-538

9. Emori T, Ohe T, Aihara N, Kurita T, Shimizu W, Kamakura S, Shimomura K: Dynamic relationship between the Q-aT-interval and heart rate in patients with long QT syndrome during 24-hour Holter ECG monitoring. Pacing.Clin.Electrophysiol. 1995;18:1909-1918

10. Homs E, Marti V, Guindo J, Laguna P, Vinolas X, Caminal P, Elosua R, Bayes-de Luna A: Automatic measurement of corrected QT-interval in Holter recordings: comparison of its dynamic behavior in patients after myocardial infarction with and without life-threatening arrhythmias. Am.Heart J. 1997;134:181-187

11. Tavernier R, Jordaens L, Haerynck F, Derycke E, Clement DL: Changes in the QT-interval and its adaptation to rate, assessed with continuous electrocardiographic recordings in patients with ventricular fibrillation, as compared to normal individuals without arrhythmias. Eur.Heart J. 1997;18:994-999

12. Walter T, Griessl G, Kluge P, Neugebauer A: QT-dispersion in surface ECG and QT dynamics in long-term ECG in patients with coronary heart disease in the chronic post-infarct stage with and without ventricular tachyarrhythmias--correlation with other risk parameters. Z.Kardiol. 1997;86:204-210

13. Stopp M, Jung J, Özbek C, Bay W, Georg T, Fries R, Schieffer H, Heisel A: Role of dynamic QT-interval analysis during 24 h Holter ECG for prediction of arrhythmic events after myocardial infarction. Herzschr. Elektrophys. 1998;53-60

14. Bruggemann T, Eisenreich S, Behrens S, Ehlers C, Müller D, Andresen D: Continuous QT-interval measurements from 24-hour electrocardiography and risk after myocardial infarction. Ann. Noninvas. Electrocardiol. 1997;2:264-273

15. Berger RD, Kasper EK, Baughman KL, Marban E, Calkins H, Tomaselli GF: Beat-to-beat QT-interval variability: novel evidence for repolarization lability in ischemic and nonischemic dilated cardiomyopathy. Circulation 1997;96:1557-1565

16. Singh J, Johnston J, Sleight P, Bird R, Ryder K, Hart G: Left ventricular hypertrophy in hypertensive patients is associated with abnormal rate adaptation of QT-interval. J.Am.Coll.Cardiol. 1997;29:778-784

17. Antimisiaris M, Sarma J, Schoenbaum M, Sharma P, Venkataraman K, Singh BN, Christenson P: Effects of amiodarone on the circadian rhythm and power spectral changes of heart rate and QT-interval: Significance for the control of sudden cardiac death. Am.Heart J. 1994;128:884-891

14. HEART RATE DEPENDENCY OF QT-INTERVAL IN CONGENITAL AND ACQUIRED PROLONGED VENTRICULAR REPOLARIZATION: LONG-TERM ANALYSIS BY HOLTER MONITORING

EMANUELA H. LOCATI AND GIUSEPPE BAGLIANI

SHORT AND LONG-TERM ANALYSIS OF VENTRICULAR REPOLARIZATION DYNAMICS

Prolonged ventricular repolarization, with abnormal configuration and increased dispersion of QT-interval duration, has been associated with an increased risk of malignant arrhythmias in congenital and acquired conditions [1,2]. The QT-interval is modulated by multiple factors, such as heart rate level, circadian rhythm and autonomic nervous system activity, that cannot fully be evaluated by a brief ECG tracing obtained in basal conditions [3]. Together with the long term analysis of heart rate variability, the long-term analysis of QT-interval dynamicity can now be explored from 24-hour ECG Holter recordings by new computerized programs, in some cases already available for routine clinical use. However, the automatic measurement of QT-interval by Holter techniques has several methodological limitations, due to the relatively low sampling rates utilized in Holter recordings, the shifting of the isoelectric baseline, the low signal-to-noise ratio, and the difficult determination of the T-wave end. To overcome such problems, it has been proposed to utilize the interval from Q-wave onset to T-wave apex (QT_{apex}), since in most cases T-wave apex can be more accurately identified than T-wave end (QT_{end}) [4]. However, QT_{apex} cannot be considered equivalent to the total QT duration, particularly in prolonged QT syndromes, where the QT

H.-H. Osterhues et al. (eds.),
Advances in Noninvasive Electrocardiographic Monitoring Techniques, 155–160.
© 2000 *Kluwer Academic Publishers. Printed in the Netherlands.*

prolongation may affect specifically the terminal components of the T-wave [2,5], whereas the early phase, QT_{apex}, should mainly account for the rate dependency of ventricular repolarization [4].

Reliable long-term automatic measurements of both QT_{apex} and QT_{end} from Holter monitoring can be obtained by *averaging procedures*, in order to obtain a low-noise ECG signal ; however averaging procedures necessarily ignore the instantaneous variations of the QT interval. In contrast, while the long-term beat-to-beat automatic analysis of QT duration can often be unreliable, short-term *beat-to-beat procedures* can explore the instantaneous fluctuations of QT duration and T-wave morphology by sophisticated analyses requiring high quality ECG tracings in controlled conditions.

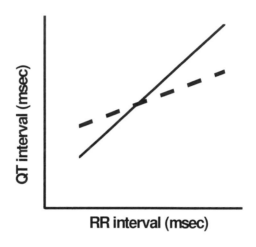

Figure 1. Schematic representation of two linear regressions (steep, solid line, and flat, dashed line) expressing two possible different relation between QT and RR-interval

LONG-TERM RELATION BETWEEN VENTRICULAR REPOLARIZATION AND HEART RATE

Among the several methods proposed to evaluate the long-term modulation of ventricular repolarization by heart rate, one standard approach is to compute the linear regression between QT-intervals and correspondent RR-intervals, both on the entire 24-hours or on pre-selected time-periods. Of note, a *steep slope* may indicate a further prolongation of the QT-interval at longer cycle lengths, whereas an adequate QT shortening at shorter cardiac cycles; conversely, a *flat slope* indicates that the QT-interval is less dependent from the cardiac cycle, and it fails to shorten at shorter cycle (Figure 1).

Recent studies demonstrated that the QT-RR relation shows typical day-night differences [3], with flatter slope during night than during day-time. Also, the QT-RR relation is steeper in females than in males in normal adult subjects, in parallel with a longer duration of the corrected QT-interval observed in adult females [6].

LONG-TERM QT-RR RELATION IN CONGENITAL LONG QT SYNDROMES.

The QT-RR relation can be impaired in conditions of congenital and acquired prolonged ventricular repolarization [4,7-10]. In patients with *congenital long QT syndrome* (LQTS), where at least three distinct genotypes (LQT1, LQT2, and LQT3) have been identified, typical gene-specific differences in rate dependency of QT duration have been recently demonstrated [7,8]. Preliminary findings indicate that patients with K+ channel abnormalities (Iks for LQT1 patients with KVLQT1 gene mutations located on chromosome 11, and Ikr for LQT2 with HERG gene-mutations on chromosome 7) may have impaired shortening of QT duration at fast heart rate, i.e. a flat slope of the QT-RR relation. In contrast, LQT3 patients, with SCN5A gene-mutations on chromosome 3, with impaired inactivation of cardiac sodium channels, tend to have further QT prolongation at longer cardiac cycles, i.e. a steep slope of the QT-RR relation [6,7]. Of note, preliminary findings indicate that distinct patterns of circadian QT-variability may also be present in LQTS patients with different genotypes. Patients with LQT3 genotype, with further QT prolongation at low heart rate, have longer corrected QT duration during sleep [11], that may account for the increased incidence of cardiac event during sleep and at rest observed in these patients [7]. In contrast, patients with LQT1 genotype appear to have longer QTc during day time, consistent with an impaired shortening of QT duration at fast heart rate, that may account for the higher incidence of cardiac events during activity or stress more often observed among these patients.

LONG-TERM QT-RR RELATION IN ACQUIRED PROLONGED VENTRICULAR REPOLARIZATION

In patients with *acquired prolonged ventricular repolarization*, the heart rate dependency of QT duration may vary according with the drug and the cardiac condition provoking the QT prolongation. Conflicting information has so far been provided concerning the heart rate dependency of the moderate QT

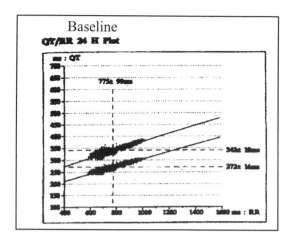

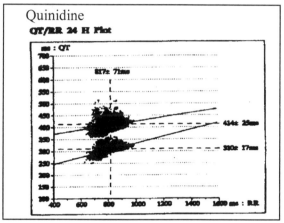

Figure 2. Plots illustrating the slopes of the linear regressions for QT_{end}/RR (upper lines) and QT_{apex}/RR relation (lower lines) in a patient at baseline (left) and after one-week Quinidine therapy (right). Analyses were performed by a dedicated Holter algorithm (Ela Medical, Inc), which automatically measured QT duration in 2880 QRST templates computed from 30-sec median beats, plotted QT against RR-interval, and calculated linear regression (QT/RR slope), correlation coefficient (r), mean RR and corrected QT (QTc, msec).

prolongation observed in patients following a myocardial infarction. Recently, patients with malignant arrhythmias were showed to have a steeper QT/RR slope than patients with coronary artery disease but with no history of malignant arrhythmias[12]. Of note, patients with coronary artery disease, when compared to normal subjects, may show lack of circadian modulation of the QT dynamics [12]. Abnormal circadian patterns of prolonged QT-interval may be associated with an increased incidence of malignant arrhythmias [13] and sudden cardiac death after myocardial infarction [14].

More consistent information is available on the rate-dependent effects of antiarrhythmic drugs prolonging QT-interval duration. A study comparing four drugs with different sensitivity of blockade for potassium channel (d-sotalol, dofetilide, E4031 or MS551) showed differential profile of rate dependence in drug-induced QT prolongation. With the exception of d-sotalol, steeper slopes were present after drug administration when compared to baseline, an effect correspondent to the "reverse-use-dependency" induced by the drugs [9]. In a more recent study, we observed that quinidine not only prolonged ventricular repolarization, but also impairs QT-interval shortenings at shorter cycle lengths, corresponding to a "use-dependent" effect [10] (Figure 2). Such lack of QT adaptation at faster heart rate, similar to what observed in LQTS patients with K+ channel abnormalities, may play a role in the genesis of proarrhythmias sometimes observed during quinidine therapy.

FUTURE PROSPECTIVES

The automatic computerized analysis of the long-term QT-interval dynamics by Holter techniques is nowadays a reliable technique that may contribute to identify conditions leading to potentially fatal cardiac arrhythmias. Further studies on larger groups of patients are still needed to explore the effect of different therapeutic interventions on different short and long-term measures of QT dynamics, including the relation between QT-interval and heart rate relation and the circadian pattern of QT duration.

The combined analysis of ventricular repolarization dynamics and heart rate variability may transform Holter monitoring in a *"non-invasive electrophysiological test"*, exploring the interaction between autonomic nervous system and myocardial substrate, in order to identify subjects at high risk of malignant arrhythmias in congenital and acquired prolonged ventricular repolarization.

REFERENCES

1. Schwartz PJ, Locati EH, Priori SG, Napolitano C. The idiopathic long QT syndrome. In: Cardiac Electrophysiology: From Cell to Bedside (DP Zipes, J Jalife, Eds, 2nd Ed.). WB Saunders Co, Philadelphia, 1995: 788-811.

2. Jackman WM, Friday KJ, Anderson JL, Aliot EM, Clark M, Lazzara R: The long QT syndromes: A critical review, new clinical observations and a unifying hypothesis. Prog Cardiovasc Dis 1988; 31: 115-72.

3. Maison-Blanche P, Catuli D, Fayn J, Coumel P : QT-interval, heart rate and ventricular arrhythmias. In: Noninvasive Electrocardiology: Clinical Aspects of Holter Monitoring. Moss AJ, Stern S, Eds. WB Saunders Co Ltd, London, 1996: 383-404.

4. Merri M, Moss AJ, Benhorin J, Locati EH, Alberti M, Badilini F: Relationship between ventricular repolarization and cardiac cycle lenght during 24-hour electrocardiographic (Holter) recordings: Findings in normals and patients with Long QT Syndrome. Circulation 1992; 85:1916-21.

5. Moss AJ, Zareba W, Benhorin J, Locati EH, Hall WJ, Robinson JL, Schwartz PJ, Towbin JA, Vincent GM, Lehmann M, Keating MT, MacCluer JW, Timothy KW: ECG T-wave patterns in genetically distinct forms of the hereditary long QT syndrome. Circulation 1995; 92: 2929-34.

6. Stramba-Badiale M, Locati EH, Martinelli A, Courville J, Schwartz PJ: Gender and the relationship between ventricular repolarization and cardiac cycle length during 24-hour Holter recordings. Eur Heart J 1997; 18: 1000-6.

7. Schwartz PJ, Priori SG, Locati EH, Napolitano C, Cantu' F, Towbin AJ, Keating MT, Hammoude H, Brown AM, Chen LK, Cotasky TJ: Long QT syndrome patients with mutations on the SCN5A and HERG genes have differential responses to Na+ channel blockade and to increase in heart rate. Implications for gene-specific therapy. Circulation 1995; 92: 3381-86.

8. Locati EH, Stramba-Badiale M, Priori SG, Napolitano C, Towbin JA, Keating MT, Vinolas X, Schwartz PJ: Gene-specific differences in the dynamic relation of QT-interval and heart rate in the congenital long QT syndrome. Eur Heart J 1996; 17 (abs suppl): 126.

9. Okada Y, Ogawa S, Sadanaga T, Mitamura H : Assessment of reverse use-dependent blocking actions of Class II antiarrhythmic drugs by 24-hour Holter monitoring. J Am Coll Cardiol 1996 ; 27 : 84-9.

10. Locati EH, Bagliani G, Meniconi L : Quinidine Impairs QT-interval Shortening at Shorter Cycle Lengths: A Long-Term Automatic Holter Analysis of Rate-Dependent QT-Interval Changes. J Am Coll Cardiol 1998 ; 31 : 265A.

11. Stramba-Badiale M, Locati EH, Priori SG, Napolitano C, Epis E, Towbin JA, Keating MT, Vinolas X, Schwartz PJ : Gene-specific differences in the circadian variation of ventricular repolarization in the long QT syndrome. Circulation 1996 ; 94 : I-450.

12. Kluge P, Walter T, Neugebauer A : Comparison of Q/RR relationship using two algorithms of QT-interval analysis for identification of high risk patients for life-threatening arrhythmias. Ann Noninvasive Electrocardiol 1997 ; 2 : 3-8.

13. Molnar J, Zhang F, Weiss J, Ehlert FA, Rosenthal JE: Diurnal pattern of QTc-interval: How long is prolonged? Possible relation to circadian triggers of cardiovascular events. J Am Coll Cardiol 1996; 27: 76-83.

14. Singh JP, Johnston J, Sleight P, Marinho MF, Kulangara S, Casadei B, Hart G : Circadian variation and waking hour dynamics of QT-interval : Implications for mechanisms underlying sudden cardiac death. Ann Noninvasive Electrocardiol 1997; 2: 242-53.

CHAPTER TWO: ECG ASPECTS INVESTIGATED BY DIFFERENT METHODS

SECTION THREE: T-WAVE ALTERNANS / REPOLARIZATION

15. MODERN APPROACHES TO ASSESSMENT OF VENTRICULAR REPOLARISATION

IRINA SAVELIEVA AND MAREK MALIK

ABSTRACT

Although experimental evidence of a significant role of myocardial repolarisation inhomogeneity in arrhythmogenesis has been grown rapidly, progress in the clinical arena has been comparatively slow. There continues to be methodological uncertainty regarding ventricular repolarisation assessment from body surface electrocardiogram. Multiple approaches are currently being investigated for this purpose, indicating that no one satisfactory method has yet been found. Despite rapid development of sophisticated computer-assisted algorithms for QT-interval and QT-dispersion measurement, low reproducibility of repeated measurements, particularly of QT-dispersion, remains a major limitation. In recent years, some progress has been made in developing alternative methods of ventricular repolarisation assessment. Suggested approaches have focused on analysis of QT-interval variability during 24-hour Holter recording (QT/RR dynamicity) and beat-to-beat changes in the repolarisation patterns (T-wave alternans) which reflect two different aspects of ventricular repolarisation: spatial and dynamic. Simultaneous assessment of both aspects is believed to be a promising tool which allows not only to identify patients at high risk of arrhythmic events but also to investigate spontaneous or triggered changes in ventricular repolarisation leading to arrhythmias. Recent studies of T-wave alternans have documented that repolarisation patterns are closely related to arrhythmic and pro-arrhythmic complications, indicating that analy-

H.-H. Osterhues et al. (eds.),
Advances in Noninvasive Electrocardiographic Monitoring Techniques, 163–175.
© 2000 Kluwer Academic Publishers. Printed in the Netherlands.

sis T and TU-wave morphology may play an important role in risk stratification.

Table I. Non-invasive methods for ventricular repolarisation assessment

- QT-interval and QT-dispersion measurement
- QT-variability, QT/RR dynamicity assessment
- T-wave alternans analysis
- T/TU-wave pattern analysis
- Body surface potential mapping

In conclusion, further development of practical approaches to quantitative assessment of ventricular repolarisation is essential for better understanding of physiological and pathophysiological processes governing this phenomenon, and for improving of arrhythmogenic risk stratification.

Key words: Ventricular repolarisation, QT-interval, QT-dispersion, QT-variability, T-wave alternans

INTRODUCTION

Experimental and clinical studies performed over the past years have confirmed that electrocardiographic patterns of myocardial repolarisation are closely linked to arrhythmogenesis and may represent a potential tool for arrhythmogenic risk stratification. Methods for non-invasive assessment of myocardial repolarisation have been developed and are currently being investigated, including QT-interval dispersion, QT-interval variability (QT/RR dynamicity), and T-wave alternans. Although noticeable success in identifying patients at high risk of lethal arrhythmic events has been achieved with these techniques, there is still a need for new technologies with better predictive accuracy. Recently, the NASPE/ISHNE Task Force on the QT-interval and T-wave have provisionally concluded that T and TU-wave patterns analysis should be further developed as it is at least as important as QT-interval measurement. Methods currently available for ventricular repolarisation assessment are summarised in Table I.

QT-INTERVAL AND QT-DISPERSION

Prolongation of QT-interval has long been known as a factor predisposing to ventricular tachyarrhythmias and sudden cardiac death [1-3]. Following the fact that prolonged QT-interval may reflect both the uniform increase in action potential duration and nonuniform recovery of myocardial excitability, Day et al [4] suggested in 1990 to use the assessment of QT interlead variability (QT-dispersion) as a measure of repolarisation inhomogeneity. Although an increased QT-dispersion have been shown to correlate with arrhythmogenesis in a variety of clinical conditions [4-9], controversies regarding many aspects remain, including the prevalence of this phenomenon, criteria for normality, and the optimal methodological approaches to detection of repolarisation abnormalities in body surface electrocardiogram (ECG). Well-known difficulties with manual measurement of the QT-interval [10,11], make many researchers advocate the use of computerised methods which are believed to be more stable and bias independent.

Currently available commercial systems offer a variety of algorithms for the automatic measurement of QT-interval and related parameters. Threshold and least-square curve fitting methods or their combination are suggested for the automatic detection of the end of the T-wave (Marquette Medical Systems, Milwaukee, Wisc.) [12]. The threshold techniques determine the T-wave end as the intersection of the T-wave or its differential with a predetermined threshold level. The least-square curve fitting method detects the end of the T-wave as the intersection of the least-square-fit line around the tangent to the downslope of the T-wave with isoelectric baseline. The accuracy of the QT-interval measurement depends largely on morhology of the T-wave. Low amplitude, biphasic, notched T-waves, and TU-wave fusion patterns may preclude precise detection of the end of the T-wave, resulting in false QT-interval and QT-dispersion abnormalities. Automatic techniques using strict algorithms for detection of the T-wave end may be substantially affected by the T-wave patterns. McLaughlin et al [13] showed that the T-wave amplitude <0.25 mV was associated with as much as twice greater error in the automatic QT-interval measurement in cardiac patients compared to normal subjects, which emphasises the fact that the performance of automatic algorithm is strongly affected by the subject group analysed.

The technical reasons for low reliability of QT-interval and, particularly, QT-dispersion measurement by automatic algorithms should also be considered. For instance, the analysis of digital ECG from the MAC VU electrocardiograph operates with 250 HZ sample rates resulting in possibility of the measurement of the QT-interval at a discrete scale with 4 ms steps. Because the values of QT-dispersion measured in precordial leads often lie within the 4 ms limits, the difference between the maximum and the minimum precordial QT-interval is precisely 1 step on the scale. Thus, the difference of ± 1 step will result in substantial increase in variability of measurements obtained from repeated ECG recordings.

Recently suggested algorithms implementing ECG signal derivatives have not justify expectations regarding preciseness of measurement. Although Bor-

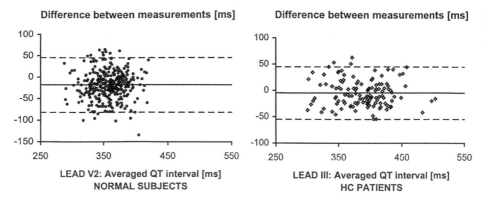

Figure 1. Bland-Altman plots for the automatic versus manual measurements of the QT-interval. In normal subjects, the best agreement between both methods ($r^2=0.25$) was observed in lead V₂; in patients with hypertrophic cardiomyopathy (HC), the highest correlation between methods ($r^2=0.67$) was observed in lead III. Solid lines represent mean of difference between the automatic and manual QT measurement; dashed lines represent values for mean ± 2SD. Reprinted from Savelieva I et al, Am J Cardiol 1998;81:471-477.

tolan et al [14] have reported satisfactory results with the threshold method applied on the derivative signal, other studies did not confirm these findings [15].

Although published data on comparison between the automatic methods and manual measurements are scarce, there is an observation that for both methods, the reproducibility of QT-interval assessment is substantially higher than that of QT-dispersion, and that the agreement between methods is low (Figure 1) [16,17]. A most likely explanation is that the automatic algorithm does not entirely copy the way of the manual measurement, which makes both methods depend in a different manner on the shape of the descending part of the T-wave. The lack of agreement between manual and automatic measurement of QT-interval suggests that clinical experience gained with manual measurement cannot be applied blindly to data obtained from modern computerised systems.

QT-INTERVAL VARIABILITY AND QT/RR DYNAMICITY

A vast number of studies show and confirm that QT-interval is largely affected by heart rate and autonomic modulations. Autonomic imbalance with an increased sympathetic activity may augment vulnerability to malignant ventricular arrhythmias [18]. This mechanism is hypothesised to operate through alteration in ventricular refractoriness, which can result in changes in the re-polarisation duration measured as QT-interval in the surface ECG. Since heart rate is also the subject to autonomic modulation, one can expect close relation between QT and RR-intervals which is, indeed, the case [19]. Attempts to avoid a confusing effect of rate correction formulae on QT-interval [20,21] through evaluating QT-interval at the same stable heart rates either from Holter recording or during atrial pacing at fixed cycle length [22,23], have led to awareness of strong interrelation between QT-interval and RR-interval variability. Observations made in patients with long QT syndrome (LQTS) [24], coronary artery disease and myocardial infarction [25,26], and hypertrophic cardiomyopathy [27] confirmed the presence of a progressive prolongation of QT-interval at slower heart rates compared to normal subjects, which may indicate pronounced inhomogeneity of ventricular repolarisation and risk of arrhythmogenesis. These studies also support a concept that the pattern of QT-interval variability may have more clinical potential than QT-interval duration itself.

Recently suggested approaches have been focused on the analysis of QT-interval variability during 24-hour Holter recording (QT/RR dynamicity) which reflects two different aspects of ventricular repolarisation: spatial and dynamic. Simultaneous assessment of both aspects is believed to be a promising tool which allows not only to identify patients at high risk of arrhythmic events but also to investigate spontaneous or triggered changes in ventricular repolarisation leading to arrhythmias. It may be speculated that these methods overcome limitations of conventional assessment of repolarisation inhomogeneity expressed by QT-dispersion. Coumel et al [28] investigated QT-interval adaptation to changes in heart rate during 24-hour Holter recording and demonstrated different diurnal patterns of QT/RR interrelation in normal subjects, patients with LQTS and patients with heart failure. It has been proposed that computerised algorithm recognising subtle dynamics in QT-interval in response to changes in heart rate can provide new insight into the effects of autonomic nervous system on myocardial repolarisation.

QT-variability from Holter recording may be investigated in two ways: by analysing changes in QT-interval corrected according to heart rate QTc [29,30] and by analysing QT-variability on beat-to-beat basis independent of heart rate [23,31,32]. Significant circadian variations in the QT-interval in patients with preserved autonomic function have uniformly been reported in these studies. Both the QT and QT_c-intervals were prolonged during sleep following by an increase in the absolute values of QT_c-interval and QT_c-variability after awakening, suggesting an enhanced autonomic imbalance, which coincides with observations of high incidence of arrhythmic events in early morning hours [33]. Gang et al of our group [30] have reported low variability of both the QT and QT_c-intervals and a significant prolongation in QT_c-interval in post-

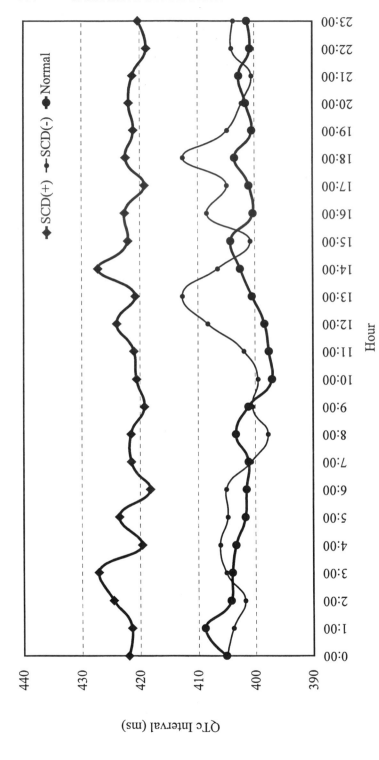

Figure 2. The mean hourly QT_C-intervals plotted against absolute time of the day for normal subjects, post-myocardial infarction patients without sudden cardiac death (SCD(-)), and post-myocardial infarction patients who developed sudden cardiac death (SCD(+)). Note a significant prolongation and decrease in variability of QT_C-interval in patients died suddenly. Reprinted from Gangy et al. Am J Cardiol 1998;81:950-956.

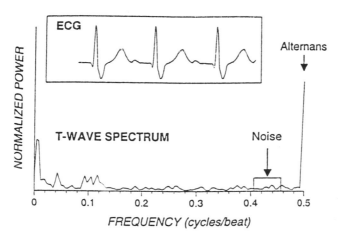

Figure 3. Spectral analysis of the T-wave reveals peak of power density at the alternans frequency (0.5 cycles/beat), in the absence of apparent changes in T-wave morphology on surface ECG. Reprinted from Rosenbaum DS et al, New Engl J Med 1994;330:235-241.

myocardial infarction patients developed sudden cardiac death during 1 year follow-up (Figure 2). The QT circadian variation is believed to result from autonomic tone modulations and from fluctuations in plasma catecholamines.

It has been advocated to use the analysis of rate-corrected QT-interval variability [29]. In contrast to beat-to-beat analysis, the method based on measurement of 5-min average templates and corresponding average RR-intervals does not depend on QT/RR "hysteresis". However, it may be speculated that these subtle and rapid changes in QT-variability in response to RR changes may be of clinical importance. Thus, signal averaging techniques while improving quality of signal, result in loss of feasibility to analyse beat-to-beat QT changes. Again, there is no agreement on which of the formulae suggested for rate correction is most appropriate [34]. In conclusion, although there is no doubt that analysis of QT-variability from long-term recording is of potential benefit, methodology of such analysis remains challengeable.

T-WAVE ALTERNANS

Over the past years a number of studies assessing electrical alternans of the heart in a variety of clinical conditions, have uniformly confirmed that T-wave alternans, defined as a consistent beat-to-beat variations in the T-wave shape during sinus rhythm is closely linked to malignant ventricular tachyarrhythmias [18-41]. Rapid changes in T-wave shape from beat to beat are the result of the multifactorial process that involves complex sequences of electrophysiological changes at the cellular level that occur under different conditions such as gene abnormalities, myocardial ischemia, and electrolyte imbalance. There is a strong evidence that increased sympathetic tone and catecholamines excess also can precipitate T-wave alternans [37]. Two hypotheses have been proposed to explain this phenomenon and to link it to arrhythmogenesis: spatial dispersion of recovery of myocardial excitability, and changes in cellular action potentials [42,43]. Both mechanisms are likely to be responsible for dispersion of myocardial refractoriness, wavefront fractionation and reentry, suggesting that detection of T-wave alternans in the surface ECG may provide a promising tool for arrhythmogenic risk assessment.

However, practical application of T-wave alternans is complicated by the technical limitations. Conventional method based on visual assessment of changes in amplitude, width and shape of the T-wave, is not useful for the detection of subtle electrical alternans that occur at microvolt level. Therefore, implementation of computerised systems has advanced prognostic role of T-wave alternans. Spectral analysis utilising Fast Fourier Transform [44] separates the useful signals responsible for alternans-type fluctuations from other signals caused by respiration and noise, and detects a spectrum power peak at the alternans frequencies in the presence of microvolt-level alternans which cannot be recognised visually (Figure 3). Complex demodulation of the T-wave based on assumption of the T-wave as a sinusoidal signal with varying amplitude and phase at the alternans frequency [45] detects microvolt changes in the T-wave morphology from non-stationary ECG signals. In analogy with previous observations, Nearing et al [45], using complex demodulation method in experimental setting, demonstrated a strong linear correlation between the magnitude of T-wave alternans and probability of ischemia-induced ventricular fibrillation. Furthermore, in recent studies, positive predictive value of T-wave alternans analysis in rest and during exercise regarding sudden cardiac death and inducibility of ventricular tachycardia was found to be 81-91% [41,46]. Despite this evidence repeatedly indicating close relationship between T-wave alternans and arrhythmogenesis in experimental and clinical settings, much remains to be learned regarding this phenomenon, optimal diagnostic techniques for its identification, and its value in arrhythmogenic risk stratification.

OTHER ASPECTS OF QUANTIFICATION OF VENTRICULAR REPO-
LARISATION

Recently T/TU-wave pattern analysis has attracted significant attention of research community. Several methods are suggested for evaluation of T-wave
shape, including principal component analysis (PCA), algebraic decomposition
of the T-wave, cluster analysis, and analysis of energy distribution in the T-
wave. PCA, allowing to evaluate the degree of complexity of the T-wave has
initially been implemented to the body surface maps in patients with LQTS by
De Ambroggi et al [47]. The sensitivity and specificity of this method regarding differentiation between normal subjects and patients with LQTS has been
reported to be 87% and 96%, respectively. Later, Priori et al [48] applied PCA
to the standard ECG with approximation of the eight vectors to their correspondence to the two axis of the T-wave loop. Compared to normal subjects,
patients with LQTS were characterised by significantly higher ratio between
the second (short axis) and the first (long axis) components of the T-wave
loop. This observation confirms the concept that analysis of the T-wave shape
may provide information different from that gained with other methods.

Three dimensional analysis of the digitised XYZ ECG applied by Badilini
et al [49] revealed an increased roundness and loss of planarity of the T-wave
loop in post-myocardial infarction patients and patients with LQTS compared
to normal subjects. Spatial characteristics of the T-wave loop correlated well
with scalar measurement of ventricular repolarisation.

Recently, QRST integral and activation recovery (AR) integral maps from
the body surface have been investigated by Lux et al [50]. QRST integrals
calculated by integrating the signal from the QRS onset to the end of the T-
wave reflect disparity of repolarisation. AR integrals measured from the time
of intrinsic deflection of the QRS defined as the time of the minimum dv/dt, to
the maximum upstroke velocity defined as the time of the maximum dv/dt,
were associated with effective refractory period and transmembrane action
potential duration obtained from endocardial electrodes.

CONCLUSION

Measurement of ventricular repolarisation from body surface ECG represent a
potential tool for arrhythmogenic risk stratification in a variety of clinical settings. Although many attempts regarding quantitative assessment of this phenomenon have been undertaken, including primitive measurement of QT-
dispersion and complex mathematical analyses, none of these technologies is
able to evaluate reliably spatial and temporal repolarisation inhomogeneity.

Multiple approaches are currently being investigated for this purpose, indicating that no one satisfactory method has yet been found. Recently suggested evaluation QT-interval variability during 24-hour Holter recording (QT/RR dynamicity) and beat-to-beat changes in the repolarisation patterns (T-wave alternans) based on automatic algorithms may provide a promising tool for better identifying patients at high risk of arrhythmic events. Analysis of the T-wave shape has recently attracted significant attention of the research community. However, further development of practical approaches to quantitative assessment of ventricular is urgently needed.

REFERENCES

1. Schwartz PJ, Wolf S. QT-interval prolongation as predictor of sudden death in patients with myocardial infarction. Circulation 1978;57:1074-1077.
2. Moss AJ, Schwartz PJ. Delayed repolarization (QT and Q-U prolongation) and malignant ventricular arrhythmias. Mod Concepts Cardiovasc Dis 1982;51:85-90.
3. Algra A, Tijssen JGP, Roelandt JRTC, et al. QTc prolongation measured by standard 12-lead electrocardiography is an independent risk factor for sudden death due to cardiac arrest. Circulation 1991;83:1888-1894.
4. Day CP, McComb JM, Campbell RWF. QT-dispersion: an indication of arrhythmia risk in patients with long QT-intervals. Br Heart J 1990;63:342-344.
5. Priori S, Napolitano C, Diehl L, Schwartz PJ. Dispersion of QT-interval. A marker of therapeutic efficacy in the idiopathic long QT syndrome. Circulation 1994;89:1681-1689.
6. Zareba W, Moss AJ, Le Cessie SI. Dispersion of ventricular repolarisation and arrhythmic death in coronary artery disease. Am J Cardiol 1994;74:550-553.
7. Fu GS, Meissner A, Simon R. Repolarization dispersion and sudden cardiac death in patients with impaired left ventricular function. Eur Heart J 1997;18:281-289.
8. Buja G, Miorelli M, Turrini P, et al. Comparison of QT-dispersion in hypertrophic cardiomyopathy between patients with and without ventricular arrhythmias and sudden death. Am J Cardiol 1993;72:973-976.
9. Gang Y, Elliot PM, Prasad K, Sharma S, et al. Computerised QT-dispersion measurement and risk stratification in patients with hypertrophic cardiomyopathy. Circulation 1997;96(Suppl): I-759
10. Lepeshkin E, Surawicz B. The measurement of the QT-interval of the electrocardiogram. Circulation 1952;6:378-388.
11. Campbell RWF, Gardiner P, Amos PA, et al. Measurement of the QT-interval. Eur Heart J 1985;6 (Suppl.D):81-83.
12. Xue Q, Reddy S. New algorithms for QT-dispersion analysis. Proceedings of the Marquette 14th ECG Analysis Seminar 1996:20-23.
13. McLaughlin NB, Campbell RWF, Murray A. Comparison of automatic QT measurement techniques in the normal 12 lead electrocardiogram. *Br Heart J* 1995;74:84-89.

14. Bortolan G, Bressan M, Cavaggion C, Fusaro S. Validation of QT-dispersion algorithms and some clinical investigation. Comp Cardiol, IEEE 1996:665-668.

15. Batchvarov V, Gang Y, Savelieva I, Camm AJ, Malik M. The first and second differential of the T-wave are less reliable than the original signal for automatic QT measurement. Ann Noninvas Electrocardiol 1998;3:S11.

16. Glancy JM, Weston PJ, Bhullar HK, et al. Reproducibility and automatic measurement of QT-dispersion. Eur Heart J 1996; 17:1035-1039.

17. Savelieva I, Gang Y, Guo X, et al. Agreement and reproducibility of automatic versus manual measurement of QT-interval and QT-dispersion. Am J Cardiol 1998;81:471-477.

18. Schwartz PJ, Priori SG. Sympathetic nervous system and cardiac arrhythmias. Chapter in DP Zipes, J Jalife (eds.): Cardiac Electrophysiology: From Cell to Bedside. Philadelphia, PA: WB Saunders, 1990:330-343.

19. Franz MR, Swerdlow CD, Liem LB, Shaefer J. Cycle length dependence of human action potential duration in vivo. Effects of single extrastimuli, sudden sustained rate acceleration and deceleration, and different steady-state frequencies. J Clin Invest 1988;82:972-979.

20. Sarma JSM, Sarma RJ, Bilitch M, et al. An exponential formula for heart rate dependence of QT-interval during exercise and cardiac pacing in humans: Reevaluation of Bazett's formula. Am J Cardiol 1984;54:103-108.

21. Todt H, Krumpl G, Krejcy K, Raberger G. Mode of QT correction for heart rate: Implications for the detection of inhomogeneous repolarization after myocardial infarction. Am Heart J 1992;124:602-609.

22. Viitasalo M, Karjalainen J. QT-intervals at heart rates from 50 to 120 beats per minute during 24-hour electrocardiographic recordings in 100 healthy men. Effects of atenolol. Circulation 1992;86:1439-1442.

23. Bexton RS, Vallin HO, Camm AJ. Diurnal variation of the QT-interval: Influence of the autonomic nervous system. Br Heart J 1986;55:253-258.

24. Merri M, Moss AJ, Benhorin J, et al. Relation between ventricular repolarization duration and cardiac cycle lenghth during 24-hour Holter recordings: Findings in normal patients and patients with long QT syndrome. Circulation 1992;85:1816-1821.

25. Kluge P, Walter T, Neugebauer A. Comparison of QT/RR relationship using two algorithms of QT-interval analysis for identification of high risk patients for life-threatening ventricular arrhythmias. Ann Noninvas Electrocardiol 1997;2:3-8.

26. Extramiana F, Huikuri HV, Neyroad N, et al. QT rate adaptation: A new index to discriminate patients with and without ventricular arrhythmias following myocardial infarction? Circulation 1997;96(Suppl.1):I-716.

27. Singh JP, Johnston J, Sleight P, et al. Left ventricular hypertrophy in hypertensive patients is associated with abnormal rate adaptation of QT-interval. J Am Coll Cardiol 1997;29:778-784.

28. Coumel P, Fayn J, Maison-Blanche P, Rubel P. Clinical relevance of assessing QT dynamicity in Holter recordings. J Electrocardiol 1994; 27 (Suppl.):62-66.

29. Molnar J, Zhang F, Weiss J, et al. Diurnal pattern of QT_c-interval: How long is prolong? Possible relation to circadian triggers of cardiovascular events. J Am Coll Cardiol 1996;27:76-83.

30. Gang Y, Guo X, Reardon M et al. Circadian variation of the QT-interval in patients with sudden cardiac death after myocardial infarction. Am J Cardiol 1998;81:950-956.

31. Browne KF, Prystowsky E, Heger LL, et al. Prolongation of the QT-interval in man during sleep. Am J Cardiol 1983;52:55-59.

32. Ahmed MW, Kadish AH, Goldberger JJ. Autonomic effects on the QT-interval. Ann Non-invas Electrocardiol 1996;1:44-53.

33. Muller JE, Tofler GH, Stone PH. Circadian variation and triggers of onset of acute cardiovascular disease. Circulation 1989;79:733-743.

34. Molnar J, Zhang F, Weiss JS, Rosenthal J. Why not Bazett's? Evaluation of 5 QT correction formulas using a new software assisted method of continuous QT measurement from 24-hour Holter recordings. PACE 1995;18:852.

35. Surawicz B. The pathogenesis and clinical significance of primary T-wave abnormalities. Chapter in RC Schlant, JW Hurst (eds.): Advances in Electrocardiography, New York, Grune and Stratton, 1972, pp.377-421

36. Schwartz PJ, Malliani A. Electrical alteration of the T-wave: Clinical and experimental evidence of its relationship with the sympathetic nervous system and with the long QT syndrome. Am Heart J 1975;89:45-50.

37. Zareba W, Moss AJ. T-wave alternans in idiopathic long QT syndrome. J Am Coll Cardiol 1994;23:1541-1546.

38. Salerno JA, Previtali M, Panciroli C, et al. Ventricular arrhythmia during acute myocardial ischemia in man. The role and significance of R-ST-T-alternans and the prevention of ischemic sudden death by medical treatment. Eur Heart J 1986;7:63-75.

39. Rozanski JJ, Kleinfeld M. Alternans of the ST-segment and T-wave. A sign of electrical instability in Prinzmetal's angina. PACE 1982;5:359-365.

40. Rosenbaum DS, Jackson LE, Smith JM, et al. Electrical alternans and vulnerability to ventricular arrhythmias. N Engl J Med 1994; 330:235-241.

41. Murda'h M, Nagayoshi H, Albrecht P, et al. T-wave alternans as a predictor of sudden death in hypertrophic cardiomyopathy. Circulation 1996;94 (Suppl.):I-669.

42. Verrier RL, Nearing BD. Electrophysiologic basis for T-wave alternans as an index of vulnerability to ventricular fibrillation. J Cardiovasc Electrophysiol 1994;5:445-461.

43. Abe S, Nagamoto Y, Fukuchi Y, et al. Relationship of alternans of monophasic action potential and conduction delay inside the ischemic border zone to serious ventricular arrythmia during acute myocardial ischemia in dogs. Am Heart J 1989;117:1223-1233.

44. Rosenbaum DS, Albrecht P, Cohen RJ. Predicting Sudden Cardiac Death from T-wave alternans of the surface electrocardiograms: Promise and Pitfalls. J Cardiovasc Electrophysiol 1996;7:1095-1111.

45. Nearing BD, Huang AH, Verrier RL. Dynamic tracking of cardiac vulnerability by complex demodulation of the T-wave. Science 1991; 252:1989.

46. Estes MNA, Zipes DP, El-Sherif N, et al. Electrical alternans during rest and exercise as a predictors of vulnerability to ventricular arrhythmias. J Am Coll Cardiol 1995; Special issue: 409A.

47. De Ambroggi L, Bertoni T, Locati E, et al. Mapping of the body surface potentials in patients with idiopathic long QT syndrome. Circulation 1986;74:1334-1345.

48. Priori SG, Mortara DW, Diehl L, et al. Quantification of ventricular repolarization: From dispersion to complexity. New Trends in Arrhythmias 1995;9 (Suppl):95-100.

49. Badilini F, Fayn J, Maison-Blanche P, et al. Quantitative aspects of ventricular repolarization: Relationship between three-dimensional T-wave loop morhology and scalar QT-dispersion. Ann Noninvas Electrocardiol 1997;2:146-157.
50. Lux RL, Green LS, MacLeod RS, Taccardi B. Assessment of spatial and temporal characteristics of ventricular repolarization. J Electrocardiol 1994;27:100-105.

16. DYNAMICITY OF T-WAVE ALTERNANS: MEASUREMENT AND ROLE IN SUDDEN CARDIAC DEATH

RICHARD L. VERRIER

INTRODUCTION

Interest in T-wave alternans, a 2:1 fluctuation in the magnitude and shape of the T-wave, has grown considerably in the past few years. Among the main factors which have contributed to this increased attention have been the demonstration, using spectral analytical methods, of the relative ubiquity of alternans in diverse pathophysiologic conditions and the clinical evidence suggesting its value in assessing risk for life-threatening cardiac arrhythmias. The goals of this brief review are: (a) to describe the most common clinical presentations of T-wave alternans; (b) to summarize the main physiologic and pharmacologic influences which affect the magnitude of T-wave alternans; (c) to discuss methodologic considerations for ambulatory monitoring of T- wave alternans.

CLINICAL PRESENTATIONS OF T-WAVE ALTERNANS

Although T-wave alternans is a distinct phenomenon, the particular pattern of oscillation varies considerably according to the underlying pathophysiologic state (1-4). For example, in patients with the long QT syndrome, the T-wave frequently alternates both above and below the isoelectric line without

177

H.-H. Osterhues et al. (eds.),
Advances in Noninvasive Electrocardiographic Monitoring Techniques, 177–189.
© 2000 *Kluwer Academic Publishers. Printed in the Netherlands.*

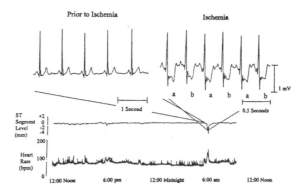

Figure 1A. Representative AECG recordings of ST-segment level, heart rate, and ECG in a patient from the Angina and Silent Ischemia Study [ASIS] using an ACS ambulatory recorder. In the absence of significant ST-segment depression, there was no visible T-wave alternans. During a bout of ischemia, as indicated by a drop in ST-segment level, there is marked T-wave alternans in the absence of R-wave alternans or other notable changes in the activation waveform. [Reprinted with permission from Futura Press from reference 10.]

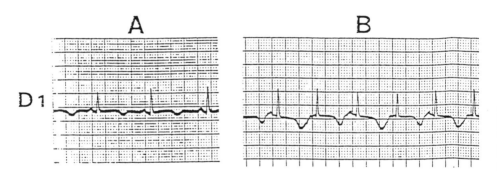

Figure 1B. Electrocardiogram of 9-year old patient affected by long QT syndrome. A: at rest. B: Alternation of T-wave appeared during unintentionally induced fear. [Reprinted with permission from the American Heart Association from reference 5.]

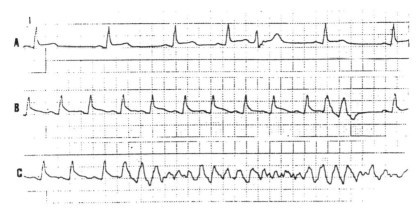

Figure 1C. Sinus tachycardia after atropine leading to ventricular fibrillation. Patient with anterior infarction, lead I. A: Sinus bradycardia [rate 55 beats/min] with ventricular ectopics. B: Record 2 min after atropine 0.6 mg, i.v. Sinus tachycardia [rate 110/min] with consecutive ventricular ectopics. C: Record 3 min after atropine showing development of ventricular fibrillation. [Reprinted with permission from Raven Press from reference 9]

concomitant ST-segment changes (5,6) (Fig. 1A). Prinzmetal's angina (7,8) and acute myocardial infarction (3,9) are characterized by transmural ischemia. In these disease conditions, the entire ST-T-segment is elevated and alternates (Fig. 1B). Ischemia is usually subendocardial in ambulatory patients with stable coronary disease. These patients experience ST-segment depression with discrete T-wave alternation primarily in the first half of the T-wave, and there are no evident R-wave changes (10) (Fig. 1C). T-wave alternans has been observed in a number of cases during ischemia induced in association with angioplasty (11) and bypass graft occlusion (12). In the general electrophysiologic patient population, including those with chronic coronary disease, dilated coronary myopathy, and heart failure, subtle, nonvisible alternation in the T-wave is evident, is detectable by spectral analytical techniques, and has predictive value in terms of arrhythmia-free survival (2,3,13,14). Collectively, these observations indicate that the physiologic basis for alternans differs considerably as a function of the pathophysiologic state, and this is a paramount consideration in evaluating electrophysiologic mechanism, as has been discussed in a number of recent reviews (1-4). The potential mechanisms involved are summarized in Table 1.

TABLE 1

ELECTROPHYSIOLOGIC BASIS FOR T-WAVE ALTERNANS AS A
FUNCTION OF DISEASE STATE

Disease or Condition	Putative Mechanism
Acute Ischemia	

1A phase 2-10 min of ischemia	Re-entrant mechanisms:
	Alternation in action potential
	  morphology
	Post-repolarization refractoriness
	Dispersion of repolarization in
	  subpopulations of cells

1B phase 10-30 min of ischemia	Non-reentrant mechanisms:
	2:1 activation block
	Derangements in impulse formation
	  (frequently triggered by abrupt changes in
	  cycle length)

Acute Myocardial Infarction	Combination of re-entrant and non-re- entrant mechanisms: Action potential morphology alternation Conduction abnormalities

EP Patient Population
  Stable, non-ischemic, but damaged
  cardiac substrate due to chronic
  coronary disease, cardiomyopathy,
  heart failure
	Re-entry around nonviable tissue
	  Dispersion of repolarization in
	  subpopulations of cells

Long QT Syndrome	Disparity in action potential duration in response to rate of stimulation and electrical restitution in subendocardial vs subepicardial fibers

Reprinted from reference 4

PHYSIOLOGIC INFLUENCES

The physiologic processes which impact on induction of T-wave alternans are numerous and highly interactive. For example, during exercise, numerous independent and countervailing influences summate to alter the pattern of the action potential, conduction properties, and ultimately the morphology of the T wave. Among the most significant factors are heart rate, autonomic changes, myocardial temperature, blood constituents, and pH. These distinct influences will be discussed first independently and then in the context of the main activities thought to influence vulnerability, namely, ischemia, exercise, behavioral stress, and pharmacologic therapy.

BASIC FACTORS

Heart Rate

In the normal heart, accelerations in sinus heart rate shorten repolarization and the QT-interval (15). Except for extremely rapid rates, when the T-wave flattens, its morphology and amplitude are relatively unaffected. However, under pathophysiologic conditions, particularly myocardial ischemia, heart rate elevations can lead to drastic changes in ST-segment and T-wave morphology. Depending on whether the ischemia is subepicardial or subendocardial, elevated heart rate can enhance the degree of ST-segment elevation or depression, respectively. Increased heart rates can predispose to increased heterogeneity of repolarization and can exacerbate myocardial ischemia by compromising diastolic coronary perfusion time, altering coronary vasomotor tone, impairing oxygen supply-demand ratio due to increased metabolic activity, and altering preload and afterload. The direct effects on cardiac electrophysiologic function include derangements in impulse formation, conduction, or both (16). During acute myocardial ischemia, sinus tachycardia induces T-wave alternans, a response largely attributed to disruption of intracellular cycling of calcium (17).

Sympathetic Nerve Stimulation

Even in the normal heart, intense sympathetic nerve stimulation can lead to detectable levels of T-wave alternans (18). The precise electrophysiologic and ionic bases for catecholamine-induced T-wave alternans are not fully elucidated. When sympathetic nerve stimulation is superimposed on myocardial ischemia, T-wave alternans magnitude is greatly enhanced. Simultaneous assessment of heart rate variability and T-wave alternans demonstrates that the maximum level of T-wave alternans during ischemia coincides with the maximum increase in reflex sympathetic nerve activity (3). This effect is attributed to disruption of intracellular cycling of calcium, as it is abolished by calcium channel blockade (17). Patients with the Long QT Syndrome, who are susceptible to recurrent episodes of syncope and torsades de pointes, exhibit marked alternation of the T-wave (5). In this syndrome, adrenergic stimulation prolongs the QT-interval due to genetically determined derangements in ion channel function (19).

Parasympathetic Nerve Stimulation

Activation of parasympathetic nerves generally exerts an effect on repolarization and T-wave morphology which is opposite to that of sympathetic nerve stimulation (20,21). Two general actions are at the root of these opposing effects: by accentuated antagonism of sympathetic nerve activity, in which acetylcholine opposes the effects of adrenergic activation by presynaptic inhibition of norepinephrine release, and by inhibiting the release of second messenger through an action at the muscarinic receptor level. Acetylcholine also alters the acetylcholine-sensitive potassium channel to affect excitable properties. It has been demonstrated in experimental animals that vagus nerve stimulation is able to suppress ischemia-induced T-wave alternans independent of a heart rate change (2). In a patient with recurring ventricular fibrillation, Navarro-Lopez and coworkers (22) demonstrated that vagus nerve activation by carotid sinus massage is capable of suppressing recurring T-wave alternans. This effect could have been due in part to baroreceptor-mediated withdrawal of sympathetic tone.

Vagus nerve stimulation moderates the magnitude of T-wave alternans during experimentally induced myocardial ischemia (2). This demonstration is consistent with the finding that vagus nerve excitation is antifibrillatory during acute myocardial ischemia (20,23). However, parasympathetic stimulation did not reduce reperfusion-induced alternans or fibrillation when heart rate was kept constant.

Temperature

Severe hypothermia results in drastic changes in repolarization and frank T-wave alternans is observed (24). The magnitude of hypothermia-induced T-wave alternans correlates with a reduction in ventricular fibrillation threshold and with increased propensity for ventricular fibrillation.

Electrolytes

Disturbances in electrolyte balance, especially those associated with disruption in plasma potassium and calcium, exert profound changes on repolarization, QT-interval, and T-wave morphology (1 S). Complex electrocardiographic changes are generated which are strongly related to the magnitude of the electrolyte imbalance. For example, hypocalcemia substantially prolongs the action potential plateau, increases the QT-interval, and can induce T-wave alternans. The role of pH has been difficult to elucidate because of the confounding influences of abnormal concentrations of potassium and ionized calcium which are usually associated with acidosis and alkalosis.

INTEGRATED RESPONSES

Ischemia and Reperfusion

Extensive experimental evidence has demonstrated that T-wave alternans tracks vulnerability to ventricular tachyarrhythmias and fibrillation during both myocardial ischemia and reperfusion. A mechanistic linkage between alternans and vulnerability is evident in the timecourse of the waxing and waning of T-wave alternans in parallel with enhanced predisposition to ventricular fibrillation. Furthermore, the magnitude of T-wave alternans during ischemia and reperfusion has been statistically related (r^2=0.98) to the probability of impending ventricular tachyarrhythmias and fibrillation (11,17,18). The underlying mechanisms are complex and appear to involve both intrinsic cardiac factors and extrinsic influences due to altered autonomic nervous system activity. The prevailing view is that ischemia-induced T-wave alternans is indicative of heterogeneity of repolarization (2,3,7,16,24,25), due to alternation in action potential duration and morphology. Action potential dispersion and electrical inhomogeneity are greatest during the early phase of repolarization, when T-wave alternans is maximum, and account for the location of the cardiac vulnerable period during the first half of the T wave (1,15,26,27). The leading current hypotheses for ischemia-induced alternans are summarized in Table 1 and reviewed in detail (2,3). The majority of evidence indicates that alternans is due to spatial and temporal unevenness of ventricular repolarization. Investigators have observed alternans in all recordings in the ischemic area, in two-thirds of recordings in the border area, and no alternans in the nonischemic area, supporting the conclusion that alternans is a "distinctive electrophysiological characteristic of the ischemic myocardium which may be causally related to arrhythmias and fibrillation." It has also been suggested that alternation in the waxing and waning of the dome portion of the epicardial action potential, which is present during simulated ischemia in isolated tissues, may be responsible for alternating T-wave patterns. Post-repolarization refractoriness, establishing the conditions for unidirectional block and reentry, has also been proposed as a basis for ischemia-induced T-wave altemans (16). The ionic bases for ischemia-induced alternans are complex but current evidence appears to indicate calcium transients and changes in potassium gradients as critical factors.

Exercise and Recovery

T-wave alternans has not been reported in normal subjects during exercise. However, there have been several reports of exercise-induced, sizeable T-wave alternans in patients with severe coronary artery disease (28,29). The phenomenon has also been reported in the post-exercise recovery phase in these patients (30).

More recently, the application of signal processing techniques has revealed that the phenomenon in its more subtle but prognostically significant forms is more prevalent during exercise than has been anticipated. Low-level T-wave alternans during moderate exercise has been reported in patients with hypertrophic cardiomyopathy (31) and the long QT syndrome (32). In patients with history of ventricular tachyarrhythmias, bicycle exercise produced a degree of T-wave alternans similar to atrial pacing (33), the index protocol (13). When data gathered both at rest and during bicycle ergometry were combined, alternans achieved a sensitivity of 89% and specificity of 75% in identifying individuals with a positive electrophysiologic test (34).

Emotions

Ambulatory monitoring of T-wave alternans, particularly during behavioral stress, may allow assessment of the impact of this important potential trigger of life-threatening arrhythmias (35). This is especially important in the context of recent evidence which indicates that the stress of anger may account for 2 to 4% of fatal and nonfatal myocardial infarctions (36). Induction of an angerlike state in canines during a confrontation paradigm produces marked shortening of QT-interval, peaking of T-waves, and T-wave alternans even in the normal heart (3). When anger was induced during coronary artery occlusion, there was an apparent synergistic effect in which alternans was more marked than the sum of the independent effects of anger and ischemia. The stress-induced changes were significantly blunted by metoprolol further implicating a primary role of beta-adrenergic receptors in sympathetically induced vulnerability and T-wave alternans. In a young patient with the long QT syndrome (5), the appearance of T-wave alternans followed an episode of fear.

Pharmacologic Interventions

The capability of several pharmacologic agents to reduce ischemia- and reperfusion-induced T-wave alternans has been tested in experimental animals. The drugs tested include beta-adrenergic receptor antagonists, calcium channel blockers, and coronary artery dilators. In parallel with their ability to suppress ventricular tachyarrhythmias, these different classes of antiarrhythmic agents have been shown to reduce the magnitude of alternans during ischemia and reperfusion (2,17) (Table 2). However, there is little or no clinical information on the use of this parameter in guiding antiarrhythmic therapy. This deficiency represents an important gap in our knowledge.

METHODOLOGIC CONSIDERATIONS FOR AMBULATORY ECG MONITORING OF T-WAVE ALTERNANS

Both technical and conceptual considerations have heretofore limited exploitation of T-wave alternans as a marker of risk for arrhythmias during ambulatory ECG monitoring. Technical difficulties have related to frequency response characteristics of the recorders and the use of appropriate analytical methods to track the dynamic changes in alternans level in daily life activities. The problem of frequency response characteristics has been reduced with contemporary AM recorders and circumvented entirely by the use of digital format (37).

Two general analytical methods have been applied to quantify T-wave alternans. The first involves Fast Fourier Transformation, which treats the alternans signal as a sine wave of constant magnitude and phase. This tech nique yields an average measure of T-wave alternans over as few as 128 beats (13,24,25). In the more recent studies, a matrix method which averages Fourier Transforms across the ST-segment and T-wave was used (13,25). This type of signal averaging generally reduces random noise in the power spectral estimate

TABLE 2
PHYSIOLOGIC AND PHARMACOLOGIC FACTORS
INFLUENCING T-WAVE ALTERNANS MAGNITUDE

Increase	Decrease
•Acute myocardial ischemia	•Beta-adrenergic blockade
•Reperfusion	•Vagus nerve stimulation
•Sympathetic nerve stimulation	•Calcium channel blockade
•Behavioral arousal, esp anger, fear	•Stellectomy
•Rapid atrial pacing	•Nitroglyccrin during myocardial
•Hypothermia	ischemia
•Exercise during ischemia	

by cancellation. The Fast Fourier Transform methods carry the general intrinsic disadvantage of requiring both a high degree of data stationarity and absence of phase changes in the alternation pattern (i.e., ABAB to BABA). Either of these conditions may occur during abrupt cycle length changes and arrhythmias. Unless adapted, these methods are not suited to tracking rapid changes in cardiac electrical stability such as those which occur during post-ischemia reperfusion and surges in autonomic activity.

The second category of techniques is comprised of dynamic methods, which are well-suited for analyzing ambulatory recordings of the transitory arrhythmogenic stimuli of daily life. The techniques include complex demodulation, estimation by subtraction, least squares estimation, auto-regressive estimation, and auto-regressive moving average estimation. The dynamic method which has been most extensively employed is complex demodulation (11,18,38). This spectral analytical technique estimates the alternans signal as a sine wave whose amplitude and phase may vary with time and thus provides a continuous measure of T-wave alternans on a beat-by-beat basis. This technique has been described in detail (38). The mathematical transformations essentially provide a measure of the changing area under successive T-waves. Complex demodulation is relatively tolerant of nonstationary data, is independent of phase-shift perturbations, and requires <30 seconds of data. These performance characteristics make it suitable for quantifying the effects of transient events, such as abrupt release-reperfusion and surges in autonomic nervous system activity, which may occur reflexly or in response to behavioral stress, and which exert a profound influence on cardiac vulnerability but may last <1 minute.

By employing digital monitoring and dynamic analytical methods, the approach to T-wave alternans analysis is optimized, particularly as the workstations for signal enhancement, noise reduction, and quantification.

A final important facet which deserves consideration is lead placement to optimize signal acquisition. With respect to myocardial ischemia, extensive studies indicate that the alternans phenomenon is regionally specific. Therefore, it is essential to monitor the precordial leads which overlie the anticipated region of myocardial ischemia. As for other conditions, in which the disease condition may be less localized, such as cardiomyopathies, heart failure, and the long QT syndrome, the optimum lead configuration remains to be determined.

CONCLUSION

T-wave alternans is a sensitive marker which is highly responsive to the main pathophysiologic influences known to be associated with life-threatening arrhythmias. Extensive experimental evidence and mounting clinical studies suggest that this parameter may be useful in stratification of risk for cardiac events. With appropriate techniques, alternans appears to be amenable to ambulatory ECG monitoring. Among the most salient considerations are the use of AM recorders with appropriate frequency response characteristics, or preferably, digital recorders, and the application of dynamic analytical methods for determining alternans level. Assessment of alternans level during daily life possesses a major conceptual advantage over resting determinations because of the potential for disclosing latent electrical instability in response to important provocative physiologic and emotional stressors (35). Ultimately, alternans detection may help to guide therapy, as there is encouraging evidence that T-wave alternans also predicts antifibrillatory efficacy of drugs and is able to disclose propensity for proarrhythmic responses.

REFERENCES

1. Surawicz B, Fisch C. Cardiac alternans: diverse mechanisms and clinical manifestations. J Am Coll Cardiol 1992;20:483-499.
2. Verrier RL, Nearing BD. Electrophysiologic basis for T-wave alternans as an index of vulnerability to ventricular fibrillation. J Cardiovasc Electrophysiol 1994;5:445-461.
3. Verrier RL, Nearing BD. T-wave alternans as a harbinger of ischemia-induced sudden cardiac death. In: Zipes DP, Jalife J, eds. Cardiac Electrophysiology: From Cell to Bedside. WB Saunders, Philadelphia, 1995.
4. Verrier RL. Physiology of electrical alternans. Cardiac Electrophysiology Review 1997;3:383-388.
5. Schwartz PJ, Zaza A, Locati E, Moss AJ. Stress and sudden death. The case of the long QT syndrome. Circulation 1991;83 [suppl 4]:I171-I190.

6. Zareba W, Moss AJ, le Cessie S, Hall WJ. T-wave altemans in idiopathic long QT syndrome. JACC 1994;23:1541-1546.

7. Salerno JA, Previtali M, Panciroli C, Klersy C, Chimienti M, Regazzi Bonora M, Marangoni E, Flacone C, Guasti L, Campana C, Rondanelli R. Ventricular arrhythmias during acute myocardial ischaemia in man. The role and significance of R-ST-T alternans and the prevention of ischaemic sudden death by medical treatment. Eur Heart J 1986;7:63-75.

8. Turitto G, El-Sherif N. Alternans ot the ST-segment in variant angina. Incidence, time course and relation to ventricular arrhythmias during ambulatory electrocardiographic recording. Chest 1988; 93:587-591.

9. Pantridge JF. Autonomic disturbance at the onset of acute myocardial infarction. In: Schwartz PJ, Brown AM, Malliani A, Zanchetti A, eds. Neural Mechanisms in Cardiac Arrhythmias, New York, Raven Press, 1978:7.

10. Verrier RL, Nearing BD, MacCallum G, Stone PH. T-wave alternans during ambulatory ischemia in patients with stable coronary disease. A.N.E. 1996; 1: 113-120.

11. Nearing BD, Oesterle SN, Verrier RL. Quantification of ischaemia-induced vulnerability by precordial T-wave alternans analysis in dog and human. Cardiovasc Res 1994;28: 1440-1449.

12. Sutton PMI, Taggart P, Lab M, Runnalls ME, O'Brien W, Treasure T. Alternans of epicardial repolarization as a localized phenomenon in man. Eur Heart J 1991;12:70-78.

13. Rosenbaum DS, Jackson LE, Smith JM, Garan H, Ruskin JN, Cohen RJ Electrical alternans and vulnerability to ventricular arrhythmia. N Engl J Med 1994;330:235-241.

14. Rosenbaum DS, Albrecht P, Cohen RJ. Predicting sudden cardiac death from T-wave alternans of the surface electrocardiogram: Promise and pitfalls. J Cardiovasc Electrophysiol 1996;7:1095-1111.

15. Surawicz B. Electrophysiologic Basis of ECG and Cardiac Arrhythmias. Williams and Wilkins, Baltimore, 1995.

16. Janse MJ, Wit AL. Electrophysiological mechanism of ventricular arrhythmias resulting from myocardial ischemia and infarction. Physiol Rev 1989;69: 1049- 1169.

17. Nearing BD, Hutter JJ, Verrier RL. Potent antifibrillatory effect of combined blockade of calcium channels and 5-HT2 receptors with nexopamil during myocardial ischemia and reperfusion in canines: comparison to diltiazem. J Cardiovasc Pharmacol 1996;27:777-787.

18. Nearing BD, Huang AH, Verrier RL. Dynamic tracking of cardiac vulnerability by complex demodulation of the T-wave. Science 1991;252:437-440.

19. Schwartz PJ, Priori SG, Locati EH, Napolitano C, Cantu F, Towbin AJ, Keating MT, Hammoude H, Brown AM, Chen LK, Colatsky TJ. Long QT syndrome patients with mutations of the SCN5A and HERG genes have differential responses to Na+ channel blockade and to increases in heart rate. Implications for gene-specific therapy. Circulation 1995;92:3381-3386.

20. Levy MN, Schwartz PJ, eds. Vagal Control of the Heart. Futura, Mt. Kisco, 1994.

21. Sicilian Gambit. Task Force of the Working Group on Arrhythmias of the European Society of Cardiology. A new approach to the classification of antiarrhythmic drugs based on their actions on arrhythmogenic mechanisms. Circulation 1991;84:1831-1851.

22. Navarro-Lopez F, Cinca J, Sanz G, Periz A, Magrina J, Betriu A. Isolated T-wave alternans. Am Heart J 1978;95:369-374.

23. De Ferrari GM, Vanoli E, Schwartz PJ. Cardiac vagal activity, myocardial ischemia, and sudden death. In Zipes DP, Jalife J, eds. Cardiac Electrophysiology: From Cell to Bedside. New York, WB Saunders, 1995, pp. 422-434.

24. Adam DR, Smith J, Akselrod S, Nyberg S, Powell AO, Cohen RJ. Fluctuations in T-wave morphology and susceptibility to ventricular fibrillation. J Electrocardiol 1984;17:209-218.

25. Smith J, Clancy EA, Valeri CR, et al. Electrical alternans and cardiac electrical instability. Circulation 1988;77:110-121.

26. Lown B, Amarasingham R, Neuman J. New method for terminating ventricular arrhythmias. JAMA 1962;182:548.

27. Bilitch M, Cosby RS, Catterky EA. Ventricular fibrillation and competitive pacing. N Engl J Med 1967;276:598-604.

28. Wayne VS, Bishop RL, Spodick DH. Exercise-induced ST-segment alternans. Chest 1983;83 :824-825.

29. Ring ME, Fenster PE. Exercise-induced ST-segment alternans. Am Heart J 1986;111: 1009-1011.

30. Belic N, Gardin JM. ECG manifestations of myocardial ischemia. Arch Intern Med 1980;140: 1162-1165.

31. Hohnloser SH, Klingenheben T, Yi-Gang L, Zabel M, Peetermans J, Cohen RJ. T-wave alternans as a predictor of recurrent ventricular tachyarrhythmias in ICD recipients: prospective comparison with conventional risk markers. J Cardiovasc Electrophysiol 1998;9:1258-1268.

32. Platt SB, Vijgen J, Albrecht P, Van Hare GF, Carlson MD, Rosenbaum DS. Occult T-wave alternans in long QT syndrome. J Cardiovasc Electrophysiol 1996;7: 144-148.

33. Hohnloser SH, Klingenheben T, Zabel M, Li Y-G, Albrecht P, Cohen RJ. T-wave alternans during exercise and atrial pacing in humans. J Cardiovasc Electrophysiol 1997;8:987-993.

34. Estes NAM, Michaud G, Zipes DP, El-Sherif N, Venditti FJ, Rosenbaum DS, Albrecht P, Wang PJ, Cohen RJ. Electrical alternans during rest and exercise as predictors of vulnerability to ventricular arrhythmias. Am J Cardiol 1997;80: 1314- 1318.

35. Verrier RL, Stone PJ. Exercise stress testing for T-wave alternans to expose latent electrical instability. J Cardiovasc Electrophysiol 1997;8:994-997.

36. Verrier RL, Mittleman MA. Life-threatening cardiovascular consequences of anger in patients with coronary heart disease. In: Deedwania PC, Tofler GH, eds. Triggers and Timing of Cardiac Events. Cardiology Clinics 1996; 14:289-307.

37. Nearing BD, Stone H, Verrier RL. Frequency response characteristics required for detection of T-wave alternans during ambulatory ECG monitoring. A.N.E. 1996;1: 103-112.

38. Nearing BD, Verrier RL. Personal computer system for tracking cardiac vulnerability by complex demodulation of the T-wave. J Appl Physiol 1993;74:2606-2612.

17. MACROVOLT T-WAVE ALTERNANS: PATHOPHYSIOLOGY AND LINK WITH REPOLARIZATION DISPERSION

MICHAEL R. FRANZ

One of the earliest electrophysiologic signs of myocardial ischemia is alternation of the T-wave in duration and magnitude from beat to beat. Although ischemia-induced T-wave alternans (TWA) has been reported previously in clinical (1) and experimental settings (2), this phenomenon recently has achieved particular significance through the demonstration that TWA is a powerful predictor of ventricular fibrillation (3,4). Because the electrocardiographic T-wave is the body surface reflection of spatial and temporal differences in ventricular repolarization, a meaningful pathophysiological approach to T-wave alternans needs to address the electrophysiological mechanisms at the myocardial tissue level, specifically abnormalities of the action potential duration (APD) response. This approach will also help to understand why ischemic T-wave alternans increases dispersion of repolarization and facilitates ventricular tachyarrhythmias (VTA). The concept that APD-alternans sets up the conditions for VTA is based on the existence of different APDs in adjacent myocardial regions which result in substantial inhomogeneities of cellular repolarization. Such differences in APD could induce regional conduction block due to regionally disparate refractoriness or result in flow of injury current, both of which may facilitate VTA (5,6).

We therefore studied in intact Langendorff-perfused rabbit hearts the relationship between APD-alternans and well-defined degrees of global ischemia. Simultaneous recordings of monophasic action potentials (MAPs) at various distinct locations of the intact heart allowed us to detect heterogeneity of electrophysiologic parameters during global ischemia. The methods used in these

H.-H. Osterhues et al. (eds.),
Advances in Noninvasive Electrocardiographic Monitoring Techniques, 191–199.
© 2000 *Kluwer Academic Publishers. Printed in the Netherlands.*

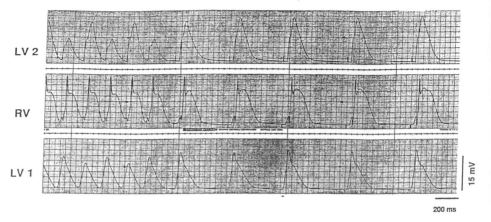

Figure 1. Original MAP tracings recorded from 3 different epicardial sites 3 minutes after onset of complete global ischemia. During pacing at 200 msec cycle length, marked alternans of MAP duration and amplitude is apparent at the 2 LV sites ("out-of-phase" alternans between the 2 LV sites in this example) but not yet at the RV site. A sudden increase in paced cycle length to 600 msec resulted in immediate dampening of alternans. From Kurz et al. (7) with permission.

studies and the obtained data have been described in detail previously (7-9). In brief, Langendorff-perfused rabbit hearts were submitted to global ischemia by lowering the perfusion by 60% to 100%. Using Franz Ag-AgCl contact electrodes (8), MAPs were recorded simultaneously from three distinct epicardial sites: the anterior portion of the right ventricle and the lateral and anterior surface of the left ventricle. The APD was determined as the interval from the steepest upstroke of the MAP to its 70% level of repolarization, taking the distance from the MAP plateau to its diastolic baseline as the total amplitude. The onset, magnitude and pattern of APD-alternans were evaluated by measurements of beat-to-beat differences in APD (7).

APD-ALTERNANS DURING ISCHEMIA: INTERDEPENDENCE OF FLOW, PRELOAD AND CYCLE LENGTH

1. Dependence of APD-alternans on the degree and duration of acute ischemia (at constant cycle length and preload).

Hearts being paced at a constant cycle length developed APD-alternans within minutes of myocardial flow reduction (Fig. 1). Alternating MAPs occurred either "in phase" or "out of phase" when compared between different recording sites. Both forms of APD-alternans sometimes transformed into one another.

Rate Dependence of Ischemic Alternans

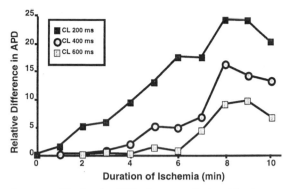

Figure 2. Development of ischemic APD-alternans during 10 minutes of total ischemia at 3 different paced cycle lengths (200, 400, and 600 msec). The values represent the relative differences in APD between two consecutive alternating MAPs, expressed as percentage of the longer one (values are means; SEM< 4% are not shown for clarity of the illustration, n=8). Abbreviations: EA: electrical alternans, APD = action potential duration, MAP = monophasic action potential, CL = cycle length, RV= right ventricle, LV1= left lateral ventricle, LV2= left anterior ventricle. Modified after Kurz et al. (7).

While ischemia was kept sustained, APD-alternans progressed gradually, resulting in an increasing difference in APD between alternating beats. In addition to this temporal dispersion, APD-alternans commenced at different time points at the different recording sites, creating increased spatial dispersion of repolarization (see below).

2. Preload dependence of APD-alternans.
The occurrence of APD-alternans under ischemic conditions was significantly impacted by ventricular preload. APD-alternans, both of duration and voltage, commenced much earlier and proceeded more rapidly in the LV as compared to the RV (8). This suggests an essential contribution of ventricular loading to the development of APD-alternans under ischemic conditions.

3. Cycle length dependence of APD-alternans (at constant perfusion and preload).
APD-alternans was highly sensitive to heart rate. At any of the 3 recording sites, while of different magnitudes between these sites, alternans developed earlier and was much more pronounced at shorter cycle lengths (Fig. 2). A higher heart rate may increase the metabolic demand of the myocardium, thereby aggravating existing ischemia. The following data suggest, however, that cycle length may in itself be a determinant of alternans, without being

ERCs During Normal Perfusion

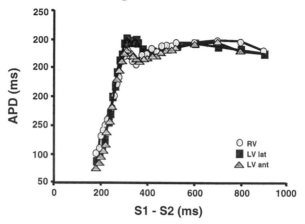

Figure 3. Example of electrical restitution curves (ERCs) recorded simultaneously at 3 different epicardial sites during normal perfusion at a basic cycle length of 500 msec. All 3 ERCs are nearly superimposable and exhibit a steep initial recovery phase with complete APD recovery at an S1 -S2-interval of approximately 300 msec, maintaining at a stable level for S1-S2-intervals up to 900 msec. Abbreviations: APD = action potential duration, ERC = electrical restitution curve, BCL = basic cycle length, RV = right ventricle, LV lat = left lateral ventricle, LV ant = left anterior ventricle, S 1-S2 = test cycle length.

ERC Changes with Global Ischemia

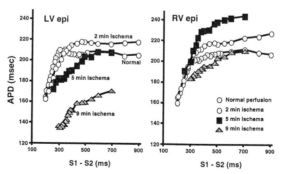

Figure 4. ERCs recorded simultaneously at 3 different epicardial sites at 5 minutes of ischemia. The time courses of the ERCs differed significantly from one another. The disparity between the ischemic ERCs increased toward shorter S1-S2-intervals and was most pronounced between the RV and either LV recording sites. APD = action potential duration, ERC = electrical restitution curve, S 1-S2 = test cycle length, RV = right ventricle, LV lat = left lateral ventricle, LV ant = left anterior ventricle.

secondary to rate-induced increase of ischemia. At long cycle lengths (600 msec), APD-alternans could not be detected within 6 minutes of complete ischemia (100% flow reduction). When the paced CL was shortened abruptly (e.g. to 200 msec), APD-alternans developed within the first 2 beats following the rate increase. Conversely, when during persistent ischemia, the cycle length was lengthened again, APD-alternans was immediately abolished (Fig. 1). This immediate onset and offset of APD-alternans could be consistently reproduced. Thus, a longer CL (i.e. 600 msec) not only prevented spontaneous APD-alternans but also abolished APD-alternans induced by a shorter CL (200, 400 msec) (Fig. 1) (7). It is highly unlikely that the metabolic situation deteriorates significantly within a single beat after the rate increase and recovers equally fast after the rate decrease. Indeed, these observations clearly underline the importance of a shorter cycle length for APD-alternans development and suggest that cycle length itself is a contributor to ischemic alternans independent of the degree of ischemia.

EFFECTS OF ISCHEMIA ON ELECTRICAL RESTITUTION

To further elucidate the role of cycle length in ischemic APD-alternans development, we determined the inter-beat dependence of APD by determining the electrical restitution curve (ERC). The ERC describes the APD dependence over a range of single cycle length changes, from the most premature beat to the one following a long pause (10). The ERC therefore is a useful means to describe the immediate effects of cycle length changes on the subsequent APD. The ERC not only relates to changes in cycle length but more specifically to changes in the electrical diastolic interval (10), which is important to consider for understanding the beat-to-beat changes in APD during APD-alternans.

ERCs recorded simultaneously at 3 different epicardial sites at a basic CL of 500 msec are shown in Figure 3. The ERCs showed a steep initial recovery phase which reached a plateau at test cycle lengths of approximately 300 msec. During normal perfusion, ERCs at the 3 different recording sites were extremely uniform (nearly superimposable) (Fig. 3). Global ischemia induced significant changes in ERCs: ischemia produced a flattening of the initial ERC slope and this flattening progressed with continuing ischemia (Fig. 4). Furthermore, with progressing ischemia, ERCs were shifted rightward (toward longer cycle lengths) and downward (toward shorter APD). Thus, the shortening response of APD to ischemia increased and also occurred at longer cycle lengths. Also, during ischemia, the time courses of the ERCs at the 3 recording sites differed significantly from each other. The disparity of the ischemic ERCs increased progressively toward shorter coupling intervals (9).

ERC and Electrical Alternans

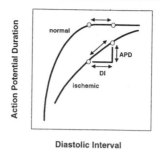

Figure 5. Schematic illustration to explain the mechanism of ischemia-related EA based on the ERC. See text for details. Abbreviations: ERC = electrical restitution curve, APD = action potential duration, CL = cycle length.

LINK BETWEEN IMPAIRED ELECTRICAL RESTITUTION AND APD-ALTERNANS (FIG. 5)

The occurrence of APD-alternans during myocardial ischemia coincided with the flattening of the time course of the ERC (7,9). The decreased slope of the initial phase of the ERC resulted in incomplete recovery of APD which attained the steady state value just shortly before the basic CL and fell short significantly of the APD reached at the same CL under non-ischemic conditions.Thus, more time is needed for APD to reach its steady state value, and therefore APD recovery becomes more dependent on the duration of the preceding diastolic interval. Since ER is a function of the electrical diastolic interval (11), the ischemia-induced delay in ER can explain the development of persistent APD-alternans. While the rapid time course of the normal ERC ensures complete APD recovery from one beat to the next even at fast heart rates, incomplete recovery of APD during ischemia sets the stage for alternating longer and shorter action potentials. Shortening of APD at a given CL entails reciprocal lengthening of the subsequent diastolic interval which in turn lengthens the subsequent APD and shortens the following diastolic interval. The slow recovery time course during ischemia, with an ERC slope of near unity, perpetuates the alternans of APD and diastolic interval as the APD moves up and down the slope of the ERC without ever reaching full recovery (Fig. 5).

Alternans During Coronary Occlusion

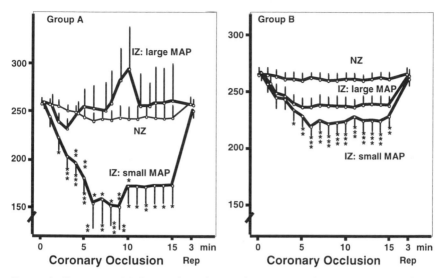

Figure 6. Alternans in MAP recordings from ischemic (IZ) and normal (NZ) zone during 15 minutes selective coronary artery occlusion and reperfusion (Rep) in dogs. Group A had a high incidence of arrhythmias while group B did not. From Abe et al. (1) with permission.

CLINICAL IMPORTANCE OF APD-ALTERNANS DURING ISCHEMIA

Electrical alternans in the setting of ischemia was first demonstrated by Hellerstein and Liebow (12) and confirmed by others (13). These authors documented a high incidence of S-T-segment and T-wave alternans of the electrocardiogram occurring early upon coronary occlusion. Investigations of the intracellular electrical activity have demonstrated alternans of both duration and amplitude of ischemic action potentials which accompany S-T-segment and T-wave alternans (5,14,15). The clinical and electrophysiologic significance of APD-alternans lies in its close relationship to ischemia-induced arrhythmias. Several groups have shown that VTA during acute myocardial ischemia is preceded immediately by a period of APD-alternans, suggesting a causal relationship between the two (1,5,14). Abe and coworkers (1) could show in canine hearts that the occurrence of arrhythmias during single coronary occlusion was much more common when there was a greater magnitude of alternans and regional dispersion of repolarization (Fig.6).

While global ischemia as in our experiments is not a common manifestation of coronary artery disease, our experiments may resemble clinical conditions such as low output heart failure, dilative cardiomyopathy or diffuse coronary artery disease. In these clinical conditions "global" reduction in perfusion may result in inhomogeneous reduction of tissue flow. This may be due to differences in wall thickness, transmural perfusion pressure, ventricular strain, and ventricular geometry. We found APD-alternans to be a sensitive parameter for ischemia, depending on both duration and severity of underperfusion and preload. The effect of cycle length on APD-alternans seems to be functionally separate from the effect of cycle length on the ischemic burden. A considerable delay in electrical restitution has been found during ischemia and may indicate a pivotal role for a disturbed mechanism controlling the normal relationship between APD and cycle length in the generation of ischemic APD-alternans. Whereas regional ischemia necessarily leads to electrophysiologic heterogeneity of the whole heart, the effects of global flow reduction - as in our experiments - were expected to develop rather uniformly. However, our experiments in intact mammalian hearts revealed a significant dispersion of electrophysiologic properties during global ischemia.

REFERENCES

1. Abe S, Nagamoto Y, Fukuchi Y et al.: Relationship of alternans of monophasic action potential and conduction delay inside the ischaemic border zone to serious ventricular arrhythmia during acute myocardial ischaemia in dogs. Am Heart J 1989; 117: 1223-1233.
2. Dilly SG, Lab MJ: Electrophysiological alternans and restitution during acute regional ischaemia in myocardium of anesthetized pig. J Physiol (Lond) 1988; 402:315-333.
3. Nearing BD, Huang AH, Verrier RL: Dynamic tracking of cardiac vulnerability by complex demodulation of the T-wave. Science 1991; 252:437-440.
4. Verrier RL, Nearing BD: Electrophysiologic basis for T-wave alternans as an index of vulnerability to ventricular fibrillation. J Cardiovasc Electrophysiol 1994; 5:445-461.
5. Janse MJ, van Capelle FJL, Morsink H el al.: Flow of "injury" current and patterns of excitation during early ventricular arrhythmias in acute regional myocardial ischemia in isolated porcine and canine hearts. Evidence for two different arrhythmogenic mechanisms. Circ Res 1980; 47: 151-165.
6. Janse MJ, Cinca J, Morena H, et al.: The "border zone" in myocardial ischemia. An electrophysiological, metabolic, and histochemical correlation in the pig heart. Circ Res 1979; 44:576-588.
7. Kurz RW, Mohabir R, Ren X-L, Franz MR: Ischaemia induced alternans of action potential duration in the intact heart: dependence on coronary flow, preload and cycle length. Eur Heart J 1993; 14:1410-1420.

8. Kurz RW, Ren X-L, Franz MR: Increased dispersion of ventricular repolarization and ventricular tachyarrhythmias in the globally ischaemic rabbit heart. Eur Heart J 1993; 14: 1561-1571.

9. Kurz RW, Ren X-L, Franz MR: Dispersion and delay of electrical restitution in the globally ischaemic heart. Eur Heart J 1994; 15: 547-554.

10. Bass BG: Restitution of the action potential in cat papillary muscle. Am J Physiol 1975; 228: 1717-1724.

11. Franz MR, Schaefer J, Schottler M et al.: Electrical and mechanical restitution of the human heart at different rates of stimulation. Circ Res 1983; 53:815-822.

12. Hellerstein HK, Liebow IM: Electrical alternation in experimental coronary artery occlusion. Am J Physiol 1950;160:366-374.

13. Hoffman BF, Suckling, EE: Effect of heart rate on cardiac membrane potentials and the unipolarelectrogram. Am J Physiol 1954; 179:123-130.

14. Lab MJ, Woollard KV: Monophasic action potentials, electrocardiograms and mechanical performance in normal and ischaemic epicardial segments of the pig ventricle in situ. Cardiovasc Res 1978; 12:555-565.

15. Hashimoto H, Suzuki K, Miyake S, Nakashima M: Effects of calcium antagonists on the electrical alternation of the ST-segment and on associated mechanical alternans during acute coronary occlusion in dogs. Circulation 1983; 68:667-672.

18. T-WAVE ALTERNANS AND VARIABILITY: PROGNOSTIC, DIAGNOSTIC, AND THERAPEUTIC IMPLICATIONS

WOJCIECH ZAREBA

PATHOGENESIS OF T-WAVE ALTERNANS AND T-WAVE VARIABILITY

Recent advances in experimental and clinical electrophysiology have provided substantial evidence for a crucial role of repolarization abnormalities in arrhythmogenic conditions precipitating ventricular tachyarrhythmias. Early afterdepolarizations, beat-to-beat variability in diastolic time, and transmural heterogeneity of repolarization contribute to an arrhythmogenic cascade of ventricular tachyarrhythmias (1). Early afterdepolarizatons may arise from Purkinje fibers, but may also originate from M cells, which are particularly prone to exhibit selective prolongation and abnormalities of refractory periods. Transmural heterogeneity of repolarization, with action potentials in M cells longer than in endo- and epicardial cells, was demonstrated to facilitate the mechanism of reentry (1-3). The same transmural heterogeneity of action potential duration and morphology was recently shown to underlie T-wave alternans, an ECG phenomenon consisting of 2:1 changes in ST-T-complex duration and morphology (4,5). T-wave alternans has been attributed to beat-to-beat changes in the kinetics of repolarizing ionic currents leading to varying degree of transmural heterogeneity (6). As shown in schematic Figure 1 (based on the recent NASPE presentation by Shimizu and Antzelevitch [4]),

H.-H. Osterhues et al. (eds.),
Advances in Noninvasive Electrocardiographic Monitoring Techniques, 201–208.
© 2000 *Kluwer Academic Publishers. Printed in the Netherlands.*

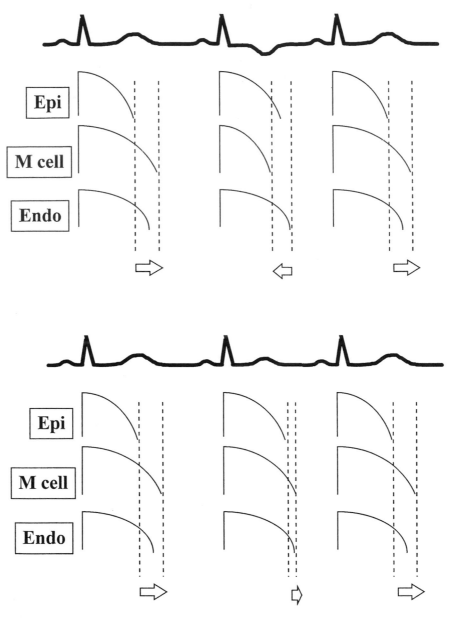

Figure 1. Schematic representation of repolarization phenomena underlying biphasic T-wave alternans (upper panel) and T-wave variability ECG phenomena flower panel. For more explanation see text.

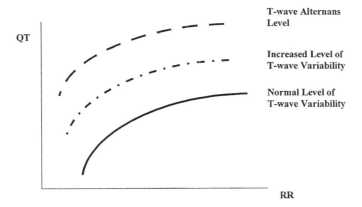

Figure 2. The dependence of T-wave alternans and T-wave variability on relationship between QT and RR-interval.

biphasic T-wave alternans is caused by the alternating "direction" of transmural heterogeneity. Odd alternating beats (negative T-waves) are caused by M cells having a shorter action potential duration than neighboring endo- and epicardial layers. The opposite is found in normal beats (with upright positive T-waves), i.e. M cells have a longer action potential duration than endo- and epicardial cells. The same concept can be applied to beat-to-beat T-wave variability which does not have a 2:1 pattern. As per analogiam shown in lower panel of Figure 1, T-wave variability is caused by beat-to-beat changes in the magnitude of transmural heterogeneity of action potential duration and morphology. Beat-to-beat variability in T-wave morphology, which can be observed in healthy subjects (7), is partially related to the regulatory function of the autonomic nervous system, but more likely it is caused by physiologic beat-to-beat variations in the kinetics of ionic channels, leading to physiologic transmural heterogeneity of repolarization. The relationship between repolarization duration (more precisely ion channel kinetics) and cycle length (QT and RR-intervals in ECG) determines the likelihood of T-wave alternans and T-wave variability occurrence (Figure 2). With a moderate elevation of the QT-RR relationship curve, one may expect to detect increased levels of T-wave variability. Further elevation of this curve may lead to 2:1 T-wave variability, known as T-wave alternans. This concept promotes the hypothesis that T-wave variability and T wave alternans are continuous manifestations of the same electrophysiologic phenomena resulting from varying degrees of transmural heterogeneity of repolarization.

T-WAVE ALTERNANS - PROGNOSTIC AND DIAGNOSTIC APPLICATIONS

Microvolt level T-wave alternans and T-wave variability can be detected automatically in digital surface ECGs. Neither the diagnostic nor prognostic significance of these ECG phenomena is yet established, however, growing evidence is being accumulated for a significant prognostic value of T-wave alternans for predicting arrhythmic events in various patient populations. In patients undergoing invasive electrophysiological testing, Rosenbaum et al. (8) found that pacing-induced microvolt T-wave alternans was able to predict arrhythmic events with a prognostic accuracy similar to that of inducible ventricular tachycardia. Recently, detection of microvolt T-wave alternans has been enabled during exercise testing (9,10). Preliminary data from the exercise-induced T-wave alternans protocols in 27 patients undergoing electrophysiological testing (10) and in 30 ventricular fibrillation survivors (11) indicate further that T-wave alternans is a promising stratifier of arrhythmic risk. Similarly, T-wave alternans evaluated in 160 patients with hypertrophic cardiomoypathy was found to improve risk stratification based on traditional clinical variables (12). Microvolt T-wave alternans can be also detected in long QT syndrome patients (6), however, its long-term prognostic value for predicting cardiac events in these patients is as yet unknown. In long QT syndrome patients, T-wave alternans detection may also have diagnostic value by improving identification of phenotypic characteristics of affected individuals (13). This diagnostic benefit of T-wave alternans detection might be of particular clinical value in identifying affected individuals among long QT syndrome family members without apparent or with borderline clinical presentation of the disease. The same concept can be applied to screening family members of patients with familial hypertrophic cardiomyopathy, arrhythmogenic right ventricular displasia, or Brugada syndrome.

T-WAVE VARIABILITY - PROGNOSTIC AND DIAGNOSTIC POTENTIAL

There is a substantial evidence that repolarization duration shows a circadian pattern with the QT-interval being longer during night than day hours (14,15,16). QTc-interval lengthening observed in 24-hour Holter monitoring was found by Marti et al. (17) to be associated with malignant ventricular tachyarrhythmias in postinfarction patients. Recently Atiga et al. (18) reported that QT-variability, measured by the QT-variability index adjusted for heart rate variability, in 95 patients undergoing electrophysiological testing, was more effective in predicting arrhythmic events than T-wave alternans, QT-dispersion, and invasive ventricular tachycardia inducibility protocol. However, obtaining reliable and reproducible measures of the QT-interval in dynamic Holter recordings creates a major problem in the practical application of this methodology. Simultaneously, experimental data (3) indicate that T-wave morphology (related to abnormalities of various ionic currents active throughout the entire repolarization process) seem to reflect transmural heterogeneity of repolarization better than just QT-interval duration. For the above methodological and electrophysiological reasons there is a need for automatic quantification of T-wave morphology without determination of accurate T-wave endpoints.

Recently, we applied the wavelet transformation technique to determine beat-to-beat variability in repolarization morphology in the predetermined ECG-segment defined by the fixed points: beginning point located 100 ms after R peak and terminal point of the evaluated segment located 220 ms prior to R peak of next beat (7). The wavelet transformation technique is a novel signal processing method allowing for decomposition of ECG signal into a set of coefficients describing its time-frequency components (19). The wavelet transformation method is able to quantify beat-to-beat variability in repolarization morphology with optimal time-frequency resolution, i.e., enhancing the varying components of T-wave. This method can be used to evaluate beat-to-beat T-wave variability in a standard 12-lead ECG, as well as in exercise testing and Holter ECGs. Our preliminary investigations (7) of wavelet-detected T-wave variability in long QT syndrome patients indicate that this method can enhance phenotypic description of ECG characteristics in this disease. Prognostic significance of wavelet-detected T-wave variability is yet unknown.

THERAPEUTIC IMPLICATIONS OF T-WAVE ALTERNANS AND T-WAVE VARIABILITY DETECTION

If the potential prognostic significance of T-wave alternans and T-wave variability is confirmed in subsequent large clinical studies it is likely that computer detection of these ECG phenomena may play a crucial role in identification of patients who are likely to benefit from antiarrhythmic pharmacological and device therapy. It is also possible that these noninvasive tests will provide an opportunity to conduct an effective guided antiarrhythmic therapy and will allow for early identification of patients developing arrhythmogenic reactions. As an anecdotal case report (Figure 3), in one of our long QT syndrome patients with the SCN5A sodium channel gene mutation,

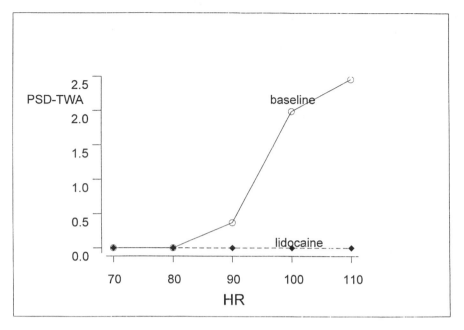

Figure 3. T wave alternans levels measured using power spectral density method (as in reference 8) in a long QT syndrome patient with the SCN5A sodium channel gene mutation during incremental atrial pacing at baseline (solid line) and after administration of lidocaine.

we were able to document that administration of lidocaine abolishes pacing-induced T-wave alternans. This effect of lidocaine can be attributed to effective shifting of QT-RR relationship (shown in Figure 2) toward a lower level of repolarization variability and heterogeneity. The above suggestions of possible therapeutic application of T-wave alternans and T-wave variability testing do not yet have support in clinical testing.

SUMMARY

Both the T-wave alternans and the T-wave variability ECG phenomena provide noninvasive insight into the magnitude of transmural (spatial) and temporal heterogeneity of repolarization. Novel computerized techniques are being developed and tested to determine the prognostic and diagnostic usefulness of these microvolt level beat-to-beat changes in repolarization morphology. There is preliminary evidence for a prognostic usefulness of T-wave alternans testing in various groups of patients at risk for ventricular tachyarrhythmias, however, further studies are needed to determine various methodological aspects and clinical benefits of this new technique. The T-wave variability field is in its infancy and requires substantial explorations. Examples of diagnostic applications of the T-wave alternans and T-wave variability testing can currently be found in identifying affected individuals among asymptomatic or borderline symptomatic family members of patients with long QT syndrome, hypertrophic cardiomyopathy, Brugada syndrome and other familial arrhythmogenic diseases. Therapeutic applications can be foreseen for identifying patients who may benefit from antiarrhythmic (pharmacological or defibrillator therapy) or those who may develop drug-related proarrhythmia.

REFERENCES

1. El-Sherif N, Caref EB, Yin H, Restivo M. The electrophysiological mechanism of ventricular arrhythmias in the long QT syndrome: tridimensional mapping of activation and recovery patterns. Circ Res 1996;79:474-92.
2. Saitoh, H, Bailey JC, Surawicz B. Alternans of action potential duration after abrupt shortening of cycle length: differences between dog purkinje and ventricular muscle fibers. Cir Res 1988;62:1027-40.
3. Shimizu W, Antzelevitch C. Sodium channel block with mexiletine in effective in reducing dispersion of repolarization and preventing torsade de pointes in LQT2 as well as LQT3 models of the long QT syndrome. Circulation 1997;96:2038-47.
4. Shimizu W, Antzelevitch C. Cellular basis for T-wave alternans in the long QT syndrome. PACE 1998; 21 (part II):856.
5. Chinushi M, Restivo M, Caref E, Nollo G, El-Sherif N. The electrophysiological basis of arrhythmogenecity of QT/T-alternans in the long QT syndrome. PACE 1998; 21 (part II):854.
6. Zareba W, Badilini F, Moss AJ: Automatic detection of heterogenous repolarization. J Electrocardiol 1994;27:65-71
7. Couderc JP, Zareba W, Moss AJ: Wavelet analysis of short-term beat-to-beat variability of repolarization in LQTS patients with SCN5A sodium channel mutation. J Am Coll Cardiol 1998;31:192A.
8. Rosenbaum DS, Jackson LE, Smith JM, Ruskin JN, Cohen RJ: Electrical alternans and vulnerability to ventricular arrhythmias. N Engl J Med 330:235,1994.
9. Hohnloser SH, Klingenheben T, Zabel M, Li YG, Albrecht P, Cohen RJ. T-wave alternans during exercise and atrial pacing in humans. J Cardiovasc Electrophysiol 1997;8:994-7.
10. Estes NA, Michaud G, Zipes DP, El-Sherif N, Venditti FJ, Rosenbaum DS, Albrecht P, Wang PJ, Cohen RJ. Electrical alternans during rest and exercise as predictor of vulnerability to ventricular arrhythmias. Am J. Cardiol 1997;80:1314-18.
11. Sticherling C, Klingenheben T, Zabel M, Haack J, Hochnloser SH. Comparison of invasive versus non-invasive risk-stratification in patients surviving primary ventricular fibrillation. PACE 1998; 21 (part II):928.

12. Murda'h MA, Yi G, Elliott P, McKenna WJ. New noninvasive electrocardiographic markers of sudden death risk in hypertrophic cardiomyopathy. G Ital Cardiol, 1998; 28 (suppl):54-56.

13. Zareba W, Burattini L, Corrielus S, Rashba EJ, Moss AJ: T-wave alternans and QT-dispersion in long QT syndrome patients with SCN5A sodium channel gene mutation. Circulation 1996:94:I-450.

14. Rasmussen V, Jensen G, Hansen JF. QT-interval analysis in 24 hour ambulatory ECG recordings from 60 healthy adult subjects. J Electrocardiol 1991;24:91-95.

15. Merri M, Alberi M, Moss AJ. Dynamic analysis of ventricular repolarization duration from 24-hour Holter recordings. IEEE Trans Biomed Eng 1993;40:1219-25.

16. Bruggemann T, Eisenreich S, Behrens S, Ehlwers C, Muller D, Anfresen D. Continuous QT-interval measurements from 24-hour electrocardiography and risk after myocardial infarction. ANE 1997;2:264-73.

17. Homs E, Marti V, Laguna P, Bayes de Luna A. Automatic QTc measurements in Holter ECG in postmyocardial infarction patients with and without life-threatening ventricular arrhythmias: mean value and circadian variation. J Amb Mionitor 1994;7:101-102.

18. Atiga WA, Calkins H, Lawrence JH, Tomaselli GF, Berger RD. A novel index of repolarization lability predicts sudden death. PACE 1997; 20 (part II):1234

19. Couderc JP, Zareba W: Wavelet contribution to noninvasive electrocardiology. ANE 1998;3:54-62.

CHAPTER THREE: FOCUS ON:

SECTION ONE: ISCHEMIC HEART DISEASE

19. NON-INVASIVE QUANTIFICATION / LOCALIZATION OF MYOCARDIAL ISCHEMIA

HIROSHI HONMA AND HIROKAZU HAYAKAWA

One of the major roles of non-invasive tests in patients with myocardial infarction (MI) is to assess the degree of myocardial damage which determines the future cardiac event rate and clinical outcome. However, it is somewhat difficult to choose clinically appropriate modalities in quantifying and localizing myocardial ischemia because of the rapid rate of recent progress of cardiac imaging methods.

TWELVE–LEAD ELECTROCARDIOGRAM

The 12-lead ECG has been used as a mean to estimate the location and infarct size. The value of deep Q and ST–segment elevation for diagnosing of acute MI is relatively high, therefore the 12-lead ECG still remains the essential method for screening patients . But its sensitivity or specificity for accurate localization of MI is not so high.

TRANSTHORACIC ECHOCARDIOGRAPHY

Transthoracic echocardiography (TTE) is one of the most advanced techniques among the non-invasive imaging modalities. Because of high quality imaging of recent equipments , sensitivity and specificity for localization of MI based on left ventricular segmental analysis are considerably good.

H.-H. Osterhues et al. (eds.),
Advances in Noninvasive Electrocardiographic Monitoring Techniques, 211–215.
© 2000 *Kluwer Academic Publishers. Printed in the Netherlands.*

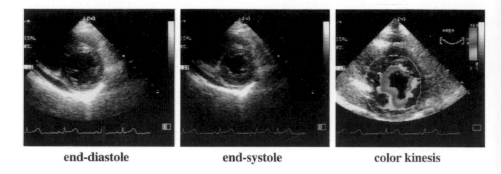

end-diastole   end-systole   color kinesis

Figure 1. 2-dimensional echocardiography with color kinesis. Instead of visual analysis of wall motion abnormality, color kinesis image clearly shows anteroseptal asynergy.

However, this technique is insensitive to small areas of infarction and to subendocardial infarction, and is difficult to determine the time course of infarction. Color kinesis based on acoustic quantification technology has been recently developed (1). By this method, the timing and magnitude of endocardial motion in real time can be clearly displayed (Fig. 1). This modality may greatly help the evaluation of myocardial ischemia.

ELECTRON BEAM COMPUTED TOMOGRAPHY

Electron beam computed tomography(EBCT) is a relatively new diagnostic modality and its images have excellent spatial and temporal resolution. Three types of scanning are available, volume mode, flow mode, and cine mode. Sensitivity and specificity for localization of MI are around 90%, 92% respectively. EBCT is non-invasive; however, there are some problems including logistic, intravenous contrast injection and radiation exposure.

MAGNETIC RESONANCE IMAGING

Magnetic Resonance Imaging (MRI) can provide soft tissue definition without exposure from radiation. Sensitivity and specificity for localization of MI by wall thinning analysis in spin-echo pulse sequence MRI imaging, compared with technetium pyrophosphate imaging, were reported as 67%, 88% respectively in recent studies. However, specificity using increased myocardial signal analysis was low. Recently, gradient recalled echo plannar magnetic resonance imaging (GRE-EPI) (2) has been developed and with the use of magnetic resonance contrast agents, the diagnostic value of localization of MI may be increasing.

One of the advantages of MRI on the detection and characterization of ischemically damaged myocardium is the identification of replacement of myocardium by fibrous scar. This suggests the possibility of differentiation between old and new MI. On the other hand, MRI sometimes cannot apply to patients with pacemakers, and so on.

ECG-GATED SINGLE PHOTON EMISSION COMPUTED TOMOGRAPHY

^{99m} Tc- pyrophosphate

Very high sensitivity and specificity of localization of MI by ^{99m} Tc-pyrophosphate imaging were reported . ^{99m} Tc- pyrophosphate is dependent on new necrosis, the presence of local coronary flow, and cellular membrane disruption. The disadvantage of this tracer is that it is dependent on the time interval between cellular damage and administration of the tracer.

Thallium-201 and ^{99m} Tc- sestamibi

Thallium-201 and ^{99m} Tc- sestamibi single photon emission tomography (SPECT) imaging are widely used at present in assessing myocardial perfusion. Good agreement and high correlation between thallium-201 imaging and postmortem location or size of MI were reported. In ^{99m} Tc-sestamibi imaging study, the final hypoperfused region correlated well with the regional wall motion score . However, perfusion defects images obtained from both tracers cannnot distinguish between acute ischemia, acute infarction, or old infarction.

^{123} I – methyl iodophenyl pentadecanoic acid

^{123} I – methyl iodophenyl pentadecanoic acid (BMIPP) is a suitable tracer for myocardial imaging , because fatty acids are a main source of energy for normal myocardium and fatty acids metabolism is altered in damaged myocardium. Usually BMIPP is injected with thallium-201 or MIBI and myocardial perfusion and metabolic abnormalities can be evaluated simultaneously. In this imaging, mismatched uptake (reduced BMIPP uptake and better thallium-201 uptake) probably indicates ischemia.

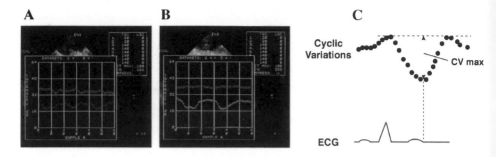

Figure 2. Cyclic variations of integrated backscatter during dobutamine stress echocardiography in a patient with acute myocardial infarction. (A) Integrated backscatter curve of anterior septal wall (upper) and of inferior wall (below) at control (B) at peak dobutamine stress (C) scheme of cyclic variation. CV max; maximum amplitude of cyclic variation. DOB; dobutamine

ASSESSMENT OF INTRAMYOCARDIAL CONTRACTILE PERFORMANCE BY INTEGRATED BACKSCATTER

Integrated backscatter, is a recently proposed technique (3), expected to be a parameter of tissue characterization. Integrated backscatter signals show cyclic variation in normal myocardium which reflects intramyocardial contractile function, while signals altered in ischemically damaged myocardium. Figure 2 shows cyclic variations of integrated backscatter in a patient with acute anteroseptal MI. Blunted or flat cyclic variation in anteroseptal region suggests that most of this area is necrotic because cyclic variation was not augumented by dobutamine stress.

We studied dobutamine (DOB) stress echocardiography and thallium-201 and ^{99m}Tc-BMIPP dual SPECT in 12 patients with AMI. Maximum amplitude (dB) of cyclic variations at control and peak of DOB and uptake of each tracer in SPECT images were compared (Table 1). Of all 24 segments, 9 segments showed mismatched uptake (reduced BMIPP uptake and better thallium uptake), and 5 showed defect in both images. In 5 defect segments, maximum amplitudes of cyclic variations were reduced and were not augumented by DOB stress (2.4 ± 0.8 vs. 2.5 ± 0.5), indicating most of those segments might be necrotic. In 9 mismatched segments, maximum amplitudes were blunted by DOB stress. Those segments might be ischemic regions.

Table 1

Assessment of Intramyocardial Contractile Function and Viability by Integrated Backscatter in Patients with AMI ; Comparison with ²⁰¹TI–¹²³I-BMIPP dual SPECT

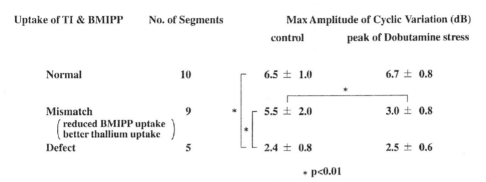

Uptake of TI & BMIPP	No. of Segments	Max Amplitude of Cyclic Variation (dB)	
		control	peak of Dobutamine stress
Normal	10	6.5 ± 1.0	6.7 ± 0.8
Mismatch (reduced BMIPP uptake / better thallium uptake)	9	5.5 ± 2.0	3.0 ± 0.8
Defect	5	2.4 ± 0.8	2.5 ± 0.6

* p<0.01

Table 1. Assessment of intramyocardial contractile function and viability by integrated backscatter in patients with acute myocardial infarction ; comparison with ²⁰¹Tl — ¹²³I-BMIPP dual SPECT

SUMMARY

Several non-invasive testings, including TTE (with or without stress), SPECT, MRI, PET, and other new techniques, have been established in evaluating myocardial necrosis and viability. Because of the high cost and little applicability, the choice of modalities should be dependent on each hospital.

REFERENCES

1. Lang RM, Vignon P, Weinert L, et al. Echocardiographic Quantification of Regional Left Ventricular Wall Motion with Color Kinesis Circulation. 93: 1877-1885, 1996.
2. Saeed M, Wendland MF, Yu KK, et al. Identification of Myocardial Reperfusion With Echo Planar Magnetic Resonance Imaging: Discrimination Between Occlusive and Reperfused Infarctions. Circulation. 90: 1492-1501, 1994.
3. Takiuchi S, Ito H. Iwakura K, et al. Ultrasonic Tissue Characterization Predicts Myocardial Viability in Early Stage of Reperfused Acute Myocardial Infarction. Circulation. 97: 356-362, 1998.

20. AMBULATORY ECG, MYOCARDIAL ISCHEMIA AND RISK STRATIFICATION

STEEN JUUL-MÖLLER AND NATASCIA PAVLIDIS

OVERVIEW

The ECG method is an accepted method for diagnosing myocardial ischemia. However, the diagnostic accuracy is highly dependent of the pre-test prevalence of coronary artery disease (CAD) in the individual patient.

The accepted criteria for this diagnosis is reversible ST-segment depression, horizontal or downsloping, of at least 0.1 millivolt, and in the case of Ambulatory ECG, for at least 1 minute (Cohn et al, Circulation 1987; 75(Suppl II): 11-51).

In order to safely diagnose reversible myocardial ischemia, a pre-test likelihood of 75% of the disease is needed to reach > 90% accuracy of CAD (Pietrowicz et al, Annals of Noninvasive Electrocardiology 1998; 3:131-138).

The ECG method generally used has by tradition been Exercise Tolerance test (ETT). For some years, Ambulatory ECG (Amb ECG) has also been used as a practical replacement for ETT, especially in screening procedures for myocardial ischemia.

The question that arises today is whether Amb-ECG may be used as a screening tool to identify apparently healthy groups with high risk for future Myocardial Infarction. If this is possible, pharmacological risk factor treatment may reduce the morbidity and mortality within this high-risk group. Also, as a consequence, and in spite of traditional cardiovascular risk factors, a low-risk group may be defined. Within this group, it will not be feasible to affect the

H.-H. Osterhues et al. (eds.),
Advances in Noninvasive Electrocardiographic Monitoring Techniques, 217–231.
© 2000 *Kluwer Academic Publishers. Printed in the Netherlands.*

cardiovascular risk factors, and thereby reduce the cost for pharmacological treatment within the group of apparently healthy high-risk individuals.

MYOCARDIAL ISCHEMIA

The prevalence of stable angina in the western world is around 3%, with a steep rise in the elderly population exceeding 60 years (men) or 70 years (women). The prevalence of silent myocardial ischemia among the apparently healthy group with an aggregation of cardiovascular risk factors is unknown. It may be as high as 12% of the middle aged population (Rautaharji et al, JACC 1986; 8:1-) and 33% in individuals with other arterial diseases such as diseases of the Carotid artery (Aronow et al, J Am Geriatr Soc 1995; 43:1272-1274).

ETT has up to now been the most generally used method in order to evaluate the prognosis in groups with cardiovascular risk factors. The risk of cardiac death among those with ST-segment depression has varied between 3-4-fold compared to those without such depressions (Rautaharji et al, JACC 1986; 8:1-. Yousuf S. In: Singh BN, ed. New York: Pergamon Press, 1988 pp 206-219).

ECG: EXERCISE TOLERANCE TEST OR AMBULATORY ECG?

Generally – but depending of the pre-test likelihood of CAD – the diagnostic specificity of reversible ST-segment depression is around 75% and the sensitivity around 70% for ETT in patients who are suspected to have CAD (Gianrossi et al, Circulation 1989; 76:237-243).

ETT however, has some drawbacks. Not everybody can perform the test, depending of other conditions such as orthopaedic diseases. The test result is dependent of fix stenosis in the coronary arteries, and does not generally reflect dynamic coronary stenosis. For safety reasons the test also requires a laboratory setting. ETT thus can not be performed at the office of a general practitioner. On the other hand, the test provides information on exercise capacity and blood pressure response. Also the method is well known and has been validated.

The most prominent drawback of Amb-ECG is that the method is not as well validated as ETT. However, it can be performed independently of a laboratory, and ECG tape-recorders may be put in the office of a general practitioner. The tape should be analysed by a highly skilled laboratory in order to secure good quality, but the tape may be transported by mail. Also, the test reflects the impact of both fix and dynamic coronary stenoses, which may explain the better prognostic impact compared to ETT ECG-results. The analysis also provides information on arrhythmias, heart rate variability and in some cases even signal-averaged ECG.

During recent years several studies have been performed in order to compare the diagnostic capacity of Amb-ECG and ETT.

In one study (Frogner and Juul-Möller, Annals of Noninvasive Electrocardiology, 1997; 2: 141-145) including 113 patients with suspected stable angina pectoris, results from coronary angiography was used as golden standard. The diagnostic accuracy was 66% (Amb-ECG) and 61% (ETT). Using both methods it rose to 71%.

In another study (Hoberg et al, Dtsch Med Wochenschr 1991; 116:441-446) it was demonstrated, that among 172 patients with suspected stable angina pectoris the diagnostic accuracy was alike (66 and 67% in Amb-ECG and ETT) for men, but that Amb-ECG showed a better accuracy for women (76%) compared to that of ETT (45%).

The prognostic impact from ETT is only moderate. Whether ETT-findings correspond to results from coronary angiography or isotope scanning has been tested in multiple studies (Paul et al, Am J Cardiol 1994; 74:991-996. Bogaty et al, JACC 1997; 29:1497-1504). The authors conclusion from these studies was, that *"The ETT indexes did not necessarily signify more severe ischemic heart disease by angiographic or scintigraphic criteria"*, and further *"Lack of concordance between the three methods* (i.e. coronary angiography, isotope investigations and ETT) *suggests that they examine different facets of myocardial ischemia, underscoring the need for caution in interpretation of their results"*.

The prognosis in patients with ST-segment depressions at Amb-ECG has been evaluated by Deedwania et al (Circulation 1990;81:748-756). In 107 patients with stable angina pectoris followed for a mean of 23 months, ST-segment depression on Amb-ECG was shown to be the most powerful risk parameter analysed, and that this finding was associated to an increased risk for heart death (p=0.02).

THE MALMÖ EXPERIENCE

Malmö in Sweden is a medium sized multiethnic city, with 250.000 inhabitants. During the last 10 years the primary health care sector has been heavily expanded, and is now based upon 15 primary health care centres. During the last 4 years each center has been offered a free ECG tape-recorder, in order to perform arrhythmia and ischemia investigations without referring the patient to the city's University hospital. This is part of a strategy to prevent unnecessary and expensive referrals to the Department of Cardiology. Thirteen of the 15 centres have accepted a recorder. Each ECG-tape is mailed to the hospital-based Laboratory for Ambulatory ECG in order to secure stable and high quality analysis. A cardiologist judges each analysis before the response is mailed to the primary health care center.

During these 4 years, the need for laboratory based ETT had decreased by 33%, while the number of Amb-ECG has increased by 77%. At the same time the number of referrals had decreased by 20%, and unnecessary referrals are now very unusual.

During the transition period, the number of patients with diagnosed angina pectoris in need for invasive or non-invasive treatment has not changed, as a rough indicator, that the change in diagnostic methods has not affected the number of patients.

RISK EVALUATION IN HEALTHY INDIVIDUALS

Two cohort studies have been performed in Malmö to investigate the prognostic power in ST-segment depressions.

The first study, "Men living in Malmö and born in 1914" was performed among all 68-years old men born on an even date. It demonstrated that in these cohort transient ST-segment depressions was found in 25%. During a 43 months follow-up period these men had a 4.4 times higher risk of myocardial infarction compared to the men without such depressions. The men with a combination of known coronary artery disease and transient ST-segment depressions had a 16-fold increased risk of myocardial infarction. Also, transient ST-segment depressions were found to predict increased cardiovascular mortality (p<0.009). The increase in mortality was independent of angina pectoris or previous myocardial infarction (Hedblad, Juul-Möller et al, European Heart J 1989, 10: 149-158).

The men were followed for a further 7 years. At the 10-years follow-up, it was found that during the first 3-4 years transient ST-segment depressions were the most important prognostic risk factor for future cardiovascular morbidity and mortality. However, at the extended follow-up, it was found, that after 10 years, men with complex ventricular arrhythmias had the highest risk for MI (1.6 times higher than in men without complex ventricular arrhythmias) and cardiovascular mortality (2.1 times higher than in men without these arrhythmias). In the men with a combination of complex ventricular arrhythmias and transient ST-segment depressions, the risk of cardiac events were 2.3 times higher than in other men, and cardiac death risk was increased by 3.5 compared to other men (Hedblad, Juul-Möller et al, European Heart J 1997; 18: 1787-1795).

In a second study a representative cohort from all 57 or 60 years old apparently healthy men in Malmö with an aggregation of cardiovascular risk factors were investigated with 48 hours Amb-ECG. The level of each risk factor (serum-cholesterol, serum-HDL, serum-Triglycerides, diastolic blood pressure and smoking habits) was such, that intervention was not indicated. The men had to be completely healthy which excluded men with diabetes mellitus, any vascular or other disease. Seventy-one per cent of the men in Malmö responded to the risk screening, and a representative sample of 154 men was invited to participate in the Amb-ECG analysis.

Thirty-four per cent had transient ST-segment depressions. The men were not informed about the result of the analysis. After 9 years of follow-up, 26% of the men with and 6% of those without ST-segment depression have had a myocardial infarction or other cardiac event. This implies a 4.4-fold increased risk for cardiac morbidity in men with ST-segment depression (range 1.9-9.9) (Juul-Möller et al, Circulation, *in press*).

CLINICAL IMPLICATIONS

In Sweden, the incidence of myocardial infarction per 100.000/year is 700 in the general grown-up population. In males this figure is 900, and in men aged 55-60 years, 600. If these men have cardiovascular risk factors, the incidence is 1450 myocardial infarctions.

Implying the risk calculations from the above mentioned study, the incidence of myocardial infarction in the 55-60 years old men with cardiovascular risk factors and transient ST-segment depressions can be calculated to be 2880, and 660 in the men without ST-segment depressions.

The incidence of MI in men with cardiovascular risk factors but without ST-segment depressions is thus at the same level as in the general population in this age group.

ECONOMIC CONSEQUENCE

According to the above mentioned results, middle aged men with an aggregation of cardiovascular risk factors but without transient ST-segment depressions at Amb-ECG does not have an increased risk for MI within the first 9 years after the ECG-analysis. This also implies that around two third of all men should not be included in a risk factor treatment program.

On the other hand, the one-third of these men (i.e. with ST-segment depression) stands a risk so high that risk factor treatment is clearly motivated.

The experience from the Woscop-study (Shephard et al, NEJM 1995; 333: 1301-1307) is, that the risk of MI among these men can be reduced by 31% if treated with 40 mg Pravastatin o.d. This would reduce the incidence of MI from 2880 to 1987 per 100.000 men/year.

According to the Woscop experience, today all middle aged men with an aggregation of cardiovascular risk factors should receive treatment in order to reduce these risk factors.

Screening cost for 100.000 men with Amb-ECG can be estimated to be 1.25 million USD. This will identify a group of 35.000 men with transient ST-segment depressions.

The saving in drug expenditure only treating 35.000 men instead of 100.000 men can (using Swedish pricing) be estimated to be 19.2 million USD/year. The Amb-ECG screening cost (1.20 million USD) has to be added, and the total saving is 18 million USD/100.000 men/year.

If these men also are treated with 75 mg of Aspirin o.d., the risk may be reduced by 30-35% further (Juul-Möller et al, Lancet 1992; 340: 1421-1425). The cost for this treatment is negligible in this context, but the risk for MI in the men with transient ST-segment depression may be reduced from 2880 to 1008 per 100.000/year, utilising a combined treatment. This is to compare with the normal risk within this cohort of 600/year.

CONCLUSION

Amb-ECG seems to possess a diagnostic precision in the same range as a maximal ETT when investigating patients for myocardial ischemia. In the group of apparently healthy middle-aged men with an aggregation of cardiovascular risk factors, transient ST-depression can define a high-risk group (one third of the men), in which risk factor treatment seems to be clearly indicated. This leaves two thirds of the men in a group with a risk of MI being so low, that intervention seems unnecessary for several years.

Leaving these low-risk men untreated may save 18 million USD/100.000 men/year. Risk factor treatment on the other hand, in combination with low dose aspirin will reduce the risk for MI to a level only somewhat higher than the average population.

21. POST THROMBOLYSIS/POST PTCA-MONITORING

ERNEST L. FALLEN

There continues to be considerable interest in post-reperfusion dynamics judging by the growing number of published reports examining the interaction between non-invasive markers and clinical outcome. It is quite a challenge to shift through the various studies each of which pose different questions, use different methodologies or experiment with a different design. Space does not permit an exhaustive review of every study and so this brief report focuses on selected studies that address questions of clinical relevance as they pertain to post-reperfusion monitoring.

WHY MONITOR?

The three most frequent objectives given for post reperfusion monitoring are: - (a) To generate a risk stratification profile (or prognostic index) based on non-invasive markers; (b) To determine if a given non-invasive marker could identify early restenosis following percutaneous coronary angioplasty (PTCA) and (c) To find a non-invasive method which reliably confirms infarct related artery patency post thrombolysis. An implicit objective in all these studies of course is to advance our understanding of the dynamic mechanisms underlying coronary artery reperfusion.

H.-H. Osterhues et al. (eds.),
Advances in Noninvasive Electrocardiographic Monitoring Techniques, 223-231.
© 2000 *Kluwer Academic Publishers. Printed in the Netherlands.*

WHAT DO WE REALLY WANT TO KNOW?

In any study it is reasonable to expect that the question posed has clinical relevance. For instance, it is well established that fatality rates are substantially increased with reocclusion post thrombolysis (1). Moreover no fewer than 4 trials (TAMI-1 (2), TIMI 2A (3), TIMI 2B (4), ECSG-V (5)) have shown that so-called "rescue" PTCA post thrombolysis is potentially harmfill in those patients whose infarct related arteries are incompletely lysed. The corollary that "rescue" PTCA may offer benefit to those with failed thrombolysis (the infarct related artery remains totally occluded) has been more or less substantiated (6). Therefore, the key question should be: which non-invasive marker yields a 100% negative predictive accuracy for identifying post-thrombolysis arterial patency?

As for post PTCA-monitoring a clinically relevant objective would be to avoid unnecessary re- catheterization by selecting a non-invasive marker that reflects adequate coronary blood flow through the dilated segment(s). Here, a Post PTCA non-invasive marker with a high sensitivity or, preferably, a high positive predictive accuracy for hemodynamically sustained nutrient blood flow would be desirable. Finally, it is as important for prognostic markers to identify the very low risk patients post-reperfusion in order to spare them unnecessary aggressive investigation or therapy as it is to identify the high risk patients for whom aggressive intervention could be life saving. To date, the majority of studies on post-reperfusion monitoring address these questions only indirectly. The following is a brief review of selected studies that perhaps come dose to acknowledging these concerns.

GENERATING A RISK STRATIFICATION PROFILE FROM POST REPERFUSION MONITORING

A. Post Thrombolysis

The use of static measurements such as demographics, baseline CK isoforms, site of MI and Killip class have generally yielded less than satisfactory predictors of outcome post thrombolysis. For instance, in the GUSTO-I trial with well over 40,000 post thrombolysed patients enrolled, the static baseline variables of age, systolic blood pressure, Killip class, anterior site of MI and heart rate accounted for 90% of the prognostic information at 30 days (7). However, the unadjusted univariate relations showed complex interactions and no attempt was made to distinguish among modes of short-term 30 day mortality let alone identify a very low risk group.

Because heart rate variability (HRV) is a powerful predictor of post MI mortality, several studies have examined the effect of thrombolysis on cardiac autonomic activity. In a non-randomized study comparing 30 patients post thrombolysis with 21 patients who did not receive thrombolysis, Pedretti et al demonstrated a significantly higher SDNN in the lysed group (8). Within 23 months follow-up, there was a significant increase in arrhythmic events in the non-lysed group independent of LV function but associated with directional changes in HRV. In another non-randomized study, Odemuyiwa et al compared the effect of thrombolysis (n=53) vs no thrombolysis (n=23) on baroreceptor sensitivity (BRS) in 76 patients at 6 days, 6 weeks and 3 months post MI (9). Again, no group differences were seen with respect to LV function (LVEF). However, BRS was improved by lysis while those with initially low BRS gradually improved over time. Caution is urged before any clinical benefit is ascribed to the "improvement" in either HRV or BRS. Although they reflect physiologic changes, they are essentially surrogate markers and while there is incontrovertible proof of a strong and independent association between HRV and prognosis post MI it has yet to be proven that simply modifying HRV or BRS confers protection against adverse outcome.

Monitoring of a physiologic time event series is a process which should capture dynamical changes in a system. Using a large database from the GISSI-II study, Zuanetti et al showed a tight relationship between time domain HRV (cut-off value for SDNN=70 ms) and subsequent mortality rates (MR) post MI thus confirming that a low HRV seen at hospital discharge remains a powerful prognostic tool in the thrombolytic era (10). However, from another large database, the GUSTO-1 trial, Singh et al failed to show a clear prognostic index derived from several time domain data (SDANN and pNN50) (11). On the other hand, they reported prognostic significance for the LF:HF ratio but, curiously, in a relationship wherein the lower the LF:HF ratio by day 2 post lysis the higher the 30 day MR. They did show that higher HRV values correlated with TIMI grade 3 flow. So, indirectly they answered a critical question on patency but provided no persuasive data on negative predictive accuracy which perhaps would have identified patients with failed reperfusion.

Another traditional predictor of post MI arrhythmic events are the fractionated electrical activity of the terminal QRS-complex known as late potentials. Breithardt recently reviewed a number of studies which focused on the association between late potentials post thrombolysis and clinical outcome post MI (12). Most of these were non-randomized in design but all demonstrated that successful post thrombolytic reperfusion significantly reduced the incidence of late potentials and thus theoretically "prevented the formation of an arrythmogenic substrate" (13-15). However, in a follow-up of 331 post MI survivors Malik et al discovered that while the positive predictive

Table 1

Predictive Values for Detection of Post Thrombolytic Patency

Study	Technique	n	% Occluded	PPV%	NPV%
Dellborg(23)	QRS Vector	21	24	94	40
Fernandez(19)	ST decrease				
	from peak	38	42	-	-
	>75%	-	-	55	100
	>25%	-	-	100	43
Hohnloser(21)	3 parameters*	82	23	-	-
	- single	-	-	97	43-64
	- all 3	-	-	97	100
Krucoff(28)	ST recovery	22	64	100	73

*PPV = Positive predictive accuracy; NPV = negative predictive accuracy. Bracketed numbers refer to references. * The 3 parameters include: - early peak CK≤ 12h; reduction in ST elevation ≥50%; reperfusion arrhythmias < 90 min.*

value for arrhythmic events based on signal averaged ECG approached 100% in patients without thrombolysis, it was only 27% for those who received the lytic therapy (16). All these studies suggest a potential mechanism by which thrombolysis improves survival (be it through restoration of cardiac autonomic balance or myocardial electrical stability). Nonetheless, until an attempt is made to randomize post reperfusion patients on the basis of altered HRV, BRS or other non-invasive monitoring parameters, the true mechanisms for improved survival post lysis will remain elusive.

B. Post PTCA

There are but scant observations on the prognostic value of non-invasive markers following PTCA. One interesting study by Bonaduce et al showed that with successful PTCA there was a relationship between reversibility of wall motion abnormality and changes in the heart rate power spectral indeces (17). This was not a prognostic study. However, Birand et al followed 51 patients post PTCA with serial measurements of HR power spectral analysis at 10 day, 30 day, and 3 mo. (18) This study was a calcium blocker trial but 25 patients served as controls. They showed no change in either the LF or HF power during any of the time intervals post PTCA.

ASSESSMENT OF REPERFUSION POST THROMBOLYSIS

A number of studies have used non-invasive monitoring to determine the reperfusion status post thrombolysis (Table 1). Single markers such as ST-segment change employing either single lead or multilead systems are partly predictive of infarct related artery patency but few studies have addressed the issue of persistent occlusion or failed thrombolysis. One of these was a study reported by Fernandez et al who used a single lead ECG system to detect reperfusion within three hours post thrombolysis in 38 patients (19). Patency was verified by early coronary angiography (60 min). ST-segment recovery was defined by the percent decrement from peak ST elevation. They showed that ST-segment recovery >50% at <10 min intervals of continuous recording was optimal to predict patency with a 100% sensitivity. Using this value, the negative predictive value for TIMI 3 flow was 94% and for TIMI 2 or 3 flow was 67%. None of the 16 patients with persistent occlusion showed more than a 50% decrease in the ST-segment from peak levels. From the GUSTO I trial, Langer et al examined the speed of ST-segment recovery post thrombolysis in relation to infarct artery patency (20). The time to 50% recovery within 30 min was assessed in 618 pts. There was no clear correlation between recovery rates and patency at 90 min. Neither was there a distinct marker that reliably identified persistent occlusion.

Hohnloser examined the influence of combined markers, namely; (a) early peak CK activity within 12 h post lysis; (b) >50% ST-segment reduction and (c) recurrence of arrhythmias in 82 first MI patients (21). Using a logistic regression model they found a 100% negative predictive accuracy for patency only when all three markers were combined.

Kelly et al investigated the relationship between post thrombolysis reperfusion and time domain HRV (22). Reperfusion was defined non-invasively by a combination of changes in ST-segment and serum myoglobin levels. Fifty-seven percent of their thrombolysed patients showed reperfusion and these had a significant increase in HRV (SDNN, SDANN, and rMSSD) compared to those who did not reperfuse. This was a small group of patients and no attempt was made to address the critical question of persistent occlusion. They did make the point that since the peak CKMB was similar in both groups the main effect on HRV was presumably related to patency of the artery and not to extent of myocardial damage. Using a trend analysis of QRS vector differences, Dellborg et al reported a 94% positive predictive accuracy for detecting post thrombolytic arterial patency among 21 patients but only two out of five patients with persistent occlusion could be identified (23).

Table 2

Predicting Restenosis Post PTCA					
Study	Technique	n	%Restenosis	PPV%	NPV%
Krucoff(25)	Multilead ST	62	31	84	?
	"fingerprint"		37	87	?
Bush(26) "fingerprint"	12 lead ST	115	7.8	100	?
Hamasaki(27)	Δ ST/Δ HR	125	38	70	94

PREDICTING RESTENOSIS POST PTCA

Several studies have used non-invasive monitoring in an attempt to identify early restenosis post PTCA (Table 2). Tseng et al studied changes in both time and frequency domain HRV one month post PTCA in 25 patients to predict restenosis defined at a 6 month follow-up coronary angiogram (24). Those patients whose LF:HF ratio improved dramatically within one month post PTCA had virtually no restenosis by 6 months. The time domain data of SDANN and rMSSD were less predictive. The numbers were small and did not permit an adequate assessment of predictive accuracies. However, of those patients whose LF:HF ratio improved (3.5 to 2.02) at one month post-PTCA, 14/14 had no evidence of restenosis.

Several investigators have used the unique approach of establishing a template or "fingerprint" of the ST changes that accompany total intraluminal occlusion during balloon inflation. The idea was to then use the same or similar ST patterns post PTCA to identify early restenosis. One such method employed by Krucoff et al used high resolution multilead ST recordings during inflation as the "fingerprint" (25). The reproducibility among repeated balloon occlusions was about 70%. During follow-up of 19 patients who developed restenosis, 16 (84%) had either an identical or related pattern within 1 month post PTCA. Bush et al compared various ECG leads to identify the most sensitive "fingerprint" pattern for ischemia during PTCA in 115 patients (26). The 12 lead system identified 90% compared to only 42% by limb lead recordings alone. In 9 patients who suffered abrupt reocclusion within 24 hr post PTCA, the ST-segment pattern was identical to that during inflation. Of interest was the observation that of the 6 patients who had no restenosis but experienced chest pain post PTCA none reproduced their ischemic "fingerprint".

Hamasaki et al used a different approach (27). They recorded a Δ ST/ΔHR index during serial exercise testing before and a few days post PTCA. Coronary angiography was performed 3-12 months later. The ΔST/ΔHR index increased in 43 of 47 patients who showed restenosis compared with only 18/78 patients without restenosis (p<0.0001). The positive predictive value was 70% and the negative predictive value was 94%. These values were more robust than either stress thallium scintigraphy or treadmill exercise testing.

CONCLUSIONS

1. Both time and frequency domain HRV values, measured early post MI, retain their prognostic power in the thrombolytic era.
2. Although of value in generating a risk stratification profile post MI, HRV measurements are less reliable for predicting either post PTCA restenosis or failed reperfusion post thrombolysis.
3. It appears, so far, that failure of ST-segment levels to recover >50% from peak levels within 30-60 min post thrombolysis is one of the signs that may be reliable in predicting persistent infarct related artery occlusion.
4. The concept of establishing a template or "fingerprint" of ST-segment changes during repetitive balloon inflations may be useful in detecting early post PTCA restenosis.

REFERENCES

1. Ohman EM, Califf RM, Topol EJ, et al. Consequences of reocclusion after successful reperfusion therapy in acute myocardial infarction. Circulation 1990; 82: 781-91.
2. Topol EJ, Califf RM, George BS, et al. A randomized trial of immediate versus delayed elective angioplasty after intravenous tissue plasminogen activator in acute myocardial infarction. N Engl J Med 1987; 317: 581-8.
3. The TIMI Research Group. Immediate vs delayed catheterization and angioplasty following thrombolytic therapy for acute myocardial infarction. TIMI II A results. JAMA 1988; 260: 2849- 58.
4. The TIMI Study Group. Comparison of invasive and conservative strategies after treatment with intravenous tissue plasminogen activator in acute myocardial infarction. Results of the Thrombolysis in Myocardial Infarction (TIMI) Phase II trial. N Engl J Med 1989; 320: 618-27.
5. Simoons ML, Betriu A, Col J, et al. Thrombolysis with tissue plasminogen activator in acute myocardial infarction: no additional benefit from immediate percutaneous coronary angioplasty. Lancet 1988; 1: 197-203.

6. Ellis SG, Ribeiro da Silva E, Heyndrick G et al. Randomized comparison of rescue angioplasty with conservative management of patients with early failure of thrombolysis for acute anterior myocardial infarction. Circulation 1994; 90: 2280-4.

7. Lee KL, Woodlief LH, Topol EJ, et al. Predictors of 30-day mortality in the era of reperfusion for acute myocardial infarction. Results from an international trial of 41 021 patients. Circulation 1995; 91: 1659-1668.

8. Pedretti RFE, Colombo E, Braga SS, et al. Effect of thrombolysis on heart rate variability and life threatening ventricular arrhythmias in survivors of acute myocardial infarction. JACC 1994; 23: 19-26.

9. Odemuyiwa O, Farrell T, Staunton A, et al. Influence of thrombolytic therapy on the evolution of baroreflex sensitivity after myocardial infarction. American Heart J 1993; 125: 285-91.

10. Zuanetti G, Neilson JMM, Latini R, et al. Prognostic significance of heart rate variability in post- myocardial infarction patients in the fibrinolytic era. The GISSI-2 Results. Circulation 1996; 94: 432-36.

11. Singh N, Mironov D, Armstrong PW, et al. Heart rate variability assessment early after acute myocardial infarction. Circulation 1996; 93: 1388-1395.

12. Breithardt G, Borggrefe M, Karbenn U. Late potentials as predictors of risk after thrombolytic treatment? Br Heart J 1990; 64: 174-6.

13. Eldar M, Leor J, Hod H, et al. Effect of thrombolysis on the evolution of late potentials within 10 days of infarction. Br Heart J 1990; 63: 273-6.

14. Gang ES, Levo,v AS, Hong M, Wang FZ, et al. Decreased incidence of ventricular late potentials after successful thrombolytic therapy for acute myocardial infarction. N Eng J Med 1989; 321: 712-6.

15. Riccio C, Cesaro F, Perrotta R, et al. Early thrombolysis, reperfusion arrhythmias and late potentials in acute myocardial infarction. New Frontiers of Arrhythmias 1990; 6: 157-61.

16. Malik M, Kulakowski P, Odemuyiwa O, et al. Effect of thrombolytic therapy on the predictive value of signal-averaged electrocardiography after acute myocardial infarction. Am J Cardiol 1992; 70: 21-25.

17. Bonaduce D, Pettretta M, Piscione F, et al. Influence of reversible segmental left ventricular dysfunction on heart period variability in patients with one-vessel coronary artery disease. JACC 1994; 24: 399-405.

18. Birand A, Kudaiberdieva GZ, Batyraliev TA, et al. Effects of trimetazidine on heart rate variability and left ventricular systolic performance in patients with coronary artery disease after percutaneous translutninal angioplasty. Angiology 1997; 48: 413-22.

19. Femandez AR, Sequeira RF, Chakko S, et al. ST-segment tracking for rapid determination of patency of the infarct-related artery in acute myocardial infarction. JACC 1995; 26: 675-83.

20. Langer A, KrucoffMW, Klootwijk P, et al. Noninvasive assessment of speed and stability of infarct-related artery reperfusion: Results of GUSTO ST-segment monitoring study. JACC 1995; 25: 1552-7.

21. Hohnloser SH, Zabel M, Kasper W, et al. Assessment of coronary artery patency after thrombolytic therapy: Accurate prediction utilizing the combined analysis of three noninvasive markers. JACC 1991; 18: 44-9.

22. Kelly PA, Nolan J, Wilson JI, et al. Preservation of autonomic function following successful reperfusion with streptokinase within 12 hours of the onset of acute myocardial infarction. Am J Cardiology 1997; 79: 203-205.

23. Dellborg M, Topol EJ, Swedberg K. Dynamic QRS-complex and ST-segment vectorcardiographic monitoring can identify vessel patency in patients with acute myocardial infarction treated with reperfusion therapy. Am Heart J 1991; 122: 943-48.

24. Tseng CD, Wang TL, Lin JL, et al. The cause-effect relationship of sympathovagal activity and the outcome of percutaneous transluminal coronary angioplasty. Jpn Heart J 1996; 37: 455-62.

25. Krucoff MW, Parente AR, Bottner RK, et al. Stability of Multilead ST-segment "fingerprints" over time after percutaneous transluminal coronary angioplasty and its usefulness in detecting reocclusion. Am J Cardiology 1988; 61: 1232-37.

26. Bush HS, Ferguson JJ, Angelini P, et al. Twelve-lead electrocardiographic evaluation of ischemia during percutaneous transluminal coronary angioplasty and its correlation with acute reocclusion. Am Heart J 1991; 121: 1591-99.

27. Hamasaki S, Arima S, Tahara M, et al. Increase in the $\Delta ST/\Delta HR$ index: A new predictor of restenosis after successful percutaneous transluminal coronary angioplasty. Am J Cardiology 1996; 78-990-95.

22. INTERACTIVE HOLTER-MONITORING OF TRANSIENT ISCHEMIC EPISODES

C. DROSTE AND G. KINNE

INTRODUCTION

Nowadays it is possible to assess myocardial ischemia in patients with coronary heart disease by using long-term Holter-ECG-instruments analyzing the electrocardiogram online over a period of 24 hours. For this purpose special algorisms had to be developed to analyze ST-segment depressions (Kennedy, 1981). Only a few attempts were made to find reliable ECG-systems being able to notify the CHD-patient by signals on the ischemic information obtained (Barry, 1987). Only few systems so far are proved to be well-suited for this purpose: online systems, like Monitor One (Qmed) and Medilog 4500 (Oxford) are technically well-equipped for resignalling coronary events in the moment of occurence (Kennedy & Wiens, 1987).

The main advantage of this interactive method is that the patient can be informed immediately about a transient ischemic episode. So parameters of anticipation and physical activity during the ischemic episode can be studied. Moreover the patients can be trained to take coronary medication or change behavior in order to cope better in daily life.

For this investigation a specially developed real time analysis system constructed by Oxford Company (Medilog FD2) was validated in various laboratory and field situations and applied to test several psychophysiological hypotheses (Kinne, 1997; Kinne & Droste, 1996; Kinne et al., in press).

H.-H. Osterhues et al. (eds.),
Advances in Noninvasive Electrocardiographic Monitoring Techniques, 233–238.
© 2000 *Kluwer Academic Publishers. Printed in the Netherlands.*

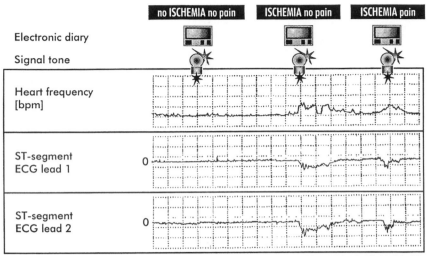

Figure 1. Symptomatic, silent and random signals

METHOD OF INTERACTIVE HOLTER-MONITORING

In cooperation with the Oxford Company the Holter-ECG was modified in a way to allow resignalling of ischemic episodes according to the 1-1-1 rule introduced by the American Heart Association using a special developed algorism. For creating a control situation the Holter-ECG randomly gives some acoustic signals during the 24 hour period without an underlying ST-segment depression. The patient is per se unable to distinguish true from random signals.

For each ischemic episode the point of depart, the moment of the maximum ST-segment depression and the end of it as well as its degree and duration are documented by an experienced cardiologist. In addition, the heart frequency is being assessed ten, five and two minutes as well as directly before the beginning of the episode at a maximum ST-segment depression and again at the end and five minutes after the episode. In order to check the reactivity with regard to the acoustic signal the heart frequency is recorded 2 minutes following this sound. For an optimal assessment of the ST-segment the two bipolar precordial leads V3 and V5 are being used (Kennedy, 1988).

The interactive Holter-ECG is supplemented by an actometer (ZAK) to assess physical activity. For an optimum synchronisation the actometer works simultaneously with the Holter ECG. Also a synchronized electronic diary (rating-box) is used for assessing setting-related subjective data (Lang et al., 1991; Ostermeier et al., 1991). When the signal of the Holter-ECG occurs the patient has to answer nine questions (and three additional optional questions regarding specification) using the rating-box for entry. The questions include the date and time of the day, the setting criteria, behaviour (the exercise performed and other activities) and psychological state (affected due to physical or psychological stress, excitement, excessive tension and nervousness) as well as the psychological state following resignalment (heart pain, perception of ischemia).

Figure 1 shows the discrimination of symptomatic, silent and random situations.

VALIDATION STUDIES

Validation using a standardized laboratory exercise situation

For a first validation of the interactive Holter-ECG ischemic ST-segment depressions were assessed in 52 CHD-patients who were examined in a standardized laboratory exercise situation with a 12-channel exercise ECG and in parallel by the Holter ECG (Kinne & Droste, 1996).

Among other factors the time of onset of ST-depression in both ECG systems was registered and compared (Fig. 2). There is a high rate of agreement (r=0.96).

All ST-segment depressions (n=29) assessed in the 12-channel ECG were resignalled by means of the Holter ECG (sensitivity 100%). In two of n=23 cases an ST-segment depression was resignalled by the Holter ECG that had not been diagnosed in the 12-channel ECG (specificity 91%).

The results show that the Holter-ECG is reliable for identifying and resignalling ST-segment depressions in patients with coronary heart disease.

Validation in the field

A monitoring system consisting of the interactive Holter-ECG, the actometer and the rating box was applied in a first field study investigating 30 male patients with an average age of 59 years (Kinne, 1997; Kinne et al., in press). Criteria of inclusion to the study consisted of the presence of a coronary heart disease (angiographic findings and/or myocardial infarct, ST-segment

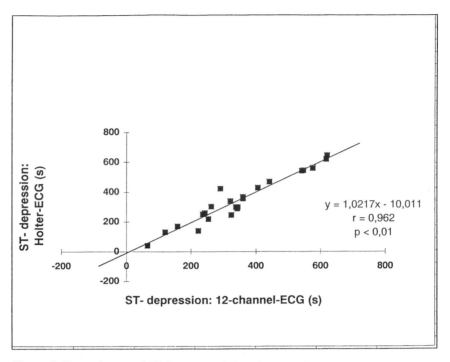

Figure 2. Time of onset of ST-depression (V3 and V5) in the 12-channel ECG and the Holter ECG

depression demonstrated by an exercise test) and evidence of transient ischemic episodes occurring in everyday life. Each patients was studied over 24-hours without coronary medication in daily life. Additionally nine patients were examined repeatedly during one year.

Physiological data (ischemic parameters, heart frequency, physical activity) and situative-psychological data (electronic diary) sampled during the ischemic episode or random signal were used to test psychophysiological hypotheses. The results show that silent and symptomatic episodes do not differ in the amount of myocardial ischaemia. But they differ in the course of heart rate during the ischemic episode. Symptomatic episodes show two minutes before the onset of ST-segment depression a significantly higher heart beat ascent than silent episodes ($p<.05$). Interestingly symptomatic and silent episodes also differ in in certain psychological context variables.

Further developments

In a running study CHD-patients fullfilling the inclusion criteria of the first field study are trained to increase their capability to perceive transient ischemic states in daily life. For this purpose the interactive Holter-ECG was improved by OXFORD Company. The apparatus now presents two different tones. A high frequency tone signals ischemic episodes or random signals as used in the first investigation. A low frequency tone serves, if activated, as a feedback tone one to four minutes after the resignallement of a transient ischemic episode. This tone allows the patient to learn the differentiation between ischemic and random episodes. First results show that patients are able to learn the perception of transient ischemic episodes by using this new method over some days.

SUMMARY

Technical developments in Holter monitoring allow us today the investigation of transient ischemic episodes online under natural conditions. Situations in dialy life that determine the apparence of ischemic episodes with and without pain can be studied more adequately by using an interactive method. So results of field studies show that situative-psychological variables influence angina pectoris pain.

Further developments of the interactive Holter-ECG make it possible to train CHD-patients to learn the perception of transient ischemic episodes. In a therapeutically sense of view situations leading to myocardial ischemia can so be avoided in order to reduce the amount of myocardial ischemia in daily life.

LITERATURE

1. Barry, J., Campell, S., Nabel, E., G., Mead, K. & Selwyn, A., P. (1987). Ambulatory monitoring of the digitized electrocardiogram for detection and early warning of transient myocardial ischemia in angina pectoris. American Journal of Cardiology, 60, 483-488.
2. Kennedy, H. L. (1988). Ambulatory electrocardiography strategies used in assesing silent myocardial ischaemia. European Heart Journal, 9 (suppl N), 70-77.
3. Kennedy, H. L. & Wiens, R. D. (1987). Ambulatory (Holter) Electrocardiography using real-time analysis. American Journal of Cardiology, 59, 1190-1195.
4. Kinne, G. (1997). Interaktives Monitoring von Myokardischämie. Frankfurt a. M.: Peter Lang.
5. Kinne, G & Droste, C (1996). Psychophysiological monitoring of transient ischemic states in patients with coronary heart disease. In: Fahrenberg, J. & Myrtek, M. (Eds.). Ambulatory

assessment. Computer-assisted psychological and psychophysiological methods in monitoring and field studies. Seattle: Hogrefe & Huber Publishers:347-363.

6. Kinne, G., Droste, C., Fahrenberg, J. Roskamm, H. (in press). Symptomatic myocardial ischaemia (heart pain) is linked to the psychological context in daily life - Implications for a clinical use of interactive monitoring. Submitted to Journal of Psychosomatic Research.

7. Lang, E.. Ostermeier, M., Forster, C. & Handwerker, H. O. (1991). Die Rating-Box - ein neues Gerät zur ambulanten Erfassung von subjektiven Variablen. Biomedizinische Technik 36, 210-212.

8. Ostermeier, M., Lang E., Pittel, M. & Forster, C. (1991). Ambulante Datenerfassung an Schmerzpatienten mittels elektronischem Schmerztagebuch. Der Schmerz, 5, 9-14.

23. SILENT ISCHEMIA: THE 1998 STATUS: NEW OBSERVATIONS ON TRIGGERS, PATHOPHYSIOLOGICAL MECHANISMS AND CIRCADIAN VARIATIONS

SHLOMO STERN

Since Heberden described the clinical picture of Angina Pectoris ("pain in the chest") in 1772, but especially since Harrick clinched the connection between pain in the chest and myocardial ischemia, this symptom became inseparable from the diagnosis of angina pectoris. Later, ST-depression in the electrocardiogram during a spontaneous attack of chest pain or provoked by exercise, became for many decades the only confirmation of the diagnosis of angina pectoris.

Episodic ST-depression during everyday activities was described by us in 1974 (1) and similar findings were described by Schang and Pepine (2) three years later. The confirmation of ischemia as a cause for such ST-depression even if unaccompanied by chest pain came from Deanfield and co-workers (3) who in 1984 documented perfusion defects on PET imaging during ST-depression even if the patient was asymptomatic.

WHY SILENT?

The question why is ischemia silent in certain patients and painful in others was the subject of several investigations. Falcone et al (4) demonstrated a higher pain threshold in the silent patients, a defective pain perception was assumed by Maseri et al (5) and high endorphine levels as a cause of silentness was assumed by Droste and Roskamm (6).

H.-H. Osterhues et al. (eds.),
Advances in Noninvasive Electrocardiographic Monitoring Techniques, 239–245.
© 2000 *Kluwer Academic Publishers. Printed in the Netherlands.*

In a more detailed study Hikita and co-workers (7) studied patients with exercise tests, Holter monitoring and during PTCA and in patients who were silent during ischemia during PTCA. They found in silent patients endorphine levels higher than in patients with pain, although exercise time and inflation time were similar among the silents and the painfuls.

Rosen and co-workers (8) performed delicate PET measurements of regional cerebral blood flow. They showed that during myocardial ischemia thalamic and cortical blood flow increased bilaterally, but in patients with silent ischemia the frontal cortical activation was decreased. This abnormal central pain-processing seems to have a role in the silentness of ischemia in these patients.

IS SILENT ISCHEMIA LESS ISCHEMIA THEN THE PAINFUL ONE?

We compared characteristics of ischemic episodes on Holter monitoring and compared the length of episodes, degree of ST-depression, etc., between silent and painful episodes all parameters were found to be similar. Moreover, a similar coronary score of the lesions was found on arteriography (9). Weiner and co-workers (10) studied the exercise test results on entering the CASS study and compared it with survival after a seven-year follow up; this was similar whether pain did or did not accompany the ST-depression on the entrance test.

Similar results were obtained when using a wall-motion abnormality score on echocardiography (11). They showed that patients with silent and symptomatic ischemia during dipyridamole-induced ischemia had similar extent of coronary events. Beller and co-workers (12) compared patients with silent vs. painful ischemia during a 201-Thallium exercise test. The exercise tolerance, hemodynamic changes, the extent of lesions on angiography and the extent of hypoperfusion on the scan, were all similar in two groups of patients. A Thallium SPECT study conducted by Manharian et al (13) showed that the extent of quantified perfusion defects was identical in patients with and without exertional chest pain. In patients undergoing PTCA a similar decrease in segmental and global LVEF and a similar duration of decrease in LV function was found in patients with or without pain during the procedure (14).

Thus, it looks now that the silentness of ischemia is not a sign of less ischemia. Pain, whether elicited by exercise or pharmocological stress does not point to a more severe ischemia than the asymptomatic one.

PATHOPHYSIOLOGICAL OBSERVATIONS

A slight, but definite heart rate increase precedes ischemia, as it was shown by Pepine et al (15), Deedwania et al (16), Andrew et al (17) and others. This points towards an increased sympathetic tone prior to the ischemic episode, with a consequent increased demand. This observation has also therapeutic consequences as for these patients beta-blockers are the therapy of choice, and only in the minority of patients without a heart rate change before the daily-life ischemic episode, would calcium blockers be the therapy of choice. Recently it was shown that not only the heart rate, but also the blood pressure rises prior to an ischemic episode in the majority of patients (18). This demonstrates the crucial role of increased oxygen demand in precipitating spontaneous ischemia. In the minority without a preceding heart rate and blood pressure rise, coronary vasoconstriction is most probably the cause of the transient myocardial ischemia.

TRIGGERS OF DAILY LIFE ISCHEMIA

Already in 1974 we (1) mentioned mental stress as one of the triggers of ischemia documented on Holter monitoring, but a systematic study documenting the importance of provoked mental stress in inducing silent ischemia was published only in 1988 by Rozanskini and co-workers (19).

An important study by Goldberg et al (20) compared mental stress vs. exercise induced ischemia. They have measured Holter ECG, nuclear ventriculography for wall-motion abnormalities, ejection fraction and cardiac output, as well as blood norepinephrine and epinephrine. Systemic vascular resistance dropped during exercise, but rose during mental stress. They documented that the hemodynamic changes during mental stress are mediated by the secretion of epinephrine. During physical exercise more norepinephrine secretion could be documented than during mental stress. The different mechanisms documented may have importance in the selection of anti-ischemic therapy. Blumenthal and co-workers (21) documented wall-motion abnormalities by different triggers for mental stress.

Thus, mental stress seems to be a most important trigger for ischemia during everyday activities and one has to consider this factor also as a very early mechanism for ischemia. This point has been stressed by Kral and co-workers (22) who studied an asymptomatic population who are siblings of a parent with premature coronary disease. Of the 152 persons studied, 15 has ischemia documented both on exercise or on Thallium perfusion studies or on both. Most interestingly these 15 persons with "preclinical coronary disease" had an exaggerated response to mental stress, provoked by the Stroop Color Word Test.

CIRCADIAN VARIATIONS OF ISCHEMIA

Several investigations documented that the greatest frequency of ambulatory ischemia is seen between 6 AM-Noon (23-25). Most interestingly, the incidence of acute myocardial infarction is also more frequent between 6AM-Noon (26), as well as the incidence of sudden cardiac death.

Other similar circadian 6AM- Noon patterns in cardiovascular system were also documented, as a higher blood pressure, a higher heart rate, increased platelet aggregability, a higher defibrillation threshold, a higher ischemic threshold (heart rate at one millimeter ST-depression) and even a better efficacy of thrombolytic therapy; all shown to be increased between 6AM-Noon.

In an ambulatory Holter study this increased 6AM-Noon ischemia was explained mainly by the sudden increase of physical and mental activities following the awakening (27). These observations were in line with the investigation of Parker et al (28) who studied in-hospital patients. They demonstrated that if the start of activities was delayed by four hours after awakening, a corresponding four-hour time lag was observed in the appearance of ischemia.

SILENT ISCHEMIA UNDER VARIOUS CLINICAL CONDITIONS.

Silent myocardial ischemia seems to be strongly associated with high blood pressure and silent ST-T changes are markers both of ischemic heart disease and of hypertension and studies have shown that ST-T changes contribute independently to coronary death in such patients.

Conflicting results were published during the past few years about frequency of silent ischemia in diabetic patients. Today, it seems to be confirmed that diabetic patients have an increased frequency of silent ischemia. The frequency of ischemic episodes seems to be somewhat less in woman (29), but the heart rate increase before ischemic episodes, the circadian variations and the ischemic thresholds were all found to be similar in men and woman (30).

Bayes de Luna (31) collected information about patients who died suddenly while wearing a Holter monitor and could show that ST changes preceded the death in 12% of the patients. In the study of Pepine and co-workers (32) on 35 patients dying while wearing Holter, in 12 ST-depression or elevation preceded the ventricular fibrillation.

CONCLUSIONS

It seems that Holter monitoring is an excellent tool to disclose ischemic episodes during daily life. These episodes are most frequent between 6AM-noon. 80-90% of the unprovoked episodes are silent. A slight increase in heart rate and in blood pressure were documented in the majority of patients to precede such episodes, pointing to an increase in sympathetic activity and consequent oxygen demand as the mechanism leading to such episodes. Mental stress is the most frequent trigger of silent ischemia during everyday activities. Provoked ischemia by exercise or pharmacological stress is also frequently silent, as demonstrated by PET, SPECT and echo studies.

REFERENCES

1. Stern S, Tzivoni D. Early detection of silent ischemic heart disease by 24-hour electrocardiographic monitoring of active subjects. *Br Heart J*. 1974;16:481-486.
2. Schang SJ, Pepine CJ. Transient asymptomatic ST-segment depression during daily activity. *Am J Cardiol*. 1977;39:396-402.
3. Deanfield JE, Maseri A, Selwyn AP et al. Myocardial ischemia during daily life in patients with stable angina: its relation to symptoms and heart rate changes. *Lancet*. 1983;1:753-758.
4. Falcone C, Sconocchia R, Guasti L, Codega S, Montemartine C, Speccchia G. Dental pain threshold and angina pectoris in patients with coronary artery disease. *J AM Coll Cardiol* 1988;12:348-52.
5. Maseri A, Chierchia S, Davies G, Glazier JJ. Mechanisms of ischemic cardiac pain and silent myocardial ischemia. *Am J Med* 1985;79(suppl 3A):7-11.
6. Droste C, Roskamm H. Experimental pain measurement in patients with asymptomatic myocardial ischemia. *J Am Coll Cardiol* 1983; 1:940-5.
7. Hikita H, Kurita A, Takase B, Satomura K, Etsuda H, Nakamura H. The role of beta-endorphin in the mechanisms of silent myocardial ischemia. *Eur H J Abst*.1997;18:56.
8. Rosen SD, Paulesu E, Nihoyannopoulos P et al. Silent ischemia as a central problem: regional brain activation compaired in silent and painful myocardial ischemia. *Ann Intern Med* 1996;124:939-49.
9. Stern S, Weisz G, Gavish A et al. Comparison between silent and asymptomatic ischemia during exercise testing in patients with coronary artery disease. *J Cardiopulm Rehabil* 1988;12:507-12.
10. Weiner DA, Ryan TJ, McCabe CH et al. Significance of silent myocardial ischemia during exercise testing in patients with coronary artery disease. *Am J Cardiol*. 1987;59:725-729.
11. Bolognese L, Rossi L, Sarasso G, et al. Silent versus symptomatic dipyridamole-induced ischemia after myocardial infarction: clinical and prognostic significance. *J Am Coll Cardiol* 1992;19:953-9.
12. Beller GA. *Clinical Nuclear Cardiology* (Philadelphia, PA: WB Saunders, 1995).

13. Mahmarian JJ, Pratt CM, Cocanougher MK, Verani MS. Altered myocardial perfusion in patients with angina pectoris or silent ischemia during exercise as assessed by quantitative thallium-201 single-photon emission computed tomography. *Circulation* 1990;82:1305-15.

14. Wohlgelertner D, Jaffe CC, Cabin HS, Yeatman LA, Cleman M. Silent ischemia during coronary occlusion produced by balloon inflation: relation to regional myocardial dysfunction. *J Am Coll Cardiol* 1987;10:491-98.

15. Pepine C, Hill J, Imperi G, Norvell N. Beta-adrenergic blockers in silent myocardial ischemia. *Am J Cardiol* 1988;29:61:18B-21B.

16. Deedwania PC, Nelson JR. Pathophysiology of silent myocardial ischemia during   daily life: Hemodynamic evaluation by simultaneous electrocardiographic and blood pressure monitoring. *Circulation* 1990;82:1296-1304.

17. Andrews TC, Fenton T, Toyosaki N et al. For the Angina and Silent Ischemia Study Group (ASIS). Subsets of ambulatory myocardialischemiabased on heart rate activity: circadian distribution and response to anti-ischemic medication. *Circulation* 1993;88:1962-72.

18. Rehman A, Zalos G, Andrews NP, Mylcahy C, Quyymi AA. Blood pressure changes during transient myocardial ischemia: insights into mechanisms. *J Am Coll Cardiol* 1997;30:1249-1255.

19. Rozanski A, Bairey CN, Krantz DS et al. Mental stress and the induction of silent myocardial ischemia in patients with coronary artery disease. *N Engl J Med.* 1988;318:1005-1012.

20. Goldberg AD, Becker LC, Bonsall R et al. Ischemic, hemodynamic, and neurohormonal responses to mental and exercise stress. Experience from the Psychophysiological Investigations of Myocardial Ischemia Study (PIMI). *Circulation* 1996;94.

21. Blumenthal JA, Jiang W, Waugh RA et al. Mental stress-induced ischemia in the laboratory and ambulatory ischemia during daily life: association and hemodynamic features. *Circulation* 1995; 92:2102-8.

22. Kral GB, Becker LC, Blumenthal RS, Aversano T, Fleisher LA, Yook RM, Becker DM. Exaggerated reactivity to mental stress is associated with exercise-induced myocardial ischemia in an asymptomatic high-risk population. *Circulation* 1997;96:4246-53.

23. Rocco MB, Barry J, Campbell S et al. Circadian variation of transient myocardial ischemia in patients with coronary artery disease. *Circulation.* 1987;75:395-400.

24. Mulcahy D, Deegan J, Cunningham Jet al. Circadian variation of total ischemic burden and its alteration with anti-anginal agents. *Lancet* 1988;II:755-9.

25. Benhorin J, Banai S, Moriel M, Gavish A, Keren A, Stern S, Tzivoni D. Circadian variation in ischemic threshold and their relation to the occurrence od ischemic episodes. *Circulation* 1993;87:808-14.

26. Muller JE, Ludmer PL, Willich SN et al. Circadian variation in the frequency of sudden death. *Circulation* 1987;75:131-8.

27. Kranz DS, Kop WJ, Gabbay FH et al. Circadian variation of ambulatory myocardial ischemia: triggering by daily activities and evidence for an endogenous circadian component. *Circulation* 1996;93:1364-71.

28. Parker JD, Testa MA, Jimenez AH et al. Morning increase in ambulatory ischemia in patients with stable coronary artery disease: importance of physical activity and increased cardiac demand. *Circulation.* 1994;89:604-614.

29. Stern S., Gottlieb S. Silent myocardial ischemia in women. In: Julian DG, Wenger NK, eds. *Woman and Heart Disease.* London: Martin Dunitz; 1997:125-33.

30. Mulcahy D, Dakak N, Zalos G et al. Patterns and behavior of transient myocardial ischemia in stable coronary disease are the same in both men and women: a comparative study. *J Am Coll Cardiol* 1996;27:1629-36.
31. Vınola X, Guindo J, Rodriguez E, Bayes de Luna A. Sudden death and myocardial ischemia. In: Stern S, ed. *Silent Myocardial Ischemia*. London: Martin Dunitz; 1998:67-83.
32. Pepine CJ, Gottlieg SO, Morganroth J. Ambulatory ischemia and sudden death: analysis of 35 cases of sudden death during ambulatory ECG monitorying. *J Am Coll Cardiol* 1991;17:63-5.

24. CIRCADIAN VARIATION IN MYOCARDIAL ISCHEMIA AND INFARCTION

ARSHED A. QUYYUMI

Several cardiovascular phenomena including heart rate (1,2), blood pressure (3), premature ventricular contractions (4,5), sudden cardiac death (6), myocardial infarction (7), transient myocardial ischemia (1,2,5,8), and stroke are distributed unevenly according to the time of day. Understanding the pathophysiology of the morning preponderance of these vascular events will doubtless lead to development of successful strategies for prevention.

CIRCADIAN RHYTHM OF TRANSIENT MYOCARDIAL ISCHEMIA AND INFARCTION

Several studies demonstrate marked circadian variation in transient myocardial ischemia with a peak in the morning hours, sometimes a second evening peak, and a trough at night, a phenomenon observed in both men and women (9, Fig.1). Muller et als' demonstration of a circadian pattern of distribution of myocardial infarction by analysis of the time of first appearance of creatine kinase in the plasma in the MILIS study (Multicenter Investigation of Limitation of Infarct Size) confirmed previous smaller observations (6) (Fig. l) The distribution of myocardial infarctions was similar to that of transient ischemia with an estimated three times increased risk in the morning hours between 7 a.m. and noon compared to the late evening. When adjusted for the time of awakening in the Worcester Heart Attack study, 26% had onset of symptoms within the first two hours of awakening (lO). However, evidence is emerging that not all subgroups of patients with myocardial infarction have a preponderance of events in the morning hours; a lack of any peak was

H.-H. Osterhues et al. (eds.),
Advances in Noninvasive Electrocardiographic Monitoring Techniques, 247–261.
© 2000 *Kluwer Academic Publishers. Printed in the Netherlands.*

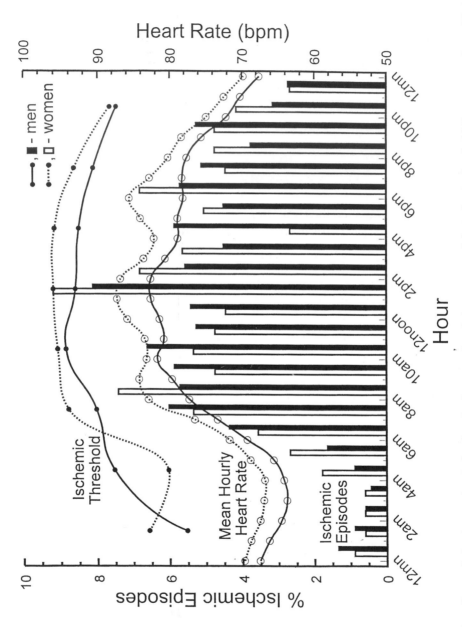

Figure 1. Circadian variation in transient ischemic episodes, mean hourly heart rate and the ischemic threshold (heart rate at 1 mm ST-depression) in men and women. Adapted from Ref. 9.

observed in those with previous infarction, two equal peaks in the morning and the late evening were noted in patients older than 70 years, smokers, diabetics, and in women. Finally, only a late evening peak was present in patients with non Q-wave myocardial infarction and those with congestive heart failure (11).

Ambulatory ST-segment monitoring in patients with stable coronary artery disease demonstrates that approximately a third have transient ischemic episodes during daily living, that more than 80% of these episodes are asymptomatic, that they are more frequent in those with severe disease, and in those with normal left ventricular function and preservation of the R-wave in the electrocardiogram (2).

PATHOPHYSIOLOGY OF TRANSIENT ISCHEMIA

There is a striking circadian variation in heart rate, blood pressure, and presumably contractility, measured indirectly from plasma catecholamine levels, that parallel the diurnal change in ischemia frequency (1-3,8) (Fig 2). In most ischemic episodes (80-90%), increases in myocardial oxygen demand, measured from heart rate and systolic blood pressure precede the development of ischemia during normal daily activities (12-16). Increases in heart rate may occur over a long period before ischemia occurs, although the major increase appears to occur in the immediate five minute period before ischemia (12,14).

The dramatic increase in ischemic activity between 7 and 8 a.m. appears to be triggered by awakening, arousal and activity, because allowing patients to arise later in the day delays the peak (17). Adjusting ischemic frequency to wake-up time shows that 24% of all episodes occur in the first 2-3 hours after awakening (8).

Apart from increases in myocardial oxygen demand, myocardial ischemia may be precipitated also by decreases in coronary blood flow. Limitation of myocardial blood supply is determined by the balance between the severity of the coronary stenosis and the state of the collateral circulation. There is overwhelming evidence that favors the role of coronary vasomotion and hence alteration in the caliber of the stenosis as a determinant for the variability in the ischemic threshold: for example, psychologic stress and exposure to cold are frequent environmental triggers for precipitation of myocardial ischemia at a lower rate-pressure product than during exercise (18,19). Variations in the heart rate ischemic threshold occur during ambulatory ST-segment monitoring; ischemia occurs not only during physical activities, but also during less intense circumstances such as eating, sleeping, or driving, and approximately 15% of episodes are not preceded by any increases in heart rate (12,14,16). A possible

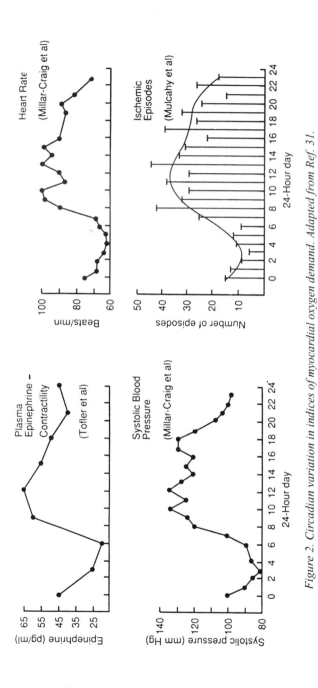

Figure 2. Circadian variation in indices of myocardial oxygen demand. Adapted from Ref. 31.

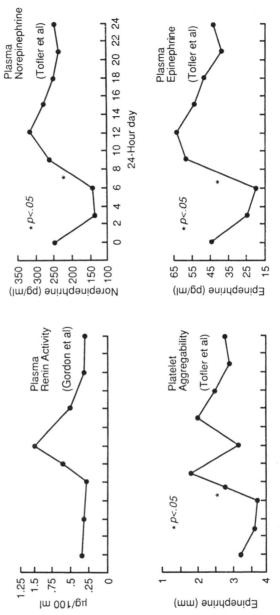

Figure 3. Circadian variation in plasma renin activity, plasma norepinephrine and epinephrine levels, and platelet aggregability. Adapted from Ref. 31.

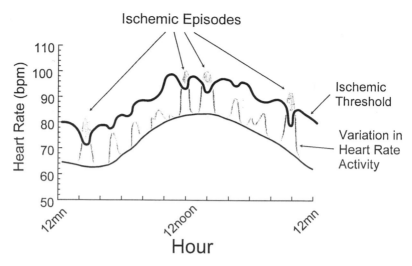

Figure 4. Proposed pattern and mechanisms of ischemia, showing circadian variation in basal heart rate, heart rate at onset of ischemia (ischemic threshold) and transient ischemic activity during both nocturnal and daytime hours. Adapted from Ref. 9.

explanation for these findings is that alterations in the caliber of the coronary arteries, particularly at the site of coronary narrowing may transiently lower coronary blood flow to such an extent that myocardial ischemia occurs with little or no change in myocardial oxygen demand.

There are systemic and local regulators of coronary and peripheral vasomotion that also have a circadian variation parralleling acute events (Fig 3). For example, catecholamine levels surge and the renin-angiotensin system is activated in the morning hours, triggered by assumption of upright posture and exercise (20,21). To investigate the possibility that the morning increase in myocardial ischemia is due not only to an increase in demand at that time, but also to an increase in coronary vasoconstrictor tone, patients were exercised four times during the day and the heart rate at onset of ST-segment depression (ischemic threshold) was measured (22). The ischemic threshold was lower in the morning and at night compared to other times of the day, a change that paralleled the simultaneous circadian variation in post-ischemic forearm vascular resistance, suggesting that there is a generalized circadian variation in coronary and peripheral vascular tone. Other studies support this concept; heart rate at onset of episodes of ischemia is significantly lower at night than it is during the day time (9,23) (Fig 1). Angiography demonstrated narrower coronary arteries in the morning (7 AM) in patients with normal coronary arteries than later in the day (24).

The contribution of sympathetic nervous system to this phenomenon has has been studied; norepinephrine-induced constriction through activation of a-1 and a-2 adrenoceptors in the human coronary circulation occurs with exercise, cold-pressor testing, and mental stress. Exercise-induced ST-segment depression, coronary flow during mental stress, and the morning increase in forearm vascular tone can be ameliorated by phentolamine, an alpha receptor antagonist (25,26). These observations may have immense therapeutic implications. Increase in exercise capacity has been reported in patients with stable coronary artery disease with an a-1 adrenergic antagonist, indoramin and further studies are warranted (27).

Figure 4 illustrates the potential mechanisms in the genesis of transient myocardial ischemia (9). The ischemic threshold is lower at night compared to the daytime as a result of the circadian variation in coronary vasomotor tone. The mean basal hourly heart rate also troughs at night, and thus the relative increase in heart rate required to produce ischemia is similar at nighttime compared with all other times of the day, despite the fact that the heart rate at which ischemia occurs is lower at night. This underscores the importance of heart rate increases in the genesis of ischemia throughout the 24 hour period, even allowing for variations in coronary tone. Additionally, every time there is an increase in heart rate, there is paradoxical vasoconstriction of the stenosis leading to a transient decrease in ischemic threshold. It appears, therefore, that constriction of stenotic coronary arteries and increases in myocardial oxygen demand occur simultaneously, and the considerable variation in heart rate threshold during different ischemic episodes may be accounted for by a variation in vasomotor tone.

PATHOPHYSIOLOGY OF MYOCARDIAL INFARCTION:

Myocardial infarction occurs as a result of thrombus formation over a ruptured or fissured atherosclerotic plaque (28). Moreover, this thrombus is more likely to develop at a site of mild atherosclerosis rather than over the most severe lesion (29). Thus, despite the parallel circadian distribution of myocardial infarction and transient myocardial ischemia, the pathophysiologic processes and the location of the responsible lesions in the coronary tree for these two events are often different.

Triggers of Myocardial Infarction

Factors that contribute to thrombus formation appear to be more prevalent in the morning hours (Fig. 3). Platelet aggregability increases after arousal and assumption of upright posture (30). Our studies demonstrate that this activation is at least partly secondary to the increase in catecholamine-mediated platelet

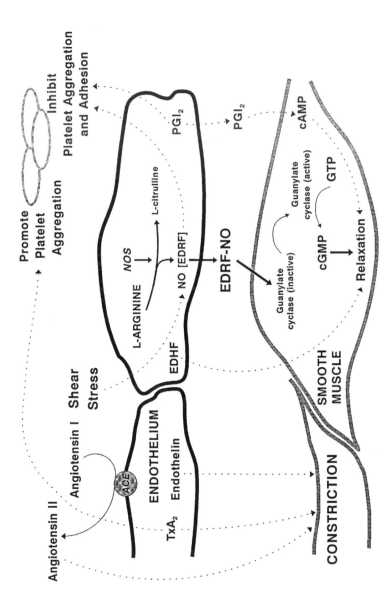

Figure 5. Factors causing endothelium-dependent vasomotion. A variety of endothelium and platelet-derived factors and shear stress can promote release of nitric oxide (NO) by stimulating nitric oxide synthase (NOS). Other dilating factors released include endothelium-derived hyperpolarizing factor (EDHF) and prostacyclin (PGI2). NO leads to relaxation by cyclic GMP (guanylate monophosphate)- dependent mechanism. PG12 causes relaxation of vascular smooth muscle cell by a cyclic AMP-dependent mechanism and both NO and PG12 inhibit platelet aggregation. Endothelium- and platelet-derived constricting factors causing smooth muscle constriction include angiotensin II, thromboxane A2 (TxA2) and endothelin. (ACE = angiotensin-converting enzyme, GTP = guanosine triphosphate, EDRF = endothelium-derived relaxing factor)

α2 receptor stimulation during assumption of upright posture. Blood fibrinolytic activity is lowest in the mornings largely due to low tissue plasminogen activator and high plasminogen activator inhibitor levels. Also blood viscosity is higher in the morning hours (31). Thus, a scenario can be constructed where the sudden sharp increase in blood pressure and heart rate on a background of increased vasoconstrictor tone in the mornings may so dramatically increase shear forces across atherosclerotic plaques, that a "vulnerable" plaque ruptures. The prothrombotic conditions prevailing during the morning hours allow propagation of the thrombus. Later in the day, when blood pressure is generally lower, the likelyhood of precipitating plaque rupture is also lowered, but in the event of plaque rupture, the propagation of thrombus may be impeded by the relative increase blood fibrinolytic activity. Investigators now hypothesize that physical or mental stress may often precipitate changes in blood pressure, heart rate, and vasoconstrictor tone which singly or together may cause a "vulnerable" atherosclerotic plaque to rupture (32). Recent evidence suggests that "vulnerable" plaques are usually lipid rich and not fibrotic. At the edge of the plaque, the relative deficiency of collagen and excess of collagenases and metalloproteinases predisposes the region to the ravages of shear stress and ultimately to cellular infiltration and plaque rupture.

External triggers for myocardial infarction have been studied extensively (33). Increased association of infarction, within a day or so, of extreme emotional stress has been reported. Between 4.5 and 7% of patients with infarction engaged in heavy physical exercise within the hour of onset of symptoms, often with pain starting during exercise. However, the risk of infarction with exertion was much higher in those who were sedentary and least in those who undertook exercise at least 5 times per week (34). Recent data also shows a marked peak in infarction in the winter months, with 53% more cases compared to summer, a finding observed in both men and women, in 5 of 10 geographic areas studied (35).

Vascular biology of Coronary Atherosclerosis
Understanding the nature of the injury to blood vessels in atherosclerosis that leads to plaque rupture and vasoconstriction during stress has evolved in recent years, with the realization that the endothelial layer regulates the vast majority of pathways in blood vessels. The endothelium is involved in the regulation of lipids, transport and permeability of solutes and fluids, participation in immune and inflammatory responses, control of cell growth and proliferation, and control of vascular smooth muscle tone and platelet function (36,37).

The endothelium regulates tone and platelet aggregation by releasing a variety of constricting and dilating substances (Figure 5). Constricting factors include arachidonic acid metabolites such as thromboxane A2, endoperoxidase, and a potent 21-amino acid peptide called endothelin. Additionally, the endothelium converts angiotensin I to angiotensin II by the membrane-bound angiotensin converting enzyme, that also metabolizes the endogenous endothelium-dependent vasodilator, bradykinin. Dilators from the endothelium include endothelium-derived relaxing factors (nitric oxide (NO) and endothelium-derived hyperpolarizing factor) and prostacyclin.

The role of constricting factors in the control of coronary vasomotor tone, their circadian variation, and their influence during physiologic stresses is poorly understood. NO, the most important and ubiquitous endothelium derived relaxing factor, is tonically produced in picomole quantities by the endothelium from L-arginine by the action of a constitutive calcium and calmodulin-dependent enzyme, nitric oxide synthase (36,37). NO is rapidly oxidized and inactivated by oxygen free radicals, an event that appears to be important in genesis of endothelial dysfunction. Tonically produced NO can be enhanced by shear stress and aggregating platelets. Other than its smooth muscle dilating action, NO also inhibits platelet aggregation (anti-thrombotic) and inhibits cell proliferation (anti-atherosclerotic) by inhibition of chemotaxis and expression of adhesion molecules.

In normal blood vessels, there is a balance between shear stress-induced endothelium- dependent relaxation and pressure or stretch-induced contraction (myogenic contraction). In patients with endothelial dysfunction (see below) the myogenic vasoconstriction would remain unopposed because of the deficient shear stress-induced release of NO, leading to constriction. Thus, in the morning hours, when vascular shear stress is increased because of increases in blood pressure and heart rate, atherosclerotic vessels are likely to constrict.

The term endothelial dysfunction refers to an inbalance between contracting and relaxing factors, between pro- and anticoagulant mediators, or between growth promoting and growth inhibiting factors. Endothelial function is impaired in patients with a variety of cardiovascular risk factors, including smoking, hypercholesterolemia, hypertension, especially in patients with left ventricular hypertrophy, diabetes and in heart failure are also accompanied by depressed endothelium-dependent vasodilation (40-42). Exposure to multiple risk factors can compound the injury to the endothelium.

Over the long-term, reduced activity of NO in the vascular wall may promote the atherogenic process. Animals on atherogenic diets and inhibitors of endothelial production of NO had significantly more rapid development of intimal thickening than those fed high cholesterol diet alone, suggesting that endothelium-derived NO prevents the development and progression of atherosclerosis (43).

Therapeutic Implications

Studies in patients with myocardial infarction have demonstrated that patients who wcrc on bcta adrenergic antagonists had an absence of the peak in myocardial infarction episodes in the morning hours (44). A similar blunting of the morning peak in myocardial infarction was observed in patients treated with aspirin (45). However, patients on calcium antagonists did not have abolition of the morning increase in myocardial infarction frequency (44). The protective value of beta blockers in reducing mortality and reinfarction after myocardial infarction has been well established (46). Whether the observed abolition of the morning increase in first myocardial infarction with beta receptor antagonists is representative of a true decrease in frequency of myocardial infarction remains to be proven. *Transient ischemia:* Beta adrenergic recieptor antagonists are able to efficiently abolish the morning increase in transient myocardial ischemia, a finding that is common to most agents without intrinsic sympathomimetic activity (1). Short-acting dihydropyridine calcium antagonists (nifedipine) fail to abolish the morning peak, however, there is blunting of the morning increase with diltiazem, long-acting nifedipine, and with verapamil (47-49).

The circadian nature of transient myocardial ischemia emphasizes the importance of 24- hour protection in patients with long-acting anti-anginal agents. It appears that agents providing chronotropic control are the most effective in attenuating myocardial ischemia. *Drugs to improve vascular function:* Treating endothelial dysfunction to stabilize the vessel wall in atherosclerotic patients and thus reduce the risk of future thrombotic events and progression has enormous potential. These approaches include tissue plasminogen activator, stable analogs of prostacyclin, NO donors such as nitroglycerin or nitroprusside that yield NO directly in smooth muscles or in the platelets. L-arginine, the substrate for endothelial NO synthesis can reverse the abnormal endothelium-dependent responses in hypercholesterolemia, heart failure, and atherosclerosis. Angiotensin converting enzyme inhibitors that antagonize vascular constriction from angiotensin II and increase bradykinin-dependent, endothelium-mediated relaxation have recently been demonstrated to reduce thrombotic events in patients with coronary artery disease and left ventricular dysfunction and also improve endothelial dysfunction (52). Increased oxidant stress in the vessel wall may be responsible for the reduced activity of NO in certain pathologic conditions (53). Antioxidants such as superoxide dismutase, oxypurinol, and vitamins C and E are being investigated as potential ways of reversing the endothelial dysfunction.

Finally, cholesterol-lowering agents, known to dramatically reduce mortality in patients with hypercholesterolemia and atherosclerosis also improve endothelial dysfunction (54). Plaque stabilization may be an important explanation for their beneficial effects, because the degree of regression in atherosclerotic lesions is negligible.

Thus, understanding the physiology and pathophysiologic role of the vascular endothelium as a modulator of smooth muscle vasomotion, intravascular thrombosis, and intimal growth, will greatly enhance future possibilities for treatment of the atherosclerotic process, and help reduce the incidence of catastrophic coronary events.

REFERENCES

1. Mulcahy D, Keegan J, Cunningham D, et al. Circadian variation of total ischaemic burden and its alteration with antianginal agents. Lancet 1988; ii: 755-59.
2. Quyyumi AA, Mockus L, Wright C, Fox KM. Morphology of ambulatory ST-segment changes in patients with varying severity of coronary artery disease: investigation of the frequency of nocturnal ischaemia and coronary spasm. Br Heart J 1985; 53: 186-93.
3. Millar-Craig MW, Bishop CN, Raftery EB. Circadian variation of blood pressure. Lancet 1978; I: 795-97.
4. Raeder EA, Hohnloser SH, Graboys TB, Podrid P, Lampert S, Lown B. Spontaneous variability and circadian distribution of ectopic activity in patients with malignant ventricular arrhythmia. J Am Coll Cardiol 1988; 12:656-61.
5. Lampert R, Rosenfeld L, Batsford W, Lee F, McPherson C. Circadian variation of sustained ventricular tachycardia in patients with coronary artery disease and implantable cardioverter defibrillators. Circulation 1994; 90: 241-47.
6. Muller JE, Ludmer PL, Willich SN, et al. Circadian variation in the frequency of sudden cardiac death. Circulation 1987; 75: 131 -38.
7. Muller JE, Stone PH, Turi ZG, et al. Circadian variation in the frequency of onset of acute myocardial infarction. N Eng J Med 1985; 313: 1315-22.
8. Rocco MB, Barry J, Campbell S, et al. Circadian variation of transient myocardial ischemia in patients with coronary artery disease. Circulation 1987; 75: 395-400.
9. Mulcahy D, Dakak N, Zalos G, Andrews NP, Proschan M, Waclawiw MA, Schenke WH, Quyyumi AA. Patterns and underlying mechanisms of transient myocardial ischemia in stable coronary artery disease are the same in both sexes: a comparative study. J Am Coll Cardiol 1996;27: 1629-36.
10. Willich SN, Lowel H, Lewis M, Amtz R, Baur R, Winther K, Keil U, Schroder R, and TRIMM Study Group. Association of wake time and the onset of myocardial infarction. Circulation 1991 ;84[suppl VI] :VI-62-VI-67.
11. Hjalmarson A, Gilpin EA, Nicod P et al. Differing circadian patterns of symptom onset in subgroups of patients with acute myocardial infarction. Circulation 1989; 80:267-275.
12. Panza JA, Diodati JG, Callahan TS, Epstein SE, Quyyumi AA. Role of increases in heart rate in determining the occurrence and frequency of myocardial ischemia during daily life in patients with stable coronary artery disease. J Am Coll Cardiol 1992; 20: 1092-98.

13. Deedwania PC, Nelson JR. Pathophysiology of silent myocardial ischemia during daily life: hemodynamic evaluation by simultaneous electrocardiographic and blood pressure monitoring. Circulation 1990; 82: 1296-1304.
14. McLenachan JM, Weidinger FF, Barry J, et al. Relations between heart rate, ischemia, and drug therapy during daily life in patients with coronary artery disease. Circulation 1991; 83: 1263-70.
15. Quyyumi AA, Wright C, Mockus LJ, Fox KM. Mechanisms of noctumal angina pectoris: importance of increased myocardial oxygen demand in patients with severe coronary artery disease. Lancet 1984; 2: 1207-9.
16. Andrews TC, Fenton T, Toyosaki N, et al. Subsets of ambulatory myocardial ischemia based on heart rate activity: circadian distribution and response to anti-ischemic medications. Circulation 1993; 88: 92-100.
17. Parker JD, Testa MA, Jimenez AH, et al. Moming increase in ambulatory ischemia in patients with stable coronary artery disease. Importance of physical activity and increased cardiac demand. Circulation 1994; 89: 604-14.
18. Deanfield JE, Selwyn AP, Chierchia S, et al. Myocardial ischaemia during daily life in patients with stable angina: its relation to symptoms and heart rate changes. Lancet 1983; I: 753-58.
19. Rozanski A, Bairey N, Krantz DS, et al. Mental stress and induction of silent myocardial ischemia in patients with coronary artery disease. N Eng J Med 1988; 318: 1005-12
20. Turton MB, Deegan T. Circadian variations of plasma catecholamine, cortisol, and immunoreactive insulin concentrations in supine subjects. Clin Chim Acta 1974; 55: 389-97.
21. Gordon RD, Wolfe LK, Island DP, Liddle GW. A diumal rhythm in plasma renin activity in man. J Clin Invest 1966; 45: 1587-92.
22. Quyyumi AA, Panza JA, Diodati JG, Lakatos E, Epstein SE. Circadian variation in ischemic threshold. A mechanism underlying the circadian variation in ischemic events. Circulation 1992; 86: 22-28.
23. Benhorin J, Banai S, Moriel M, et al. Circadian variation in ischemic threshold and their relation to the occurrence of ischemic episodes. Circulation 1993; 87: 808-14.
24. Yasue H, Omote S, Takizawaw A, Nagao M, Miwa K, Tanaka S. Circadian variation of exercise capacity in patients with Prinzmetals variant angina: role of exercise-induced coronary arterial spasm. Circulation 1979; 59: 938-48.
25. Berkenboom GM, Abramowicz M, Vandermoten P, Degre SG. Role of alpha-adrenergic coronary tone in exercise-induced angina pectoris. Am J Cardiol 1986; 57: 195-198.
26. Dakak N, Quyyumi AA, Eisenhoffer G, Goldstein DS, Cannon RO III. Sympathetically-mediated effects of mental stress on cardiac microcirculation of patients with coronary artery disease. Am J Cardiol 1995;76:125-130
27. Collins P, Sheridan D. Improvement in angina pectoris with alpha adrenoceptor blockade. Br Heart J 1985; 53: 488-492.
28. Davies MJ, Thomas AC: Thrombosis and acute coronary artery lesions in sudden cardiac ischemic death. N Engl J Med 1984:310: 1137-1140.
29. Little WC, Constatinescu MS, Applegate RJ, et al. Can coronary angiography predict the site of subsequent myocardial infarction in patients with mild-to-moderate coronary artery disease? Circulation 1988; 78: 1157-66.

30. Brezinski DA, Tofler GH, Muller JE, et al. Moming increase in platelet aggregability: Association with assumption of the upright posture. Circulation 1988; 78: 35-40.

31. Quyyumi AA, Circadian rhythms in cardiovascular disease. Am Heart J 1990; 120: 726-33.

32. Muller JE, Tofler GH, Stone PH. Circadian variation and trigger of onset of acute cardiovascular disease. Circulation 1989; 79:733-743.

33. Willich SN, Lewis M, Lowel H, Amiz HR, Schubert F, Schroder R. Physical exertion as a trigger of acute myocardial infarction. N Eng J Med 1993;328: 1686- 1690.

34. Mittleman MA, Maclure M, Tofler GH, Sherwood JB, Goldberg RJ, Muller JE. Triggering of acute myocardial infarction by heavy physical exertion. N Eng J of Med 1993 329:1677-83.

35. Spencer FA, Goldberg RJ, Becker RC, Gore JM. Seasonal distribution of acute myocardial infarction in the second national registry of myocardial infarction. J Am Coll Cardiol 1998;31:1226-33.

36. Snyder SH, Bredt DS. Biological roles of nitric oxide. Sci Am 1992; 266: 68-71, 74-7.

37. Moncada S, Higgs A. The L-arginine-nitric oxide pathway. N Eng J Med 1993; 329: 2002-12.

38. Dzau VJ. Vascular wall renin angiotensin pathway in control of the circulation. Am J Med 1984; 77: 31-6.

39. Vanhoutte PM, Shimokawa H. Endothelium-derived relaxing factor and coronary vasospasm. Circulation 1989; 80: l-9.

40. Vita JA, Treasure CB, Nabel EG, et al. Coronary vasomotor response to acetylcholine relates to risk factors for coronary artery disease. Circulation 1990;81 :494-7.

41. Quyyumi AA, Dakak N, Andrews NP, Husain S, Arora S, Gilligan DM, Panza JA, Cannon RO m. Nitric oxide activity in the human coronary circulation: Impact of risk factors for coronary atherosclerosis. J Clin Invest 1995;95: 1747-1755.

42. Quyyumi AA, Mulcahy D, Andrews NP, Husain S, Panza JA, Cannon RO m. Coronary vascular nitric oxide activity in hypertension and hypercholesterolemia: comparison of acetylcholine and substance P. Circulation 1997;95:104-110.

43. Garg UC, Hassid A. Nitric oxide-generating vasodilators and 8-bromo-cyclic guanosine monophosphate inhibit mitogenesis and proliferation of cultured rat vascular smooth muscle cells. J Clin Invest 1989; 83: 1774-1777.

44. Willich SN, Linderer T, Wegscheider K, Leizorowicz A, Alamercery I, Schroder R. Increased morning incidence of myocardial infarction in the ISAM study: absence with prior beta-adrenergic blockade. Circulation 1989; 80: 853-58.

45. Kidker PM, Manson JE, Buring JE, Muller JE, Hennekens CH. Circadian variation of acute myocardial infarction and the effect of low-dose aspirin in a randomized trial of physicianss. Circulation 1990;82:897-902.

46. Yusuf S, Peto R, Lewis J et al. Beta blockade during and after myocardial infarction: an overview of the randomized trials. Prog Cardiovasc Dis 1985; 27: 335-371.

47. Quyyumi AA, Crake T, Wright CM, Mockus LJ, Fox KM. Medical treatment of patients with severe exertional and rest angina: double blind comparison of B blocker, calcium antagonist, and nitrate. Br Heart J 1987; 57: 505- 11.

48. Parmley WW, Nesto RW, Singh BN, Deanfield J, Gottlieb SO, N-CAP Study Group. Attenuation of the circadian patterns o myocardial ischemia with nifedipine GITS in patients with chronic stable angina. J Am Coll Cardiol 1992;19:1380-9.

49. Stone PH, Gibson RS, Glasser SP, DeWood MA, Parker JD, Kawanishi DT, Crawford MH, Messineo FC, Shook TL, Raby K, Curtis DG, Hoop RS, Young PM, Braunwald E, ASIS Study Group. Comparison of propranolol, diltiazem, and nifedipine in the treatment of ambulation ischemia in patients with stable angina: differential effects on ambulatory ischemia, exercise performance, and anginal symptoms. Circulation 1990;82: 1962-1972.

50. Drexler H, Zeiher AM, Meinertz T, Just H. Correction of endothelial dysfunction in coronary microcirculation of hypercholesterolemic patients by L-arginine. Lancet 1991; 338: 1546-50.

51. Quyyumi AA, Dakak N, Diodati J, Gilligan DM, Panza JA, Cannon RO m. Effect of L-arginine on human coronary endothelium-dependent and physiologic vasodilation. J Am Coll Cardiol 1997;30: 1220-7

52. Mancini GBJ, Henry GC, Macaya C, O'Neill BJ, Pucillo AL, Carere RG, Wargovich TJ, Mudra H, L• scher TF, Klibaner MI, Haber HE, Uprichard ACG, Pepine CJ, Pitt B. Angiotensin-converting enzyme inhibition with quinapril improves endothelial vasomotor dysfunction in patients with coronary artery disease: the TREND (Trial on Reversing ENdothelial Dysfunction) Study. Circulation 1996;94:258-265.

53. Minor RL Jr, Myers PR, Guerra R Jr, Bates JN, Harrison DG: Diet-induced atherosclerosis increases the release of nitrogen oxides from rabbit aorta. J Clin Invest 1990;86:2109-2116.

54. Scandinavian Simvistatin Survival Study Group. Randomized trial of cholesterol lowering in 4444 patients with coronary heart disease: the Scandinavian Simvistatin Survival Study (4S). Lancet 1994; 344: 1383-89.

25. CHRONOPHARMACOLOGY - IMPLICATIONS FOR DIAGNOSIS AND TREATMENT

BJÖRN LEMMER

INTRODUCTION

Circadian rhythms have been documented throughout the plant and animal kingdom at every level of eukariotic organization. Circadian rhythms are endogenous in nature, driven by oscillators or clocks (Aschoff 1963), and persist under free-running (e.g. constant darkness) conditions. The genes expressing the biological clock have been identified in various species (*Drosophila melongaster, Neurospora, Mouse, Golden hamster*). The endogenous clock in man does not exactly runs at a frequency of 24 hours but somewhat slower, environmental Zeitgebers (Aschoff 1965) such as the alternation of light and darkness entrain the circadian rhythm to a precise 24-hour period. The important feature of endogeneous biological rhythms is their anticipatory character. Thus, rhythmicity inherent to all living systems, allows them to adapt more easily and to better survive under changing environmental conditions during the 24 hours of a day as well as during varying conditions of the changing seasons.

Day-night variations in heart rate and/or blood pressure have already been described since the 17th century (see Lemmer 1996a,b), the recent development of easy-to-use devices to continuously monitor blood pressure and heart rate in man (ABPM = ambulatory blood pressure monitoring) demonstrated that blood pressure in normotensive and in hypertensive patients are clearly dependent on the time of day (see Lemmer 1996a). Different forms of hypertension may exhibit different circadian patterns: In normotension as well as in primary hy-

H.-H. Osterhues et al. (eds.),
Advances in Noninvasive Electrocardiographic Monitoring Techniques, 263–278.
© 2000 *Kluwer Academic Publishers. Printed in the Netherlands.*

Biological Rhythms and Pharmacokinetics

[oral drug application]

Liberation	Absorption GI-Tract	Distribution	Metabolism Liver	Elimination Kidney
{Time-specified release programmable}	Perfusion	Perfusion	Perfusion	Perfusion
	Gastric pH	Blood Distribution	First-Pass-Effect	Renal Plasmaflow
	Acid Secretion	Periph. Resistance		Glom. Filtration
	Motility	Blood Cells	(Enzyme Activity)	Urine Excretion
	Gastric Emptying	Serum Proteines		Urine pH
		Protein Binding		Electrolytes
	Rest - Activity	Rest - Activity		

Figure 1. Biological rhythms and pharmacokinetics (From Lemmer 1997).

pertension there is in general a nightly drop in blood pressure, those patients are called "dippers" (see Figure 3). In secondary hypertension due to e.g. renal disease, gestation, Cushing's disease, the rhythm in blood pressure is in about 70% of the cases abolished or even reversed with highest values at night ("non-dippers"; Cugini et al. 1989; Middeke and Schrader 1994; Lemmer 1995, 1996b; for review see Lemmer and Portaluppi 1997). This is of particular interest since the loss in nocturnal blood pressure fall (non-dippers) correlates with increased end organ damage in cardiac, cerebral, vascular and renal tissues (Verdecchia et al., 1990; see Lemmer and Portaluppi 1997).

The rhythms in heart rate and blood pressure are the best-known periodic functions in the cardiovascular system, however, other parameters have been shown to exhibit circadian variations as well, e.g. stroke volume, cardiac output, blood flow, peripheral resistance, parameters of ECG recordings, in the plasma concentrations of pressor hormones such as noradrenaline, renin, angiotensin, aldosterone, in atrial natriuretic hormone and plasma cAMP concentration, in blood viscosity, aggregability and fibrinolytic activity, etc (Lemmer 1989, 1996b; Lemmer and Portaluppi 1997). These observations clearly demonstrate that all parts of the cardiovascular system are highly organized in time, including the 24 hours of a day.

RHYTHMS IN CARDIOVASCULAR EVENTS

Pathophysiological events within the cardiovascular system do also not occur at random (for review see Willich and Muller 1996; Lemmer and Portaluppi 1997). Thus, the onset of non-fatal or fatal myocardial infarction predominates around 08.00h - 12.00h. A similar circadian time pattern has been shown for sudden cardiac death, stroke, ventricular arrhythmias and arterial embolism. Symptoms in coronary heart diseased patients such as myocardial ischemia, angina attacks or silent ischemia are also significantly more frequent during the daytime hours than at night, whereas the onset of angina attacks in variant angina peaks around 04.00h during the night (Lemmer, 1989, 1996b).

During the early morning hours not only cardiovascular events predominate but there is also the rapid rise in blood pressure, a rapid increase in sympathetic tone and in the concentrations of pressor hormones and the highest values in peripheral resistance (see Lemmer 1996b). Interestingly, patients suffering from office hypertension have a steeper increase in the early morning rise in systolic blood pressure together with a higher excretion of catecholamines (Middeke and Lemmer, 1996). Thus, it appears that the early morning hours are the **hours of highest cardiovascular risk**.

Drug	Dose [mg] & duration	Cmax [ng/ml] Morning	Cmax [ng/ml] Evening	tmax [h] Morning	tmax [h] Evening	References
Digoxin	0.5, sd	3.6*	1.8	1.2	3.2	Bruguerolle et al., 1988
Enalaprilat						
Enalapril	10, sd	33.8	41.9	4.4	4.5	Witte et al., 1993
Enalapril	10, 3w	46.7	53.5	3.5*	5.6	
IS-5-MN i.r.	60, sd	1605.0	1588.0	0.9*	2.1	Scheidel & Lemmer, 1991
IS-5-MN s.r.	60, sd	509.0	530.0	5.2	4.9	Lemmer et al., 1991a
Molsidomine	8, sd	27.0	23.5	1.7	1.9	Nold & Lemmer, 1998
Nifedipine i.r.	10, sd	82.0*	45.7	0.4*	0.6	Lemmer et al., 1991b,c
Nifedipine s.r.	2x20, 1w	48.5	50.1	2.3	2.8	Lemmer et al., 1991b,c
Oxprenolol[a]	80, sd	507.0	375.0	1.0	1.1	Koopmans et al., 1993
Propranolol	80, sd	38.6*	26.2	2.5	3.0	Langner & Lemmer, 1988
Verapamil s.r.	360, 2w	389.0	386.0	7.2*	10.6	Jespersen et al., 1989
Verapamil	80, sd	59.4*	25.6	1.3	2.0	Hla et al., 1992

Table 1. Pharmacokinetic parameters of some cardiovascular active drugs determined in cross-over studies. At least two dosing times (around 6.00-8.00h and 18.00-20.00h) were studied, sometimes up to 6 circadian times were included. Only the parameters Cmax = peak drug concentration, and tmax = time-to-Cmax, are given. sd = single dose, w = week s , i.r. = immediate-release preparation, s.r. = sustained-release preparation. *p morning versus evening at least <0.05; [a] significant difference in half-life.

CHRONOPHARMACOLOGY OF HYPERTENSION

Having in mind the organization in time of living systems including man it is easy to conceive that not only must the *right* amount of the *right* substance be at the *right* place, but also this must occur at the *right* time. This is the more important when an organism or individual itself has to act or react in favorable biotic or environmental conditions which by themselves are highly periodic. Thus, it is easy to understand that exogenous compounds including drugs may differently challenge the individual depending on the *time* of exposition.

Drug treament of hypertension includes various types of drugs such as diuretics, β- and α-adrenoceptor blocking drugs, calcium channel blockers, converting enzyme inhibitors, AT_1-receptor blockers and others which differ in their sites of action. Since the main steps in the mechanisms regulating the blood pressure are circadian phase-dependent it is not a surprise that also antihypertensive drugs may display a circadian time-dependency in their effects and/or their pharmacokinetics (Lemmer and Bruguerolle 1994; Table 1).

Pharmacokinetics deals with absorption, distribution, metabolism and elimination of drugs. The different steps in pharmacokinetics are determined and influenced by physiological functions of the body. Pharmacokinetic parameters such as peak drug concentration [Cmax], time-to-Cmax [tmax], volume of distribution [Vd], area under the curve [AUC], bioavailability, plasma protein binding and elimination half-life [t½] are conventionally *not* considered to be influenced by the time of day at which a drug is administered. However, an increasing number of recently published studies convincingly gave evidence that this paradigm may not be unanimously correct (see Lemmer and Bruguerolle 1994) since bodily functions, including those which are known to influence the pharmacokinetics, are not constant in time, even not within 24-hours of a day as described above. In Figure 1 main biological rhythms in bodily functions are shown which may influence the kinetics of drugs. In addition, these drugs differ in their half-life, galenic formulations and, thus, in dosing interval. Despite of the great number of studies published in evaluating antihypertensive drug efficacy the time of day of drug application was only scarcely a specific point of investigation.

BETA-ADRENOCEPTOR BLOCKING DRUGS

In hypertensive patients no morning versus evening cross-over study with β-adrenoceptor antagonists has been published. From studies performed without time specified drug dosing it is difficult to draw definite conclusions on the

Drug	Dose mg/d	Duration Dosing time	Patients (n) Diagnose	Effect on 24-h Blood Pressure Day	Night	24h-Profile	Reference
Amlodipine	5	4 wks - a.m. - p.m.	20, EH	++ ++	++ ++	preserved preserved	Mengden et al., 1992
Amlodipine	5	3 wks - 08.00 - 20.00	12, EH	+ +	+ +	preserved preserved	Nold et al., 1998
Isradipine	5	4 wks - 07.00h - 19.00h	18, EH	++ ++	++ ++	preserved preserved	Fogari et al., 1993
Nifedipine GITS	30	1 or 2 wks - 10.00h - 22.00h	10, EH	++ ++	++ ++	preserved preserved	Greminger et al., 1994
Nitrendipine	20	4 wks - 07.00h - 19.00h	41, EH	+ +	+ +	preserved preserved	Meilhac et al., 1992
Nitrendipine	10	3 days - 06.00h - 18.00h	6, EH	++ +	++ ++	preserved changed	Umeda et al., 1994
Isradipine	5	4 wks - 08.00h - 20.00h	16, RH[a]	++ +	++ +++	not normalised normalised	Portaluppi et al., 1995
Nifedipine i.r.	10	single dose - 08.00h - 19.00h	12, NT	+ +	++ +	preserved preserved	Lemmer et al., 1991c

Table 2. Effects of calcium channel blockers on the 24-hour pattern in blood pressure. Table includes only data from cross-over studies. EH = essential (primary) hypertensives, RH = renal (secondary) hypertensives, NT = normotensives. [a] = abolished 24-hour blood pressure profile .

Drug	Dose		Patients (n) Diagnose	Effect on 24-h Blood Pressure			Reference
	mg/d	Duration Dosing time		Day	Night	24h-Profile	
Benazepril	10	single dose - 09.00h - 21.00h	10, EH	+++ +	++ ++	preserved changed	Palatini et al., 1993
Enalapril	10	single dose - 07.00h - 19.00h	10, EH	++ ++	+ +++	preserved changed	Witte et al., 1993
		3 wks - 07.00h - 19.00h		++ +	+ ++	preserved changed	
Quinapril	20	4 wks - 08.00h - 22.00h	18, EH	++ ++	+ ++	preserved preserved	Palatini et al., 1992
Ramipril	2.5	4 wks - 08.00h -20.00h	33, EH	+ (+)	(+) +	preserved preserved	Myburgh et al. 1995
Perindopril	2	4 wks - 09.00h - 21.00h	18, EH	++ +	+ ++	preserved changed	Morgan et al. 1997

Table 3. Effects of ACE inhibitors on the 24-hour pattern in blood pressure. Table includes only data from cross-over studies. EH = essential (primary) hypertensives.

importance of the circadian time of drug dosing for the antihypertensive drug efficacy. A resume of 20 „conventionally" performed studies (Stanton and O'Brien 1994) showed that β-adrenoceptor antagonists do either not affect or reduce or even abolish the rhythmic pattern in blood pressure. In general, however, there is a tendency for β-adrenoceptor antagonists to predominately reduce daytime blood pressure levels and not to greatly affect night-time values, being less/not effective in reducing the early morning rise in blood pressure. Consistently, the decrease in heart rate by β-adrenoceptor antagonists is more pronounced during daytime hours. In healthy subjects a cross-over study with propranolol similarly showed a more pronounced decrease in heart rate and blood pressure during daytime hours than at night (Langner and Lemmer 1988). Interestingly, the agent with partial agonist activity, pindolol, even increase heart rate at night (Quyyumi et al. 1984).

In conclusion, clinical data indicate that β-adrenoceptor mediated regulation of blood pressure dominates during daytime hours and is of less or minor importance during the night and the early morning hours.

CALCIUM CHANNEL BLOCKERS

The effects of calcium channel blockers were also analysed mainly by visual inspection of the blood pressure profiles. In primary hypertensives, t.i.d. dosing of non-retarded verapamil did not greatly change the blood pressure profile being, however, less effective at night (Gould et al. 1982). A single morning dose of a sustained-release verapamil showed a good 24-hour blood pressure control (Jespersen et al. 1989), whereas a sustained-release formulation of diltiazem was less effective at night (Lemmer et al. 1994). Dihydropyridine derivatives, differing in pharmacokinetics, seem to reduce blood pressure to a varying degree during day and night, however, drug formulation and dosing interval may play an additional role. Eight studies with calcium channel blockers using a cross-over design have been published (Table 2). In essential hypertensive patients drugs such as amlodipine, isradipine and nifedipine GITS and in normotensives immediate-release nifedipine did not differently affect the 24-h blood pressure profile after once morning or once evening dosing, whereas with nitrendipine the profile remained unaffected or slightly changed after evening dosing (Table 2). In primary hypertensive patients twice-daily nifedipine was also able to lower the blood pressure throughout a 24-hour period (Lemmer et al. 1991b,c). Most interestingly, the greatly disturbed blood pressure profile in non-dippers due to renal failure was only normalised, i.e. transformed into dippers, after evening but not after morning dosing of isradipine (Portaluppi et al. 1995).

A time-of-day effect was also described for the kinetics of various calcium channel blockers (see Table 1). However, the BP lowering effect seems not to be greatly dependent from the drugs` chronopharmacokinetics.

CONVERTING ENZYME INHIBITORS

Five cross-over studies (morning vs evening dosing) with single-daily dosing of converting enzyme inhibitors in essential hypertensive patients were published (Table 3). They demonstrate that evening dosing in contrast to morning dosing of benazepril, enalapril and perindopril resulted in a more pronounced nightly drop and the 24-h BP profile was distorted by evening enalapril. Evening dosing of quinapril also resulted in a more pronounced effect than morning dosing, the BP pattern, however, was not greatly modified. In the light of a reduced cardiac reserve of patients with hypertension at risk (Perloff et al. 1983; Pringle et al. 1992) a too a pronounced nightly drop in BP after evening dosing might be a potential risk factor for the occurrence of ischemic events (Mancia 1993).

A circadian phase-dependency was also described for the kinetics of the ACE-inhibitor enalapril (Table 1). As already described for other antihypertensive drugs the chronokinetics of the active metabolite of enalapril, enalaprilat, does not seem to be of importance for the daily variation in the drug's antihypertensive effects (Witte et al. 1993).

DURATION OF THE ANTIHYPERTENSIVE EFFECT

Ambulatory blood pressure monitoring has been widely used to evaluate the duration of action of antihypertensive drugs. In general, ABPM is performed for a single 24 hour span. However, the restriction of ABPM to 24 hours may cause potential pitfalls as can be demonstrated from several studies: A four weeks treatment of hypertensive patients with the $beta_1$-selective adrenoceptor blocking drug bisoprolol showed that the duration persisted up to 48 hours after cessation of therapy (Asmar et al. 1987). Similarly, after chronic morning dosing of the β-adrenoceptor blocking drug atenolol the BP lowering effect was no longer observed 20-24 hours after the last dose (Figure 2). However, ABPM being continued for 48 hours revealed that the reduction in BP was observed again on the next day off therapy (Figure 2; Gould and Raftery 1991). About the same findings were reported after a 3 weeks once-a-day morning or once-a-day evening administration of the ACE-inhibitor enalapril when the BP profile was monitored for 48 hours after the last dose (Figure 3; Witte et al.

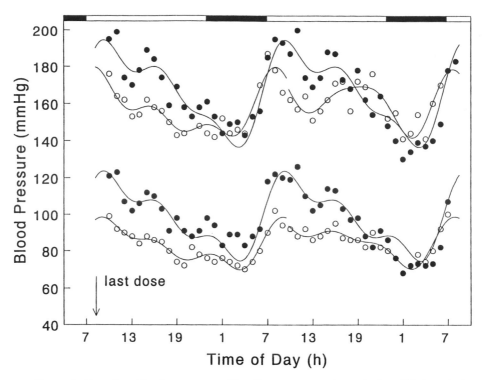

Figure 2. Circadian blood pressure profile of hypertensive patients before (filled circles) and after once-a-day treatment with atenolol (100 mg/d) for 6 weeks (open circles). (a) Ambulatory blood pressure data during last day of treatment, (b) 48-hour ambulatory blood pressure data after last dose. Note the convergence of blood pressure data curves at night and separation again during day 2. Data from (Gould and Raftery 1991) were submitted to a non-linear rhythm analysis by ABPM-FIT (Zuther et al. 1996) and redrawn accordingly (from Lemmer 1997).

1993). Conversely, the duration of the antihypertensive effect of a three weeks treatment with a sustained-release preparation of diltiazem, was restricted to about 18 hours when the BP was monitored by ABPM for 48 hours after the last dose (Lemmer et al. 1994).

These data show that the conventional method to estimate the duration of an antihypertensive effect by the peak-to-trough-ratio within 24 hours can be misleading. The peak-to-trough-ratio does not consider that regulatory mechanisms of the blood pressure rhythm predominate at certain times of day and are of minor importance at other times (see Lemmer, 1996a). β-Adrenergic tone, e.g. is higher during the daytime activity phase than at night; β-adenoceptor blockers are therefore less active at night (see above). Panza et al. (1991) showed that the vascular tone is higher in the morning and decreases thereafter leading to a more pronounced reduction of the peripheral resistance by the α-

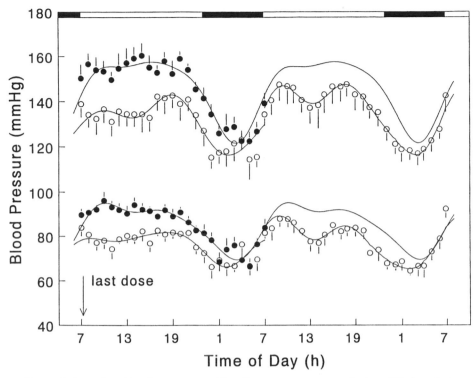

Figure 3. Circadian blood pressure profile of hypertensive patients before (filled circles) and after once-a-day morning treatment with enalapril (10mg/d) for 3 weeks (open circles). (a) Ambulatory blood pressure data on the last day of treatment, (b) 48-hour ambulatory blood pressure data after last dose. Note that the antihypertensive effect reappears again on the second day off therapy. Solid lines represent nonlinear fitting of ABPM data to partial Fourier series (Zuther et al. 1996), data from (Witte et al. 1993) (from Lemmer 1997).

adrenoceptor blocking drug phentolamine in the morning than at other times of day. As a consequence it may be worthwhile to not restrict the ABPM to a 24h span in order to avoid false conclusions on the duration of action of an antihypertensive drug.

CONCLUSION

Various functions of the cardiovascular system, including the blood pressure and heart rate, are well organized in time. There is also good evidence that a disease is able to disturb, reverse or even destroy a rhythmic pattern. At least in the rat the rhythms in systolic and diastolic blood pressures are mainly endogenous in nature, i.e. driven by an internal pacemaker (Lemmer et al. 1993; Witte and Lemmer 1995), such data is lacking for humans.

Moreover, it has been shown that different cardiovascular active compounds such as propranolol, oral nitrates and the calcium channel blocker nifedipine can display higher peak drug concentrations (Cmax) and/or a shorter time-to-peak concentration (tmax) after morning than evening oral drug dosing, at least when non-retarded formulations were used. In the case of sustained-release formulation of IS-5-MN and nifedipine, however, no circadian phase-dependency in their pharmacokinetics were found (Table 1). Since these drugs are mainly absorbed by passive diffusion the underlying mechanisms responsible for their chronokinetics can be explained by a faster gastric emptying time in the morning (Goo et al. 1987) and - more important - a higher gastro-intestinal perfusion in the morning (Lemmer and Nold 1991) resulting in higher Cmax and/or shorter tmax in the morning than in the evening.

There is some evidence that in hypertensive dippers antihypertensive drugs should be given at early morning hours, whereas in non-dippers it can be necessary to add an evening dose or to even apply a single evening dose in order not only to reduce high blood pressure but also to normalize a disturbed 24 hour blood pressure profile. However, since the pharmacokinetics can be circadian phase-dependent, the galenic formulation and/or the indiginous half life of a drug has to be considered in order to come to a final recommendation concerning to most appropriate dosing time within 24 hours.

In conclusion, these studies clearly demonstrate that the effects as well as the kinetics of cardiovascular active drugs can be dependent on the circadian phase, i.e. time of day. However, possible daily variation in the kinetics seem to be of minor importance for the degree in the circadian time dependent effects of the compounds. Nevertheless, the data published in respect to time-of-day of cardiovascular active drugs clearly demonstrate that the dose-response relationship can be circadian phase dependent. This has also been convincingly demonstrated in animal experiments in spontaneously hypertensive and transgenic hypertensive rats investigating by telemetry the dose-response relationship and the circadian phase-dependency of amlodipine, doxazosin, enalapril and losartan on the 24h-blood pressure profile (Mattes and Lemmer 1991; Lemmer et al. 1994; Schnecko et al. 1995; Lemmer and Witte 1997).

REFERENCES

1. Aschoff J 1963 Gesetzmäßigkeiten der biologischen Tagesperiodik. Dtsch med Wschr 88: 1930.

2. Aschoff J 1965 Circadian Clocks. North-Holland Publ. Comp., Amsterdam.

3. Asmar R, Hughes Ch, Pannier B, Daou J, Safar ME 1987 Duration of action of bisoprolol after cessation of a 4 weeks treatment and its influence on pulse wave velocity and aortic diameter: a pilot study in hypertensive patients. Eur Heart J 8 (Suppl M):115-120.

4. Bruguerolle B, Bouvenot G, Bartolin R, Manolis J 1988 Chronopharmacocinétique de la digoxine chez le sujet de plus de soixante-dix ans. Therapie 43, 251-253.

5. Cugini P, Kawasaki T, DiPalma L, Antonicoli S, Battisti P, Coppola A, Leone G 1989 Preventive distinction of patients with primary or secondary hypertension by discriminant analysis of chronobiologic parameters on 24-h blood pressure patterns. Jpn Circ J 53:1363-1370

6. Fogari R, Malocco E, Tettamanti F, Tettamanti F, Gnemmi AE, Milani M 1993 Evening vs morning isradipine sustained release in essential hypertension: a double-blind study with 24 h ambulatory monitoring. Br J clin Pharmac 35: 51-54.

7. Goo RH, Moore JG, Greenberg E, Alazraki NP 1987 Circadian variation in gastric emptying of meals in humans. Gastroenterology 93:515-518.

8. Gould BA, Mann S, Kieso H, Balasubramanian V, Raftery EB 1982 The 24-hour ambulatory blood pressure profile with verapamil. Circulation 65:22-27.

9. Gould BA, Raftery EB 1991 Twenty-four-hour blood pressure control: an intraarterial review. Chronobiol Int 8:495-505.

10. Greminger P, Suter PM, Holm D, Kobelt R, Vetter W 1994 Morning versus evening administration of nifedipine gastrointestinal therapeutic system in the management of essential hypertension. Clin Investig 72:864-869.

11. Hla KK, Latham AN, Henry JA 1992 Influence of time of administration on verapamil pharmacokinetics. Clin Pharmacol Ther 51:366-370.

12. Jespersen CM, Frederiksen M, Hansen JF, Klitgaard NA, Sorum C 1989 Circadian variation in the pharmacokinetics of verapamil. Eur J Clin Pharmacol 37:613-615.

13. Koopmans R, Oosterhuis B, Karemaker JM, Weiner J, van Boxtel CJ 1993 The effect of oxprenolol dosage time on its pharmacokinetics and haemodynamic effects during exercise in man. Eur J Clin Pharmacol 44:171-176.

14. Langner B, Lemmer B 1988 Circadian changes in the pharmacokinetics and cardiovascular effects of oral propranolol in healthy subjects. Eur J Clin Pharmacol 33: 619-624.

15. Lemmer B 1989 Temporal aspects in the effetcs of cardiovascular active drugs. In: Lemmer B (ed) Chronopharmacology - Cellular and Biochemical Aspects. Marcel Dekker, New York Basel, pp 525-542.

16. Lemmer B 1995 Timing of cardiovascular medications - pitfalls and challenges. Brit J Cardiol 2:303-309.

17. Lemmer B 1996a Differential effects of antihypertensive drugs on circadian rhythm in blood pressure from the chronobiological point of view. Blood Pressure Monitoring 1:161-169.

18. Lemmer B 1996b Circadian rhythm in blood pressure: Signal transduction, regulatory mechanisms and cardiovascular medication. In: Lemmer B (ed) From the Biological Clock to Chronopharmacology. medpharm Publ. Stuttgart, pp 91-117.

19. Lemmer B 1977 Chronopharmacological aspects of PK/PD-modelling. Int J Clin Pharmacol Ther 35:458-464.

20. Lemmer B, Bruguerolle B 1994 Chronopharmacokinetics - are they clinically relevant? Clin Pharmacokinet 26: 419-427.

21. Lemmer B, Mattes A, Böhm M, Ganten D 1993 Circadian blood pressure variation in transgenic hypertensive rats. Hypertension 22:97-101.

22. Lemmer B, Nold G 1991 Circadian changes in estimated hepatic blood flow in healthy subjects. Br J clin Pharmacol 32: 627-629.

23. Lemmer B, Nold G, Behne S, Kaiser R 1991c Chronopharmacokinetics and cardiovascular effects of nifedipine. Chronobiol Int 8: 485-494.

24. Lemmer B, Portaluppi F 1997 Chronopharmacology of cardiovascular diseases. In: Redfern P, Lemmer B (eds). Handbook of Experimental Pharmacology, Vol 125: Physiology and Pharmacology of Biological Rhythms. Springer, Heidelberg, New York, 251-297.

25. Lemmer B, Witte K 1997 Telemetric data acquisition of cardiovascular functions in biology and pharmacology. In: van Zutphen LFM, Balls M (eds), Animal Alternatives, Welfare and Ethics. Elsevier, Amsterdam, New York, pp 311-320.

26. Lemmer B, Sasse U, Witte K, Hopf R 1994 Pharmacokinetics and cardiovascular effects of a new sustained-release formulation of diltiazem. Naunyn-Schmiedeberg's Arch Pharmacol 349:R141.

27. Lemmer B, Scheidel B, Behne S 1991b Chronopharmacokinetics and chronophar-macodynamics of cardiovascular active drugs: propranolol, organic nitrates, nifedipine. Ann NY Acad Sci 618: 166-181.

28. Lemmer B, Scheidel B, Blume H, Becker HJ 1991a Clinical chronopharmacology of oral sustained-release isosorbide-5-mononitrate in healthy subjects. Eur J Clin Pharmacol 40: 71-75.

29. Lemmer B, Witte K, Makabe T, Ganten D, Mattes A 1994 Effects of enalaprilat on circadian profiles in blood pressure and heart rate of spontaneously and transgenic hypertensive rats. J Cardiovasc Pharmacol 23:311-314.

30. Mancia G 1993 Autonomic modulation of the cardiovascular system during sleep. N Engl J Med 328:347-349.

31. Mattes A, Lemmer B 1991 Effects of amlodipine on circadian rhythms in blood pressure, heart rate and motility - a telemetric study in rats. Chronobiol Internat 8: 526-538.

32. Meilhac B, Mallion JM, Carre A, Chanudet X, Poggi L, Gosse P, Dallochio M 1992 Étude de l'influence de l'horaire de la prise sur l'effet antihypertenseur et la tolérance de la nitrendipine chez des patients hypertendus essentiels légers à modérés. Therapie 47:205-210.

33. Mengden T, Binswanger B, Gruene S 1992 Dynamics of drug compliance and 24-hour blood pressure control of once daily morning vs evening amlodipine. J. Hypert. 10 (Suppl 4):S136.

34. Middeke M, Lemmer B 1996 Office hypertension: abnormal blood pressure regulation and increased sympathetic activity as compared with normotension. Blood Pressure Monitoring 1:403-407.

35. Middeke M, Schrader J 1994 Nocturnal blood pressure in normotensive subjects and those with white coat, primary, and secondary hypertension. Brit Med J 308:630-632.

36. Morgan T, Anderson A, Jones E 1997 The effect on 24 h blood pressure control of an angiotensin converting enzyme inhibitor (perindopril) administered in the morning or at night. J Hypertens 15:205-211.

37. Myburgh DP, Verho M, Botes JH, Erasmus ThP, Luus HG 1995 24-Hour pressure control with ramipril: comparison of once-daily morning and evening administration. Curr Ther Res 56.1298-1306.

38. Nold G, Strobel G, Lemmer B 1998 Morning versus evening dosing of amlodipine: effect on circadian blood pressure profile in essential hypertensive patients. Blood Pressure Monitoring 3:17-25.

39. Nold G, Lemmer B Pharmacokinetics of sustained-release molsidomine after morning versus evening application in healthy subjects. Naunyn-Schmiedeberg's Arch Pharmacol 357: R173, 1998.

40. Palatini P, Mos L, Motolese M, Mormino P, DelTorre M, Varotto L, Pavan E, Pessina AE 1993 Effect of evening versus morning benazepril on 24-hour blood pressure: a comparative study with continuous intraarterial monitoring. Int J Clin Pharmacol Ther Toxicol 31:295-300.

41. Palatini P, Racioppa A, Raule G, Zaninotti M, Penzo M, Pessina AC 1992 Effect of timing of administration on the plasma ACE inhibitory activity and the antihypertensive effect of quinapril. Clin Pharmacol Ther 52:378-383.

42. Panza JA, Epstein SE, Quyyumi AA 1991 Circadian variation in vascular tone and its relation to alpha-sympathetic vasoconstrictor activity. N Engl J Med 325:986-990.

43. Perloff D, Sokolow M, Cowan R 1983 The prognostic value of ambulatory blood pressures. JAMA 249:2792-2798.

44. Portaluppi F, Vergnani L, Manfredini R, degli Uberti EC, Fersini C 1995 Time-dependent effect of isradipine on the nocturnal hypertension of chronic renal failure. Am J Hypertens 8:719-726.

45. Pringle SD, Dunn FG, Tweddel AC, et al. 1992 Symptomatic and silent myocardial ischaemia in hypertensive patients with left ventricular hypertrophy. Br Heart J 67:377-382.

46. Quyyumi AA, Wright C, Mockus L, Fox KM 1984 Effect of partial agonist activity in ß blockers in severe angina pectoris: a double blind comparison of pindolol and atenolol. Br Med J 289:951-953.

47. Scheidel B, Lemmer B 1991 Chronopharmacology of oral nitrates in healthy subjects. Chronobiol Int 8: 409-419.

48. Schnecko A, Witte K, Lemmer B 1995 Effects of the angiotensin II receptor antagonist losartan on 24-hour blood pressure profiles of primary and secondary hypertensive rats. J Cardiovasc Pharmacol 26:214-221.

49. Stanton A, O'Brien E 1994 Auswirkungen der Therapie auf das zirkadiane Blutdruckprofil. Kardio 3:1-8.

50. Umeda T., S. Naomi, T. Iwaoka, Inoue J, Sasaki M, Ideguchi Y, Sato T 1994 Timing for administration of an antihypertensive drug in the treatment of essential hypertension. Hypertension 23 (Suppl. I);I211-I214.

51. Verdecchia P, Schillaci G, Guerrieri M, Gatteschi C, Benemio G, Boldrini F, Porcellati C 1990 Circadian blood pressure changes and left ventricular hypertrophy in essential hypertension (see comments). Circulation 81;528-536.

52. Willich SN, Muller JE (eds) 1996 Triggering of acute coronary syndromes. Kluwer Academic Publ., Dordrecht, The Netherlands.

53. Witte K, Lemmer B 1995 Free-running rhythms in blood pressure and heart rate in normotensive and transgenic hypertensive rats. Chronobiol Int 12:237-247.

54. Witte K, Weisser K, Neubeck M, Mutschler E, Lehmann K, Hopf R, Lemmer B 1993 Cardiovascular effects, pharmacokinetics and converting enzyme inhibition of enalapril after morning versus evening administration. Clin Pharmacol Ther 54:177-186.
55. Zuther P, Witte K, Lemmer B 1996 ABPM and CV-SORT: an easy-to-use software package for detailed analysis of data from ambulatory blood pressure monitoring. Blood Pressure Monitoring 1:347-354.

26. BETA BLOCKERS FOLLOWING ACUTE MYOCARDIAL INFARCTION

PETER F. COHN

Since their introduction into clinical use several decades ago, the beta blockers have proven enormously successful anti- ischemic, anti-hypertensive and anti-arrhythmic agents. They have been especially useful in improving morbidity and mortality after acute myocardial infarctions (MI).

The results of the placebo-controlled Norwegian Multicenter Study (with timolol),[1] the American Beta Blocker Heart Attack Trial (BHAT; with propranolol),[2] and the Goteborg Metoprolol Trial,[3] showed for the first time that medical treatment started after onset of MI can decrease total mortality. The timolol and propranolol studies, which were started 1-2 weeks after onset of acute MI and had a follow-up of approximately 2 years, showed a reduction in total mortality of 36% and 26%, respectively. In the Goteborg Metoprolol Trial, in which the beta blocker was given to patients with suspected acute MI shortly after hospital arrival, mortality at 3 months was decreased by 36%. Many other small studies have also been published, and today data are available from 24 long-term trials that included approximately 25,000 patients. The average reduction in mortality in these trials was approximately 20% over about 2 years of follow-up.

Two large trials, MIAMI[4] and ISIS-1,[5] which included about 6,000 and 16,000 patients, respectively, assessed the possibility of reducing mortality within 1-2 weeks of MI. Cardiovascular mortality was decreased by 14% after 7 days in the ISIS-1 trial and total mortality by 13% after 15 days in the MIAMI trial (a nonsignificant difference).

The reduction in the incidence of sudden cardiac death is particularly noteworthy. In the BHAT, death occurring within 1 hour after the onset of symptoms was reduced by 28% in propranolol-treated patients; in the trials using

H.-H. Osterhues et al. (eds.),
Advances in Noninvasive Electrocardiographic Monitoring Techniques, 279–281.
© 2000 *Kluwer Academic Publishers. Printed in the Netherlands.*

timolol and metoprolol, sudden death (defined as death within 24 hours after the onset of symptoms) was reduced by 40-50% by beta blocker therapy. Although ISIS-1 and MIAMI, did not report the incidence of sudden cardiac death, both reported a major effect on early cardiac rupture within 24 hours, which could also have been a cause of sudden cardiac death, especially during the short-term follow-up after acute MI.

Patients at highest risk seemed to benefit most from beta blocker therapy. Patients with congestive heart failure at onset of treatment experienced about twice as much total mortality and sudden death as patients without heart failure. In the BHAT, propranolol therapy after acute MI decreased total mortality and the incidence of sudden cardiac death more markedly in patients with congestive heart failure than in patients without it. The reduction in sudden cardiac death was about 50% in the patients with congestive heart failure. Similarly, in the 2 early intervention trials with metoprolol, the Goteborg Metoprolol and MIAMI trials, mortality reduction was more marked in patients at high risk. Based on risk factors existing before the start of blind treatment with either metoprolol or placebo, such as age, congestive heart failure, history of cardiovascular disease, or diabetes, patients were classified into high- and low-risk groups. Mortality after 15 days was 2.5 times higher in the older and/or sicker patients than in younger or previously healthy individuals. In the high-risk groups, metoprolol therapy reduced mortality by 30-45%.

Even when other medications are given, the addition of beta blockers is still important. In the Thrombolysis in Myocardial Infarction (TIMI) phase IIB study,[6] all patients underwent thrombolytic therapy and were considered for revascularization. Intravenous beta blocker therapy started shortly after hospital admission resulted in a 48% lower rate of nonfatal reinfarction within 6 days than that of beta blockade deferred for one week. The Thrombolysis Early in Acute Heart Attack Trial (TEAHAT)[7] addressed the question of whether recombinant tissue-type plasminogen activator (rt-PA) is effective in the presence of optimal therapy that includes intravenous or oral metoprolol. Intravenous metoprolol was given to 63% of the patients; in one-third of them, therapy was started before hospitalization by means of mobile coronary care. The best effect of rt-PA on infarct size limitation was seen in patients given metoprolol. The results of TIMI-2B and TEAHAT show that beta blockade and thrombolytic therapy have an additive cardioprotective effect, due to a combination of decreased heart work and metabolic demand and improved coronary blood perfusion.

The postinfarction studies with ACE inhibitors in patients with left ventricular dysfunction report that about one-third of the patients received beta blockers. In the Survival and Ventricular Enlargement (SAVE) trial,[8] for example, captopril had a better effect on mortality when given concomitantly with beta blockers. Since ACE inhibitors have a limited effect on sympathetic activity, and it is necessary to block not only the renin-angiotensin system but also the sympathetic nervous system in patients with left ventricular dysfunction, beta blockers appear to play an important role. In the US Carvedilol Heart Failure Study,[9] most patients were given ACE inhibitors in optimal dosages, yet the beta blocker carvedilol still decreased the incidence of sudden cardiac death by 50%.

REFERENCES

1. The Norwegian Multicenter Study Group. Timolol-induced reduction in mortality and reinfarction in patients surviving acute myocardial infarction. N Engl J Med 1981; 304:801-807.

2. Beta-Blocker Heart Attack Trial Research Group. A randomized trial of propranolol in patients with acute myocardial infarction, I: mortality results. JAMA 1982; 247:1407-1414.

3. Hjalmarson A, Elmfeldt D, Herlitz J, Holmberg S, Malek I, Nyberg G, Ryden L, Swedberg K, Vedin A, Waagstein F, Waldenstrom A, Waldenstrom J, Wedel H, Wilhelmsen L, Wilhelmsson C. Effect on mortality of metoprolol in acute myocardial infarction: a double-blind randomised trial. Lancet 1981; ii:823-827.

4. The MIAMI Trial Research Group. Metoprolol in Acute Myocardial Infarction (MIAMI): a randomised placebo-controlled international trial. Eur Heart J 1985; 6:199-226.

5. ISIS-1 (First International Study of Infarct Survival) Collaborative Group. Randomized trial of intravenous atenolol among 16,027 cases of suspected acute myocardial infarction: ISIS-1. Lancet 1986; ii:57-66.

6. The TIMI Study Group. Comparison of invasive and conservative strategies after treatment with intravenous tissue plasminogen activator in acute myocardial infarction: results of the Thrombolysis in Myocardial Infarction (TIMI) phase II trial. N Engl J Med 1989; 320:618-627.

7. Risenfors M, herlitz J, Bergh C-H, Dellborg M, Gustavsson G, Gottfridsson C, Lomsky M, Swedberg K, Hjalmarson A. Early treatment with thrombolysis and beta-blockade in suspected acute myocardial infarction: results from the TEAHAT Study. J Intern Med 1991; 229(suppl 734):35-42.

8. Pfeffer MA, Braunwald E, Moye LA, Basta L, Brown EJ Jr., Cuddy TE, Davis BR, Geltman EM, Goldman S, Flaker GC, Klein M, Lamas GA, Packer M, Rouleau J, Rouleau JL, Rutherford J, Wertheimer JH, Hawkins CM, on behalf of the SAVE Investicators. Effects of captopril on mortality and morbidity in patients with left ventricular dysfunction after myocardial infarction: results of the Survival and Ventricular Enlargement trial. N Engl J Med 1992; 327:669-677.

9. Packer M, Bristow MR, Cohn JN, Colucci WS, Fowler MB, Gilbert EM, Shusterman NH, for the US Carvedilol Heart Failure Study Group. The effect of carvedilol on morbidity and mortality in patients with chronic heart failure. N Engl J Med 1996; 334:1249-1355.

27. THE UNITED STATES MULTICENTER STUDY OF ENHANCED EXTERNAL COUNTERPULSATION (MUST-EECP)

PETER F. COHN

Enhanced external counterpulsation (EECP) is a noninvasive ECG-timed procedure that employs sequential balloon inflation and deflation in the lower extremities to provide diastolic augmentation and systolic unloading.[1] Open clinical trials conducted at the University Hospital and Medical Center, State University of New York at Stony Brook, demonstrated that treatment with EECP resulted in a significant decrease in anginal frequency, improved cardiac flow in radionuclide scans and increased exercise tolerance.[1] These results, however, were achieved without the benefit of a control population against which to conpare results of treatment. MUST-EECP, the first national, randomized, placebo- controlled trial of EECP, was conducted to provide such a control group and to evaluate EECP results at study centers other than Stony Brook.

MUST-EECP was conducted at seven cardiology centers across the United States from May 1995 to July 1997. The study investigators and institutions were Richard Nesto, MD (Beth Israel Deaconess Medical Center, a teaching affiliate of Harvard Medical School); Rohit Arora, MD (Columbia University College of Physicians & Surgeons at the Columbia-Presbyterian Medical Center in New York); Bruce Fleishman, MD (Grant/Riverside Methodist Hospitals in Columbus, Ohio); Thomas McKiernan, MD (Loyola University Medical Center in Maywood, Illinois); Tony Chou, MD (University of California, San Francisco); Lawrence Crawford, MD (University of Pittsburgh Medical Center); and Diwaker Jain, MD (Yale University School of Medicine in New Haven). Stony Brook served as the Data and Coordinating Center.

H.-H. Osterhues et al. (eds.),
Advances in Noninvasive Electrocardiographic Monitoring Techniques, 283–285.
© 2000 *Kluwer Academic Publishers. Printed in the Netherlands.*

Although the design was similar to that established by the U.S. Food and Drug Administration for pharmaceutical therapies, it is considered unique for a medical device in that it included randomization, double-blinding, a sham group and the use of objective endpoint measures to validate clinical results.

A total of 139 patients (average age 63) suffering from chronic angina pectoris on maximal medication, and in many of whom revascularization had failed, were randomly assigned to the treatment or sham (control) group. Neither patients nor physicians knew the tests used for endpoints to which group a participant belonged. This randomization process was applied to ensure the validity of the study and see that bias was eliminated from results. MUST-EECP enrollment criteria included documented coronary artery disease (CAD), Canadian Cardiovascular Society Classes I, II and III for angina pectoris and a positive exercise stress test within a four week baseline period. Exclusion criteria included unstable angina, myocardial infarction or bypass surgery three months prior, cardiac catheterization two weeks prior, greater than 50% stenosis in the left main coronary artery, electrocardiogram ECG abnormalities that would interfere with the interpretation of stress tests and overt congestive heart failure, or inability to provide consent or cooperate with the study protocol for the duration of the trial.

MUST-EECP measured four prespecified endpoints to determine the treatment's safety and efficacy in treating angina pectoris:

- Time to exercise-induced cardiac ischemia: Exercise-induced cardiac ischemia was determined by the depression of the ST-segment by a least one millimeter over baseline on ECG readings
- Exercise duration: Exercise duration was determined by the length of time a patient could walk on a treadmill during a standard exercise protocol before the test was terminated due to chest pain or fatigue
- Symptoms of anginal attacks as reported by test subjects: Symptoms were determined by study participants' diaries and verbal accounts of such experiences and were reported by nursing staff
- Consumption of oral nitroglycerin: Oral nitroglycerin consumption was determined by study participants' diaries and verbal reports in a manner similar to that by which angina attacks were recorded.

Treatment was administered in one hour sessions over a four-to-seven week period until patients had completed 35 hours of treatment. Overall, treatment with EECP was well tolerated during the study; no significant adverse experiences were reported.

A summary of MUST-EECP findings, as presented at the American Heart Association Meeting in November 1997[2] and the American College of Cardiology meeting in March 1998[3] are as follows:

- Exercise duration: There was a statistically significant increase in exercise duration from baseline in both groups. For patients receiving treatment, exercise duration increased 10% (p=.001) whereas exercise duration for those in the sham group increased 6% (P=.026). The between group difference was not significant.

- Time to ST-segment depression: This measurement also increased significantly in the EECP group, but no change was observed in the control group and the between-group comparisons were significant.
- Symptoms of anginal attacks as reported by test subjects: A significant decrease in the number of angina attacks was observed only for participants treated with EECP. The between group difference was significant.
- Consumption of oral nitroglycerin: Usage of on-demand nitrates remained unchanged between groups. (This finding is considered by the investigators to be related to patients' tendencies to take nitroglycerin prophylactically in anticipation of angina-inducing events).

In conclusion, significant benefits were demonstrated in patients who received EECP compared to a control patient population. Both groups were also receiving maximal medication but the latter underwent sham treatment. While MUST-EECP evaluated the immediate clinical benefits of EECP, previous open trials at Stony Brook assessed long-term benefits. The Stony Brook trials also found a persistent reduction in myocardial ischemia and symptomatic improvement as much as three years following treatment with EECP. Preliminary one year follow-up results from MUST-EECP show a similar trend in regard to decreased symptoms.[3]

REFERENCES

1. Cohn PF, Lawson WE, Burger L, Hui JCK. Enhanced external counterpulsation: A new therapeutic option for patients who have failed coronary angioplasty and/or bypass surgery. Cardiovas Rev and Reports 1997; 18:10-21.

2. Arora RR, Chou TM, Jain D, Nesto RW, Fleishmar. B, Crawford L, McKiernan T: Results of the multicenter study of enhanced external counterpulsation (MUST-EECP): EECP reduces anginal episodes and exercise-induced myocardial ischemia. Circulation 1997; 96(suppl I):I-466-I-468 (abstract).

3. Arora R, Chou T, Jain D, Nesto R, Fleishman B, Crawford L, McKiernan T for the MUST-EECP Investigators. Results of the multicenter study of enhanced external counterpulsation (MUST- EECP): Clinical benefits are sustained at a mean follow-up time of one year. JACC 1998; 31(Supp 2):214A (abstract).

CHAPTER FOUR: METHODS

SECTION ONE: QUALITY CONTROL AND STANDARDIZATION OF
MONITORING TECHNIQUES

28. HEART RATE VARIABILITY: A SIMPLE METHODOLOGY WITH SEVERAL UNRECOGNISED TECHNICAL AND METHODOLOGICAL PROBLEMS

FEDERICO LOMBARDI, ANDREA COLOMBO AND
CESARE FIORENTINI

In the last 10 years several groups of clinical and experimental cardiologists have demonstrated that the analysis of heart rate variability is unprecedented tool capable of providing relevant information on autonomic modulation of sinus node as well as on patients' prognosis in a variety of clinical conditions such as acute myocardial infarction, cardiac failure and diabetes (1). Nevertheless, despite its apparent simplicity, this methodology is still surrounded by several unresolved methodological and technical issues that have prevented not only an unique and correct interpretation of the results but also a more extensive utilisation of this non invasive technique in the clinical setting.

In this article some of the most relevant aspects due to different duration of the recordings as well as to the use of customised or commercial instrumentation will be discussed in relation to the physiological interpretation of spectral components and to the prognostic value of a reduced heart rate variability.

SHORT VERSUS LONG TERM RECORDINGS

It is well known that heart rate variability can be analysed by considering short term electrocardiographic recordings performed under controlled conditions and 24 hour Holter recording of unrestricted patients. The Task Force on heart rate variability of the European Society of Cardiology and of the North American Association of Pacing and Electrophysiology has clearly pointed out

H.-H. Osterhues et al. (eds.),
Advances in Noninvasive Electrocardiographic Monitoring Techniques, 289–295.
© 2000 *Kluwer Academic Publishers. Printed in the Netherlands.*

(1) that results obtained with these two different methodologies are poorly comparable. Indeed, spectral analysis of short term recordings(5-10 minute duration), allows a better quantification of the two principal components at low (LF~0.10 Hz) and high (HF~0.25 Hz) frequency that characterise the variability signal recorded under controlled conditions and are known to reflect autonomic modulation of sinus node (1-4). In the analysis of short term recordings, moreover, the energy below 0.03Hz, which corresponds to the very low (VLF) frequency component accounts for less than 50% of total power. The amount of energy present in the VLF range, however, is dependent on the processing of the RR-interval time series required by the algorithm utilised to perform spectral analysis: for example detrending or resampling of the time series are associated with a significant reduction in the VLF power. Also the computation of absolute power of LF and HF within the same RR-interval time series may vary in relation to the use of FFT or Autoregressive algorithm. In the first case the power of each component is the sum of all the energy included in the preselected frequency range. By using autoregressive algorithm is instead possible to estimate with greater precision the energy attributed to the identified spectral components which is considered as LF or HF in relation to its centre frequency (1).

CONDITIONS OF RECORDINGS

Additional problems may arise by comparing recordings obtained during free or controlled respiration. It is well known that respiration synchronised to a fixed frequency profoundly affect the spectral profile (1,3-6). During free breathing in normal subjects during resting conditions LF is generally slightly predominant over HF. As a result the value LF/HF ratio (the most commonly used index of sympatho-vagal interaction) is 1 or slightly above 1. During controlled respiration at a fixed rate the respiration related component becomes predominant and the LF/HF ratio is less than 1 when the respiratory rate is within the physiological range (15-20 respiratory acts /min) but may become much greater than 2 when the respiratory rate is very low and the centre frequency of the respiration related component is collocated in the LF range. It is self evident that in this latter case a LF/HF ratio greater than 2 cannot be considered to reflect a shift of sympatho-vagal balance toward a sympathetic activation and a reduced vagal tone as it has been reported, for example, in most of the patients after an acute myocardial infarction (1,7-9).

ABSOLUTE VERSUS NORMALISED UNITS:

An additional point which has to be taken into consideration is the use of absolute versus normalised units to express the power of spectral components (1,3,4,10). This issue has been previously discussed and the advantages of using either absolute or normalised units have been published elsewhere. Nevertheless, it is our opinion that the normalisation procedure may facilitate the appraisal of reciprocal changes in LF and HF components even in presence of relevant differences in total power within the same subject or when comparing different population. It must be recalled that information derived by the use of normalised units are similar to those derived by the use of LF/HF ratio a parameter universally accepted by all investigators.

24 HOUR VERSUS 10 MINUTE RECORDINGS

The presence of relevant difference in the analysis of short term recordings anticipates the critical aspect of comparing short and long term recordings. The use of 24 hour Holter tapes for the analysis of heart rate variability derives from the fact that Holter recordings are commonly performed in patients with an acute myocardial infarction to evaluate the presence of ventricular and supraventricular arrhythmias. The processing necessary to obtain a time domain analysis of heart rate variability is quite simple and available in almost all of the commercial instrumentations. After the initial observation of Kleiger and co-workers (11) a reduced standard deviation of normal RR-intervals has been confirmed as one of the most powerful predictor of increased cardiac mortality after myocardial infarction (1, 12,13). More controversial is instead the interpretation of data derived by applying spectral methodology to the entire 24 hour period. When considering a 24 hour autospectrum, most of the energy is distributed within the ultra (ULF) and VLF frequency band. As a result LF and HF components account for less than 10% of total power. In this setting the interpretation of the physiological significance of these component is hard to define as several environmental factors such as for example the level of physical activity or the respiratory rate may affect the energy distribution within the LF and HF frequency range. For these reasons it is not surprising that the power of LF or HF measured on a 24 hour recordings is significantly correlated with the power of the ULF and VLF components as well as with total power (1,12). On the other hand, the comparison of fractional distribution of power within individual components between long and short term recordings appears problematic.

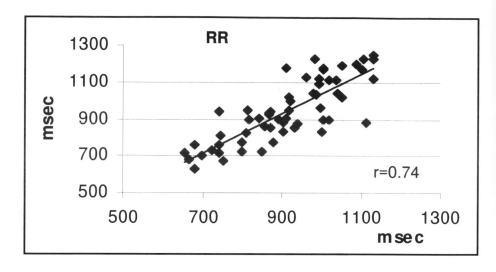

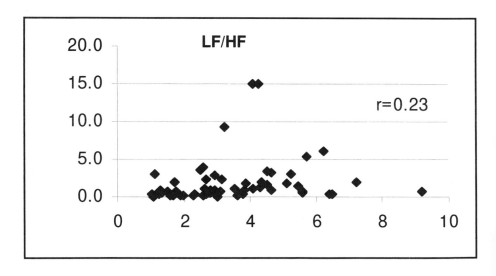

Relationship between mean RR-interval (top) or LF/HF ratio (bottom panel) measured on long (entire 24 hour period) and short (10 minute resting controlled condition) term recordings after acute myocardial infarction. A significant correlation between the two measures of the same parameter is present only for mean RR-interval.

Table. Correlation between of time and frequency domain parameters of heart rate variability measured on long (24 hours) and short (10 minutes) recordings

RR 24vs10	SDNNvsRRV	LF24vs10	HF24vs10	LF/HF 24vs10
ı−0.74	r=0.77	r=0.18	r=0.37	r=0.23
p<0.000	p<0.000	p=0.22	p=0.02	p=0.13

This issue is of particular importance in view of the capability of time and frequency domain measures of total power to identify patient at risk after myocardial infarction as well as to the possibility of obtaining information on the autonomic profile by using the same recordings (1). We are actually addressing this issue by comparing the results of spectral analysis of the entire 24 hour recordings with those obtained by the analysis of short term recordings carried out within the same day but under controlled resting conditions. In a group of 59 patients before discharge after the first acute myocardial infarction we analysed time and frequency domain parameters of heart rate variability The following parameters were considered for both long (24 hours) and short term (10 minutes) recordings: mean RR-interval, SDNN (24 hours) and RR variance (10 minutes) as measures of total power, LF and HF components in normalised and absolute units and LF/HF ratio. Linear regression analysis was used to examine the relationship between each pair of parameters. As indicated in the Table, whereas mean RR-interval and total variability were significantly correlated, no relationship between LF/HF ratio as well as the fractional distribution of energy within LF and HF components was present when comparing values derived from short and long term recordings. Thus, the analysis of short term recordings seems to provide information similar to those derived from Holter recordings for those time domain parameters known to predict mortality, while maintaining its accuracy in the characterisation of autonomic profile after an acute myocardial infarction. On the contrary, the analysis of 24 hour recording needs to be interpreted with caution in order to obtain information on individual autonomic profiles in addition to those which can be derived by considering instantaneous heart rate and its total variability (14).

NON LINEAR DYNAMICS

A new interest for long term recordings derives from the possibility of applying methods for the study of non linear dynamics to the heart rate variability signal (15). The analysis of the slope of the relationship between frequency and power expressed in logarithmic scale appears as the most promising approach. Indeed the computation of the 1/f slope appears suitable to evaluate the fractal like characteristics of the variability signal and of characterise the energy distribution within the VLF range. A significant different value of 1/f slope has been reported in post myocardial infarction patients with a reduced ejection fraction (16), in post-myocardial infarction patients prone to develop malignant ventricular arrhythmias(17) as well as in patients with implantable cardioverter defibrillator before the onset of ventricular tachycardia or fibrillation (18).

CONCLUSIONS

A proper evaluation of the technical and methodological aspects related to the use of this apparently simple non invasive methodology is necessary in order to extract completely all the information hidden in the variability signal. This issue is even more relevant when comparing results obtained with commercial instrumentation. A comparison as well a standardisation of the different methodologies employed in the analysis of heart rate variability is not only desirable but also necessary for an appropriate utilisation of this technique (1).

REFERENCES

1. Task Force of the European Society of Cardiology and the North American Society of Pacing and Electrophysiology. Heart Rate Variability. Standards of measurement, physiological interpretation, and clinical use. Circulation 1996;93:1043-1065.
2. Akserold S, Gordon D, Ubel FA, Shannon DC, Barger AC, Cohen RJ: Power spectrum analysis of heart rate fluctuations: a quantitative probe of beat-to-beat cardiovascular control. Science 1981;213:220-222.
3. Pagani M, Lombardi F, Guzzetti S, Rimoldi O. Furlan R, Pizzinelli P, Sandrone G, Malfatto G, Dell'Orto S, Piccaluga E, Turiel M, Baselli G, Cerutti S, Malliani A: Power spectral analysis of heart rate and arterial pressure variabilities as a marker of sympathovagal interaction in man and conscious dog. Cir Res 1986;59:178-193.
4. Malliani A, Pagani M, Lombardi F, Cerutti S: Advances Research Series: Cardiovascular Neural Regulation Explored in the Frequency Domain. Circulation 1991;84:482-492.
5. Pomeranz B, Macaulay RJB, Caudill MA, Kutz I, Adam D, Gordon D, Killborn KM, Barger AC, Shannon DC, Cohen RJ, Benson H. Assessment of autonomic function in humans by heart rate spectral analysis. Am J Physiol 1985;248:H151-H153.
6. Brown TE, Beightol LA, Koh J, Eckberg DL. Important influence of respiration on human RR-interval power spectra is largely ignored. J Appl Physiol 1993;75:2310-2317.
7. Lombardi F, Sandrone G, Perpruner S, Sala R, Garimoldi M, Cerutti S, Baselli G, Pagani M, Malliani A: Heart rate variability as a an index of sympathovagal interaction after acute myocardial infarction. Am J Cardiol 1987,60:1239-1245

8. Lombardi F, Malliani A, Pagani M, Cerutti S. Heart rate variability and its sympatho-vagal modulation. Cardiovasc Res 1996;32:208-216.

9. Lombardi F, Sandrone G, Spinnler MT, Torzillo D, Lavezzaro GC, Brusca A, Malliani A. Heart rate variability in the early hours of an acute myocardial infarction. Am J Cardiol 1996;77:1037-1044.

10. Malliani A, Lombardi F, Pagani M. Power spectrum analysis of heart rate variability: a tool to explore neural regulatory mechanisms. Br Heart J 1994;71:1-2.

11. Kleiger RE, Miller JP, Bigger JT, Moss AR, Multicenter Post-Infarction Research Group: Decreased heart rate variability and its association with increased mortality after acute myocardial infarction. Am J Cardiol 1987;59:256-262.

12. Bigger JT, Fleiss J, Steinman RC, Rolnitzky LM, Kleiger RE, Rottman JN. Frequency domain measures of heart period variability and mortality after myocardial infarction. Circulation 1992;85:164-171.

13. Farrell TG, Bashir Y, Cripps T, et al. Risk stratification for arrhythmic events in post-infarction patients based on heart rate variability, ambulatory electrocardiographic variables and signal averaged electrocardiogram. J Am Coll Cardiol 1991;18:687-697.

14. Lombardi F. Heart rate variability: a contribution to better understanding the clinical role of heart rate. Eur Heart J. 1998;19 in press.

15. Goldberger AL,. Non-linear dynamics for clinicians: chaos theory, fractals, and complexity at the bedside. The Lancet 1996;347:1312-1314.

16. Lombardi F, Sandrone G, Mortara A, Torzillo D, La Rovere MT, Signorini MG, Cerutti S, Malliani A. Linear and nonlinear dynamics of heart rate variability after acute myocardial infarction with normal and reduced left ventricular ejection fraction. Am J Cardiol 1996;77:283-1288.

17. Bigger JT, Steinman RC, Rolnitzky L, Fleiss JL, Albrectht P, Cohen RJ. Power law behaviour of RR-interval variability in healthy middle-aged persons, patients with recent acute myocardial infarction, and patients with heart transplants. Circulation 1996;21:2142-2151.

18. Lombardi F, Marzegalli M, Santini M, Favale S, Proclemer A, Ochetta E, De Rosa A. Linear and non-linear dynamics of heart rate variability before arrhythmic events in patients with implantable cardioverter defibrillator. Eur Heart J 1998;19:pp246 (a).

29. QUALITY CONTROL AND STANDARDIZATION: HIGH RESOLUTION ECG

R. HABERL AND P. STEINBIGLER

Studies have shown that abnormalities in high resolution electrocardiography are correlated to future arrhythmic events in patients after myocardial infarction [1,5]. Mainly, there are two approaches to detect these abnormalities: analysis of the filtered QRS-complex in the time domain [2,4,9,13] and analysis of the spectral composition of the QRS-complex [2,6,7,8,11,12], especially at its transition to the ST-segment. What means quality in this setting? Major prerequisites are standardisation of the method, reproducibility, availability, and last but not least effectiveness. Most obviously, the latter point is the most critical. Originally, the concept was that high resolution electrocardiography detects late potentials and late potentials are associated with increased risk of ventricular tachycardia and sudden death. Newer insights reveal that this might not be true. Comparative studies have shown that time domain measures (Simson method) are the least sensitive and specific to detect late potentials, however, have proven the most efficient in predicting clinical events. Spectrotemporal mapping has been designed and is the most sensitive and specific to detect late potentials at the end of QRS, but correlation to major arrhythmic events is less strong. The term signal averaging must not be applied as a synonym of late potential analysis. High resolution electrocardiography stratifies risk by measuring a parameter that still is not clearly identified. It is hard to define criteria of quality control, if scientific work is still in progress.

Standardisation can reasonably be supposed for time domain analysis and reproducibility is good. These landmarks of quality, however, might turn to the opposite, when reviewing recent publications: late potentials as biological signals arising from arrhythmogenic substrate are variable in morphology and extent (and thereby not at all ideal signals for signal averaging) and they are

H.-H. Osterhues et al. (eds.),
Advances in Noninvasive Electrocardiographic Monitoring Techniques, 297–302.
© 2000 *Kluwer Academic Publishers. Printed in the Netherlands.*

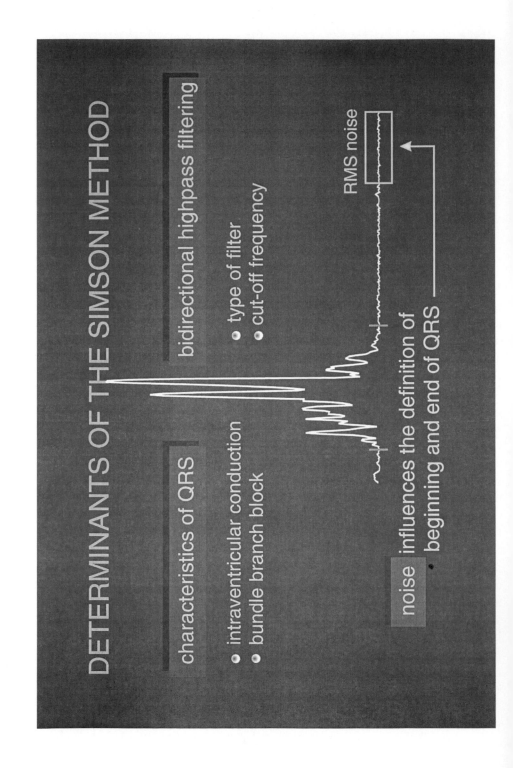

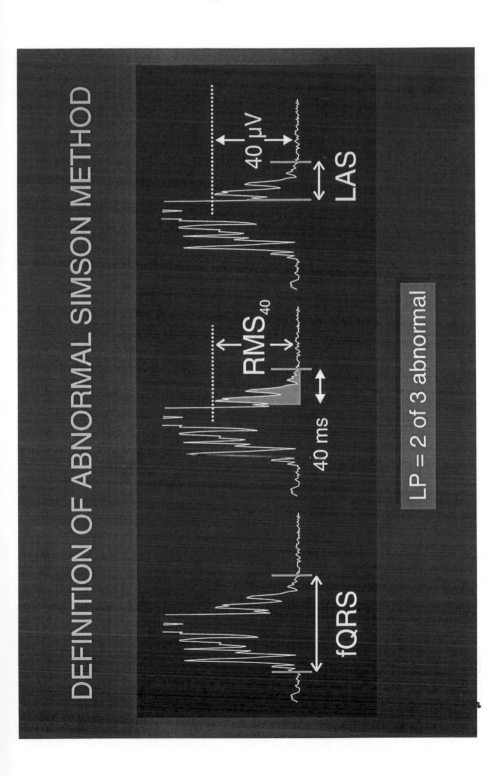

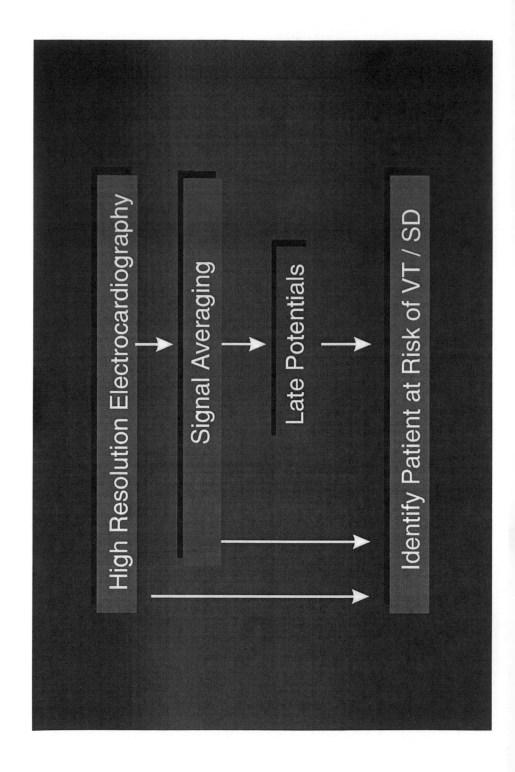

modified by drugs, changes in heart rate and ischemia.[8,14,15] As myocardial infarction is treated more effectively, a fixed arrhythmogenic substrate heartwiring reentry as a cause of sustained monomorphic ventricular tachycardia does not play a major clinical role anymore. Sudden death based on ventricular fibrillation or rapid ventricular tachycardia is the predominant clinical problem, but in this case the arrhythmogenic substrate is inconstant and viable to modulating factors such as ischemia. To this problem there are three approaches: spectral analysis of the entire cardiac cycle [3], spectral turbulence analysis[10] and functional late potential analysis with spectrotemporal mapping [8,14,15]. None of these methods is tested in large clinical studies nor is standardisation available.

In conclusion, standard risk stratification in the time domain is validated, standardised, reproducible, but its positive predictive value is too low for therapeutic decisions. On the spectral field there is scientific work in progress that offers promise for a more accurate risk stratification, however, it is too early to ask for quality control.

REFERENCES

1. Breithardt, G., Becker, R., Seipel, L., Abendroth, R. R., and Ostermeyer, J. Non-invasive detection of late potentials in man--a new marker for ventricular tachycardia. Eur Heart J 2(1), 1-11. 1981.
2. Cain ME, Ambos HD, Witkowski FX, Sobel BE: Fast-Fourier transform analysis of signal-averaged electrocardiograms for identification of patients prone to sustained ventricular tachycardia. *Circulation* 1984;69(4):711-720
3. Cain ME, Ambos HD, Markham J, Lindsay BD, Arthur RM: Diagnostic implications of spectral and temporal analysis of the entire cardiac cycle in patients with ventricular tachycardia. Circulation 1991;83(5);1637-1648
4. El Sherif N, Mehra R, Gomes JA, Kelen GJ: Appraisal of a low noise electrocardiogram. *J.Am.Coll.Cardiol.* 1983;1(2 Pt 1):456-467
5. Gomes, J. A., Winters, S. L., Martinson, M., Machac, J., Stewart, D., and Targonski, A. The prognostic significance of quantitative signal-averaged variables relative to clinical variables, site of myocardial infarction, ejection fraction and ventricular premature beats: a prospective study. J Am Coll Cardiol 13(2), 377-384. 1988
6. Haberl R, Jilge G, Pulter R, Steinbeck G: Comparison of frequency and time domain analysis of the signal-averaged electrocardiogram in patients with ventricular tachycardia and coronary artery disease: methodologic validation and clinical relevance. *J.Am.Coll.Cardiol.* 1988;12(1):150-158
7. Haberl R, Jilge G, Pulter R, Steinbeck G: Spectral mapping of the electrocardiogram with Fourier transform for identification of patients with sustained ventricular tachycardia and coronary artery disease. *Eur.Heart J.* 1989;10(4):316-322

8. Haberl R, Moroder E, Steinbigler P, Steinbeck G: Die funktionelle Spätpotentialanalyse. *Herzschr Elektrophys* 1998;9:15-19

9. Hombach V, Kebbel U, Hopp HW, Winter U, Hirche H: Noninvasive beat-by-beat registration of ventricular late potentials using high resolution electrocardiography. *Int.J.Cardiol.* 1984;6(2):167-188

10. Kelen GJ, Henkin R, Starr AM, Caref EB, Bloomfield D, el Sherif N: Spectral turbulence analysis of the signal-averaged electrocardiogram and its predictive accuracy for inducible sustained monomorphic ventricular tachycardia. *Am.J.Cardiol.* 1991;67(11):965-975

11. Lindsay BD, Ambos HD, Schechtman KB, Cain ME: Improved selection of patients for programmed ventricular stimulation by frequency analysis of signal-averaged electrocardiograms. *Circulation* 1986;73(4):675-683

12. Meste O, Rix H, Caminal P, Thakor NV: Ventricular late potentials characterization in time-frequency domain by means of a wavelet transform. *IEEE Trans.Biomed.Eng.* 1994;41(7):625-634

13. Simson, M. B. Use of signals in the terminal QRS-complex to identify patients with ventricular tachycardia after myocardial infarction. Circulation 64(2), 235-242. 1981

14. Steinbigler P, Haberl R, Jilge G, Steinbeck G: Single-beat analysis of ventricular late potentials in the surface electrocardiogram using the spectrotemporal pattern recognition algorithm in patients with coronary artery disease. *Eur Heart J* 1998;19:435-446

15. Steinbigler P, Haberl R, Moroder E, Steinbeck G: Spätpotentiale im Langzeit-EKG: Anwendung und Grenzen. *Herzschr Elektrophys* 1998;9:20-25

CHAPTER FOUR: METHODS

SECTION TWO: EXERCISE ECG

30. DIAGNOSIS OF MYOCARDIAL VIABILITY: CONTRIBUTION OF THE ECG

U. SECHTEM AND C.A. SCHNEIDER

The detection of infarct-related viability is of clinical importance to plan therapeutic strategies in an individual patient because revascularisation of dysfunctional but viable myocardium may improve left ventricular function [18]. Several imaging techniques were shown to be highly successful in detecting myocardial viability and these include angiographic [17], scintigraphic [5], echocardiographic [16] and magnetic resonance [1] techniques. This chapter will review the available evidence how easily obtainable information from the ECG can be used to diagnose myocardial viability and predict recovery of dysfunctional myocardium following revascularisation.

RESTING ECG

The presence or absence of Q-waves in infarct related leads has long been equated with transmural and non-transmural scar, respectively. However, although elaborate QRS scoring systems correlate well with scar size as measured by thallium-201 perfusion scintigraphy [9], autopsy data have shown that the ECG lacks sufficient sensitivity and specificity to permit reliable distinction of transmural from subendocardial infarcts. This is because patients with transmural infarcts may not develop Q-waves, especially when the infarct is located in the lateral wall, and Q-waves may be seen in patients with autopsy evidence of a subendocardial (nontransmural) acute myocardial infarct [22].

Nevertheless, a crude categorisation of patients into Q-wave and non-Q-wave infarcts based on the ECG is useful because Q-wave acute myocardial infarcts are usually associated with more ventricular damage, a greater ten-

305

H.-H. Osterhues et al. (eds.),
Advances in Noninvasive Electrocardiographic Monitoring Techniques, 305–316.

dency to infarct expansion and remodelling and a higher mortality rate. It has, however, been shown that in a significant percentage of patients with Q-wave infarcts viable myocardium can be detected in the myocardium supplied by the infarct related artery [3]. Therefore, one should not rely solely on the analysis of the QRS-complex in the resting ECG for making clinical decisions about revascularisation of an infarct related artery but make use of other pieces of information contained in the ECG. These are described below.

ST-ELEVATION IN INFARCT-RELATED LEADS DURING EXERCISE STRESS TESTING

ST-segment-elevation and T-wave pseudonormalisation are often seen during exercise testing in ECG leads related to an infarcted area. However, from a diagnostic view point, these changes are usually disregarded because they are generally assumed to be caused by bulging of the necrotic area [4,23] rather than induced by transient ischemia arising from perinecrotic, potentially salvageable myocardium.

Margonato and coworkers [12] were the first to challenge this view. They studied 25 consecutive patients with recent myocardial infarction (< 6 months old) who, on exercise testing, exhibited ST-segment elevation (≥ 0.1 mV at the J-point and 80 ms after) or normalisation of inverted T-waves in the infarct-related leads, or both. Half of their patients had effort angina. All patients but one had Q-waves in the infarct-related leads and all but the one without Q-waves had fixed perfusion defects on thallium perfusion scintigraphy. However, this defect was partially reversible in 16 of 17 (94%) patients with ST-elevation during the stress test and in 4 out of 8 (50%) in those with exercise induced in T-wave normalisation.

This surprising finding is clearly at odds with textbook teaching as well as with the results of several studies from the era before thrombolysis was employed on the broad basis. Dunn and coworkers [6] found reversible ischemia in patients with exercise-induced ST-segment elevation in infarct-related leads in only 52% and Lahiri and coworkers [10] detected reversible ischemia even in only 36% of patients with exercise-induced ST-segment elevation. Possible explanations for the deviating findings include that in the series of Dunn [6] antianginal treatment was not withdrawn before the exercise test and that in the series of Lahiri nearly all patients had total occlusion of the infarct-related coronary artery with no collateral flow. In contrast, 95% of the subjects in the study of Margonato had either a patent vessel or angiographically visible collateral flow to the infarcted area. Finally, one third of the patients in the study of Margonato had undergone early intravenous thrombolytic therapy which may have increased the likelihood of finding viable myocardium in the infarct area.

As planar exercise-redistribution thallium scintigraphy may not be the gold standard for detection of viable myocardium [5], Margonato and coworkers extended their observations by comparing ECG findings during exercise to fluorine-18 fluorodeoxiglucose (FDG) positron emission tomography in patients with chronic myocardial infarcts [13]. A group of 18 patients had exercise-induced ST-segment elevation and 16 patients did not. Uptake of F-18 FDG within the infarcted area was present in 18 of 18 patients in group A but only in 9 in group B (p < 0,01). In patients with anterior infarction, the sensitivity, specificity and predictive accuracy of exercise-induced ST-segment elevation for detection of residual viability were 82 %, 100 % and 86 %, respectively. Approximately half of the patients in both groups had received intravenous thrombolytic therapy within 4 hours from the onset of chest pain. Interestingly, 14 of the 18 patients with exercise induced ST-segment elevation had occluded infarct related arteries but retrograde filling of the occluded vessel by collateral flow was evident in 13 of these 14 patients (93%). In the remaining 4 patients with ST-segment elevation, the infarct-related artery was open with critical residual narrowing.

Further credibility to the results of ECG exercise stress testing for the detection of myocardial viability was given by a study of Lombardo and coworkers [11]. This group found evidence of contractile reserve in akinetic and/or dyskinetic regents in 10 of 15 patients with ST-segment elevation and in 14 of 20 patients with T-wave pseudonormalisation during low-dose dobutamine echocardiography. In contrast, only 1 of 26 patients without contractile reserve had T-wave pseudonormalisation during the test and none had ST-segment elevation.

Another recent study by Lekakis and co-workers who used dobutamine stress confirms the acceptable sensitivity of stress-induced ST-segment elevation in infarct-related leads of the ECG. 73 % of patients showed viability by thallium-201 in the infarct zone in this study, whereas patients without ST-segment elevation had only an incidence of 34% viability in this area.

Only one study by Ricci and co-workers [19] did not confirm the usefulness of stress induced ST-segment elevation in infarct related leads. These authors examined 391 patients after an acute myocardial infarct with dobutamine stress echocardiography. This study differs from the others in so far as patients were included very early after the infarct (mean 10+-2 days after a first uncomplicated acute infarct). Patients with dobutamine-induced ST-segment elevation had a similar incidence and extent of myocardial viability and homozonal ischemia as those without ST-segment elevation. Consequently, the sensitivity, specificity and accuracy of dobutamine-induced ST-segment elevation for detecting residual homozonal ischemia were only 51%, 55% and 54%, respec-

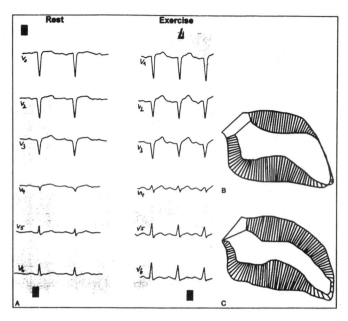

Figure 1. Patient with chronic anterior wall myocardial infarction and exercise-induced ST-elevation in the infarct region. A: Electrocardiographic tracing (leads V1 to V6) during rest and during peak. ST-segment elevation is observed during exercise in leads V1 to V3. B: Regional wall motion analysis by the centreline method before revascularisation of the LAD. C: Regional wall motion analysis after successful revascularisation of the LAD. Ejection fraction increased by 20% from 52 % before to 72% after revascularisation (reprinted from Schneider CA et al Am J Cardiol 1998; 82:148-53 with permission of the publisher and the authors).

tively, in patients with anterior wall acute myocardial infarction and 42 %, 68 % and 58 %, respectively, in patients with inferior wall infarcts. These authors feel that ST-segment elevation induced by dobutamine does not represent a clinically reliable discriminator for selecting patients for coronary angiography and possible revascularisation procedures. Thus, it is possible that the finding of ST-segment elevation provoked by exercise or dobutamine stress testing is mainly helpful in patients beyond the acute infarct phase.

ST-T-SEGMENT ELEVATION AND RECOVERY FOLLOWING REVAS-CULARISATION

The effect of revascularisation on exercise-induced ST-T-segment elevation was initially examined by Fox and co-workers [8]. Although myocardial viability was not demonstrated by an imaging technique before revascularisation and coronary angiography and left ventricular angiography were not performed after revascularisation (to demonstrate patency of the artery related to the region of interest and recovery of function), they showed that exercise-induced ST-T-segment elevation disappeared after revascularisation. They felt that this was compatible with improved myocardial blood flow to jeopardised myocardium.

A recent study from our institution [20] confirmed and extended the observations of Margonato and Fox. In this study, only patients with Q-wave myocardial infarcts with an infarct age ≥ 4 months were included. Of 64 consecutive patients who were able to undergo maximum physical exercise testing 20 patients had to be excluded from the study because of complete right or left bundle branch block (n=4), digitalis therapy (n=7), or significant ST-segment depression during the exercise electrocardiogram (n=9). Another 10 patients had to be excluded because they presented with restenosis or occlusion of the infarct related artery at repeat coronary angiography 4 months after revascularisation. Patients were restudied at that point in time because it was felt to be important to document that ST-elevation during exercise not only pointed to the presence of viable myocardium but also indicated the potential for recovery of left ventricular function. Thus, patients with restenosis of the infarct-related artery could be excluded because restenosis and reocclusion could have resulted in failure of viable myocardium to recover despite a correct diagnosis by exercise stress ECG. Of the remaining 34 patients 14 formed group I who had exercise-induced ST-segment elevation or T-wave pseudonormalisation. Figure 1 shows a typical patient with exercise induced ST-elevation in the leads showing Q-wave infarction. The remaining 20 patients (group II) had no exercise induced changes of the ST-T-segment. Individual values for the changes of left ventricular ejection fraction (LVEF) as assessed by angiography at base line and 4 months after revascularisation of patients with (group I) and without (group II) exercise-induced changes of the ST-segment are shown in figure 2. Ejection fraction increased by 12 +- 8% in group I and decreased in group II by 1 +- 6%. Similarly, average wall motion abnormality in the central infarct region as well as in the entire infarct region improved significantly only in group I. The sensitivity and specificity of ST-segment changes for the prediction of significant improvement of left ventricular ejection fraction was 80% (12 of 15) and 89% (17 of 19).

Elhendy and co-workers[7] also found a good predictive value of ST-T-segment elevation using dobutamine stress echocardiography for the detection of viable myocardium. The presence of ST-segment elevation during dobutamine stress had a sensitivity of 83 % and a specificity of 73 % to predict improved function in a subgroup of 23 patients who underwent revascularisation of the infarct-related artery. The slightly better sensitivity and specificity values in the study from our group may reflect the fact that patients with severe

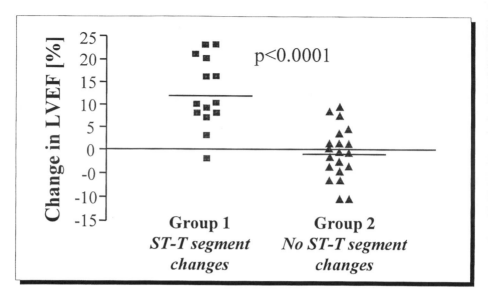

Figure 2. Individual values for the changes of LV ejection fraction (LVEF) assessed by angiography at base line and 4 months after revascularisation of patients with (group I) and without (group II) exercise-induced changes of the ST-T-segment (reprinted from Schneider CA et al. Am J Cardiol 1998; 82:148-53 with permission of the publisher and the authors).

restenosis at control angiography were excluded leading to a more homogeneous study population than that of Elhendy.

In conclusion, ST-T-segment elevation elicited by exercise or dobutamine infusion seems to be an excellent predictor of myocardial viability in most studies but patient selection may influence the accuracy of the technique. Notably, almost one third of patients cannot be adequately studied using the stress ECG because of bundle branch block, digitalis or concomitant ST-T-segment depression. This is a clear limitation of the method and these patients definitely need imaging studies in order to define the presence of viable myocardium. Another potential limitation of all the studies mentioned is that most patient populations had only moderately depressed left ventricular ejection fraction and these results cannot necessarily be directly translated to the group of patients with severely reduced global left ventricular ejection fraction who need viability tests most.

QT-DISPERSION AND MYOCARDIAL VIABILITY

A significant reduction of postinfarct QT-dispersion was shown in patients with acute myocardial infarction and successful thrombolysis [14]. These data suggested that QT-dispersion may be influenced by the extent of myocardial damage after myocardial infarction because successful thrombolysis and a patent infarct artery are associated but smaller infarct sizes and improved left ventricular function [15]. As the exact relationship between the extent myocardial scar, persisting viability in the infarct region, recovery of function and QT-dispersion after myocardial infarction was unknown, we recently examined 44 consecutive patients with chronic Q-wave myocardial infarcts [21]. All patients had positron emission tomography with F-18 FDG and underwent revascularisation of the infarct-related coronary artery. Left ventricular function was assessed by angiography at baseline and 4 months after revascularisation. QT-dispersion values were analysed in patients with and without improvement in function. Consequently, the value of QT-dispersion both for the detection of viable myocardium as defined by FDG positron emission tomography and for prediction of functional recovery after revascularisation could be assessed [21]. QT-dispersion was calculated from a standard 12-lead ECG on the day of admission. Revascularisation of the infarct-related vessel was performed independent of the results of the positron emission tomography study. An example of how QT-dispersion was determined is shown in figure 3 in a patient with anterior infarction.

QT-dispersion was significantly lower in patients with evidence of a substantial amount of viability in the infarct region as compared to patients without such evidence (figure 4). Similarly, values for QT standard deviation (calculated from QT values in the resting ECG) and QTc-dispersion (as calculated using Bazett's formula: $QTc = QT/RR^{1/2}$) were lower in patients with viability of the infarct region. There was no significant correlation between the ejection fraction and QT-dispersion. However, QT-dispersion was significantly correlated to FDG defect size and average FDG uptake (figure 5). QT-dispersion of ≤ 70 ms had the best sensitivity (85%) and specificity (82%) to predict viable myocardium in the infarct region as demonstrated by FDG positron emission tomography. Parameters of QT-dispersion as assessed on the baseline ECG were significantly lower in patients with improvement a function as compared to patients with unchanged left ventricular function. The sensitivity and specificity of QT-dispersion $\leq 7o$ ms for predicting improvement of left ventricular function was 83 % and 71 %, respectively. For comparison, sensitivity and specificity of an average FDG uptake ≥ 50 % of normalised maximum FDG uptake to predict improvement of left ventricular function were 59 % and 79 %, respectively.

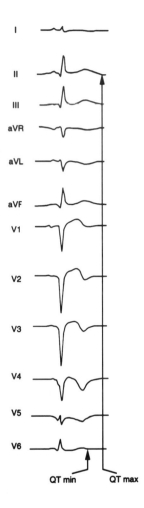

Figure 3. In this patient with chronic anterior wall myocardial infarction QT-dispersion was increased to 110 ms. The average FDG uptake in the infarct region was 31 % of maximum FDG uptake. At repeated angiography, left ventricular ejection fraction had not improved (baseline, 42%; at control 4 month later, 42%). Reprinted from Schneider CA et al. Circulation 96:3913-20, 1997 with permission of the authors and the American Heart Association.

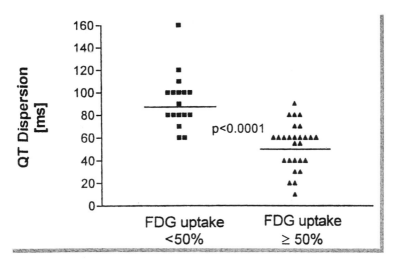

Figure 4. Column scatter graph of QT-dispersion in patients exhibiting an average FDG uptake of <50% or ≥50% of maximum FDG uptake in the infarct region. Reprinted from Schneider CA et al. Circulation 96:3913-20, 1997 with permission of the authors and the American Heart Association.

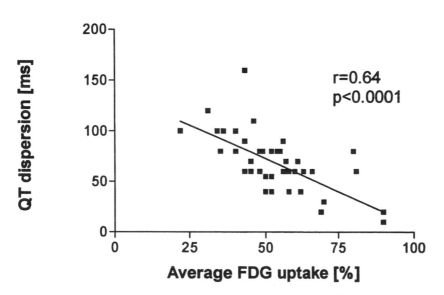

Figure 5. Correlation of QT-dispersion and average FDG uptake in the infarct region. Average FDG uptake is given in percent of maximum FDG uptake in the polar map. Reprinted from Schneider CA et al. Circulation 96:3913-20, 1997 with permission of the authors and the American Heart Association.

The study of Schneider et al. showed for the first time that the duration of QT-dispersion is reduced if viable myocardium is present in the infarct region. In comparison to the more time consuming and expensive scintigraphic-techniques using F-18 FDG, thallium-201 or technetium markers, this simple and inexpensive ECG method for estimating the extent of viable myocardium is obviously clinically attractive. But this is not only a simple and inexpensive method, but also compares favourably with the capabilities of the more expensive techniques [2]. In patients with QT-dispersion values of less than 60 ms, the probability of a larger extent viable myocardium being present in the infarct region despite the presence of Q-waves was 100%. In contrast, patients with a QT-dispersion >90 ms had a probability of 0% of having a larger extent of viable myocardium in the infarct region. In these patients, additional viability tests may not be indicated. In the intermediate range of QT-dispersion (60-90 ms), the diagnostic accuracy of the technique was between 80% and 84%. In this patient population, further viability tests with higher diagnostic accuracy may therefore be useful.

An explanation for the increased QT-dispersion values in patients with larger infarcts could be the presence of larger amounts of fibrous tissue, which may influence the duration and homogeneity of repolarisation. In addition, larger infarcts may lead to more pronounced mechanical stretch to the myocardial wall, which may further increase repolarisation inhomogeneity and may contribute to longer QT-dispersion values. These mechanisms may also be operative in patients with fatal arrhythmias or sudden cardiac death after myocardial infarction, conditions known to be associated with increased QT-dispersion values and with larger infarcts.

In summary, measuring QT-dispersion from the resting ECG may be useful for obtaining a low-cost rapid estimate of the presence of viable myocardium following myocardium infarction. It is easy and cheap to obtain this information and yet recovery of function after revascularisation can be predicted with high sensitivity and specificity in postinfarct patients showing Q-waves in the resting ECG.

REFERENCES

1. Baer F.M., Theissen P., Schneider C.A., et al. (1998) Dobutamine magnetic resonance imaging predicts contractile recovery of chronically dysfunctional myocardium after successful revascularization. J Am Coll Cardiol 31:1040-1048.
2. Bax J.J., Wijns W., Cornel J.H., et al. (1997) Accuracy of currently available techniques for prediction of functional recovery after revascularization in patients with left ventricular dysfunction due to chronic coronary artery disease: Comparison of pooled data. J Am Coll Cardiol 30:1451-1460.

3. Brunken R., Tillisch J., Schwaiger M., et al. (1986) Regional perfusion, glucose metabolism, and wall motion in patients with chronic electrocardiographic Q-wave infarctions: evidence for persistence of viable tissue in some infarct regions by positron emission tomography. Circulation 73:951-63.

4. Chahine R.A., Raizner A.E., Ishimori T. (1976) The clinical significance of exercise-induced ST-segment elevation. Circulation 54:209-13.

5. Dilsizian V., Rocco T.P., Freedman N.M.T., Leon M.B., Bonow R.O. (1990) Enhanced detection of ischemic but viable myocardium by the reinjection of thallium after stress-redistribution imaging. New Engl J Med 323:141-146.

6. Dunn R.F., Bailey I.K., Uren R., Kelly D.T. (1980) Exercise-induced ST-segment elevation: correlation of thallium-201 myocardial perfusion scanning and coronary arteriography. Circulation 61:989-95.

7. Elhendy A., Cornel J.H., Roelandt J., et al. (1997) Relation between ST-segment elevation during dobutamine stress test and myocardial viability after a recent myocardial infarction. Heart 77:115-121.

8. Fox K.M., Jonathan A., Selwyn A. (1983) Significance of exercise induced ST-segment elevation in patients with previous myocardial infarction. Br Heart J 49:15-19.

9. Juergens C.P., Fernandes C., Hasche E.T., et al. (1996) Electrocardiographic measurement of infarct size after thrombolytic therapy. J Am Coll Cardiol 27:617-624.

10. Lahiri A., Balasubramian V., Millar-Craig M.W., Crawley J., Raftery E.B. (1980) Exercise-induced ST-segment elevation: electrocardiographic, angiographic and scintigraphic evaluation. Br Heart J 43:582-8.

11. Lombardo A., Loperfido F., Pennestri F., et al. (1996) Significance of transient ST-T-segment changes during dotubamine testing in Q-wave myocardial infarction. J Am Coll Cardiol 27:599-605.

12. Margonato A., Ballarotto C., Bonetti F., et al. (1992) Assessment of residual tissue viability by exercise testing in recent myocardial infarction: Comparison of the electrocardiogram and myocardial perfusion scintigraphy. J Am Coll Cardiol 19:948-952.

13. Margonato A., Chierchia S.L., Xuereb R.G., et al. (1995) Specificity and sensitivity of exercise-induced ST-segment elevation for detection of residual viability: Comparison with fluorodeoxyglucose and positron emission tomography. J Am Coll Cardiol 25:1032-1038.

14. Moreno F.L., Villanueva M.T., Karagounis L.A., Anderson J.L. (1994) Reduction in QT-interval dispersion by successful thrombolytic therapy in acute myocardial infarction. Circulation 90:94-100.

15. Morgan C.D., Roberts R.S., Haq A., et al. (1991) Coronary patency, infarct size and left ventricular function after thrombolytic therapy for acute myocardial infarction: Results from the tissue plasminogen activator: Toronto (TPAT) placebo-controlled trial. J Am Coll Cardiol 17:1451-1457.

16. Pierard L.A., De Landsheere C.M., Berthe C., Rigo P., Kulbertus H.E. (1990) Identification of viable myocardium by echocardiography during dobutamine infusion in patients with myocardial infarction after thrombolytic therapy: Comparison with positron emission tomography. J Am Coll Cardiol 15:1021-31.

17. Popio K.A., Gorlin R., Bechtel D., Levine J.A. (1977) Postextrasystolic potentiation as a predictor of potential myocardial viability: Preoperative analysis compared with studies after coronary bypass surgery. Am J Cardiol 39:944-53.

18. Rahimtoola S.H. (1989) The hibernating myocardium. Am Heart J 117:211-21.
19. Ricci R., Bigi R., Galati A., et al. (1997) Dobutamine-induced ST-segment elevation in patients with acute myocardial infarction and the role of myocardial ischemia, viability, and ventricular dyssynergy. Am J Cardiol 79:733-737.
20. Schneider C.A., Helmig A.K., Baer F.M., et al. (1998) Significance of exercise-induced ST-segment elevation and T-wave pseudonormalization for improvement of function in healed Q-wave myocardial infarction. Am J Cardiol 82:148-53.
21. Schneider C.A., Voth E., Baer F.M., et al. (1997) QT-dispersion is determined by the extent of viable myocardium in patients with chronic Q-wave myocardial infarction. Circulation 96:3913-20.
22. Schoen F.J. The heart. In: Cotran RS, Kumar V, Robbins SL, eds. Pathologic basis of disease. Philadelphia: W. B. Saunders Company, 1994: 517.
23. Weiner D.A., McCabe C., Klein M.D., Ryan T.J. (1978) ST-segment changes post infarction: predictive value for multivessel coronary disease and left ventricular aneurysm. Circulation 58:887-91.

31. EXERCISE TESTING FOR RISK STRATIFICATION

VICTOR FROELICHER

INTRODUCTION

The use of exercise testing for risk stratification of patients with stable heart disease will be discussed in this chapter. This information will be evidence-based by following the ACC/AHA guidelines for Exercise Testing. [1]

Prognostic Use of the Exercise Test

There are two principal reasons for estimating prognosis. First, to provide accurate answers to patient's questions regarding the probable outcome of their illness. Though discussion of prognosis is inherently delicate, and probability statements can be misunderstood, most patients find this information useful in planning their affairs regarding work, recreational activities, personal estate, and finances. The second reason to determine prognosis is to identify those patients in whom interventions might improve outcome.

While improved prognosis equates with increased quantity of life, quality of life issues must also be taken into account. In that regard, it is apparent that in certain clinical settings, catheter or surgical interventions provide better therapy than medication. However, these interventions when misapplied can have a negative impact on the quality of life (inconvenience, complications, and discomfort), as well as creating a financial burden to the individual and to society.

H.-H. Osterhues et al. (eds.),
Advances in Noninvasive Electrocardiographic Monitoring Techniques, 317–329.

Risk Stratification Methods

Prognosis or the risk of adverse outcomes can be estimated in two ways: first, by following patients who underwent testing and identifying those who die or have heart attacks and second, by using severe angiographic coronary disease as a surrogate for death or MI. There are advantages and disadvantages for each approach. Follow up studies are more difficult and require adequate sample size and a sufficiently long follow up period for enough events to accrue. Follow up studies can be confounded by other causes of death and by interventions such as medications or bypass surgery. In fact, because of the high prevalence of interventions that have become part of standard clinical practice some experts feel that such "natural history studies" no longer can be performed. While the surrogate endpoint of coronary angiographic findings has the advantage of being the target for coronary artery surgery or catheter intervention, there is a patient selection problem. This problem is known as work up bias and means that only those patients with high risk exercise test results or clinical histories end up in the catheterization lab and are those pre-selected for inclusion in the study. These studies never allow us to see how the exercise test performs on all patients presenting to the clinician but only in those selected for angiography.

The ACC/AHA Guidelines for the Prognostic Use of the Standard Exercise Test

Indications for Exercise Testing to Assess Risk and prognosis in patients with symptoms or a prior history of coronary artery disease:

Class I. Conditions for which there is evidence and/or general agreement that the standard exercise test is useful and helpful to assess risk and prognosis in patients with symptoms or a prior history of coronary artery disease (ie, appropriate use)

- Patients undergoing initial evaluation with suspected or known CAD. Specific exceptions are noted below in Class IIb.
- Patients with suspected or known CAD previously evaluated with significant change in clinical status.

Class IIb. Conditions for which there is conflicting evidence and/or a divergence of opinion that the standard exercise test is useful and helpful to assess risk and prognosis in patients with symptoms or a prior history of coronary artery disease but the usefulness/efficacy is less well established (maybe appropriate).

- Patients who demonstrate the following ECG abnormalities:

- Pre-excitation (Wolff-Parkinson White) syndrome;
- Electronically paced ventricular rhythm;
- More than one millimeter of resting ST-depression; and
- Complete left bundle branch block.
- Patients with a stable clinical course who undergo periodic monitoring to guide management

Class III. Conditions for which there is evidence and/or general agreement that the standard exercise test is not useful and helpful to assess risk and prognosis in patients with symptoms or a prior history of coronary artery disease and in some cases may be harmful (not appropriate).

- Patients with severe comorbidity likely to limit life expectancy and/or candidacy for revascularization.

Part of the Basic Patient Evaluation

Per the published guidelines, patients with known or suspected coronary disease are usually evaluated initially after a careful cardiac history and physical exam with an exercise test. It can be performed safely and inexpensively and even accomplished in the physician's office. In addition to diagnostic information, the test gives practical and clinically valuable information regarding exercise capacity and response to therapy. Patients with clinical data and exercise test responses considered abnormal or associated with a high enough probability for cardiac events or of having severe coronary disease are frequently evaluated further by coronary angiography. A study evaluating the appropriateness of the performance of coronary angiography in clinical practice, considered angiography to be inappropriate nearly a quarter of the time due to the failure to obtain an exercise tests.[2]

FOLLOW UP STUDIES

As summarized previously,[3] nine studies have utilized clinical, exercise test, and catheterization data to predict prognosis in patients with coronary artery disease. All used multivariate survival analysis techniques and the variables chosen are listed in order of predictive power. Two of the nine found a history of congestive heart failure, two found exercise SBP, and one found resting ST-depression to be associated with death. Three found exercise-induced ST-depression and six of the nine found poor exercise capacity to be predictive of death. Age is not chosen by most of the studies because of the narrow age range for patients submitted to cardiac catheterization. All studies had to deal

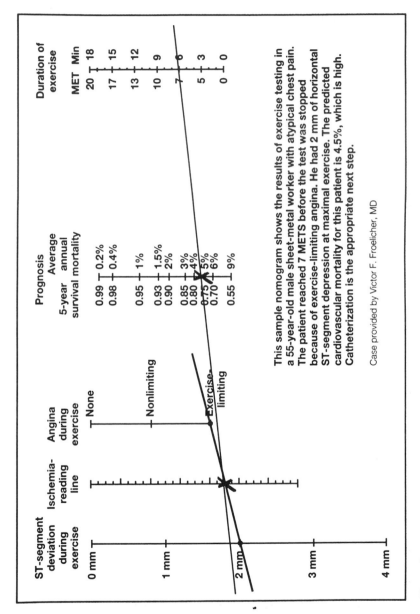

Figure 1.

with interventions that alter the natural history but each censored on them except for the earlier VA CABS study. The following study was an evolutionary improvement on these earlier studies.

The Duke Nomogram

Mark et al studied 2,842 consecutive patients who underwent cardiac catheterization and exercise testing and whose data was entered into the Duke computerized medical information system.[4] The median follow up for the study population was 5 years and 98% complete. All patients underwent a Bruce protocol exercise test and had standard ECG measurements recorded. A treadmill angina index was assigned a value of 0 if angina was absent, 1 if typical angina occurred during exercise, and 2 if angina was the reason the patient stopped exercising.

A score was calculated as: exercise time - (5 × ST maximum net deviation) - (4 × angina index) where exercise time is measured in minutes and ST deviation in millimeters. The treadmill score contained prognostically important information even after the information provided by clinical and catheterization data was considered. The score can be expressed as the nomogram below (Figure 1). This nomogram is considered by many to be the major advance in exercise testing in the past 10 years as is demonstrated by it's inclusion in all of the major guidelines.

Work-Up Bias

All of the above studies selected patients by requiring that they also underwent coronary angiography. To evaluate the effect of this selection process, the Duke group repeated their analysis in an outpatient population that did not undergo cardiac catheterization.[5] The same variables were chosen in their Cox model and the same equation was derived. Similarly, we analyzed 2,546 male patients who underwent noninvasive evaluation for coronary artery disease including exercise testing.[6] Over a mean follow-up period of 2.8 years, there were 119 cardiovascular deaths and 44 non-fatal myocardial infarctions. The Cox proportional hazard model demonstrated the following characteristics to have a significant independent hazards ratio: history of congestive heart failure and/or taking digoxin, exercise-induced ST-depression, exercise capacity in METs, and the response of SBP during exercise. A simple score based on these four factors stratified patients from low risk (annual cardiac mortality of less than 1%) to high risk (annual cardiac mortality of 7%). In addition, the Duke treadmill score was calculated for each of our Veteran patients and did nearly as well as our score validating it's portability.

PREDICTING SEVERE ANGIOGRAPHIC CORONARY DISEASE

Meta-Analysis of Studies Predicting Severe Angiographic Coronary Disease

To evaluate the variability in the reported accuracy of the exercise ECG for predicting severe coronary disease, Detrano et al applied meta analysis to 60 consecutively published reports comparing exercise-induced ST-depression with coronary angiographic findings.[7] The 60 reports included 62 distinct study groups comprising 12,030 patients who underwent both tests. Both technical and methodologic factors were analyzed. Wide variability in sensitivity and specificity was found (*mean sensitivity 86%* [range 40% to 100%, SD 12%]; mean *specificity 53%* [range 17% to 100%, SD 16%]) for left main or triple vessel disease. All three variables found to be significantly and independently related to sensitivity were methodologic (the exclusion of patients with right bundle branch block, the comparison with another exercise test thought to be superior in accuracy and the exclusion of patients taking digitalis). Exclusion of patients with right bundle branch block and comparison with a "better" exercise test were both significantly associated with sensitivity for the prediction of triple vessel or left main coronary artery disease.

Hartz et al compiled results from the literature on the use of the exercise test to identify patients with severe coronary artery disease.[8] Pooled estimates of sensitivity and specificity were derived for the ability of the exercise test to identify three-vessel or left main coronary artery disease. *One millimeter criteria averaged a sensitivity of 75% and a specificity of 66%* while *two millimeters* criteria averaged a *sensitivity of 52% and a specificity of 86%.* There was great variability among the studies examined in the estimated sensitivity and specificity of a given criterion for severe coronary artery disease and neither could these reviewers explain the reported variation.

Multi-variable Scores

Since the seminal work of Ellestad and colleagues[9] demonstrated that the accuracy of the test could be improved by combining other clinical and exercise parameters along with the ST responses, many clinical investigators have published studies proposing multivariable equations to enhance the accuracy of the standard exercise test. Studies utilizing modern statistical techniques have demonstrated that combinations of clinical and exercise test variables could more accurately predict the probability of angiographic coronary artery disease than the standard ST-depression criteria. While the statistical models proposed have proven to be superior, the available equations have differed as to the variables and coefficients chosen. Furthermore, the definitions or criteria for variables or for angiographic interpretation have not been standardized. Unfortunately, these uncertainties exist at a time when managed care providers are trying to apply cost-containment algorithms to health care.[10]

Over a 15-years period from 1980 through 1995, there were 30 articles published that used multivariable statistical analysis for the diagnosis of the presence of any or of severe angiographic coronary artery disease.[11] Since some did both, there were 24 studies that predicted presence of angiographic coronary artery disease and 13 studies that predicted disease extent or severe angiographic coronary artery disease.

STUDIES PREDICTING SEVERE ANGIOGRAPHIC CORONARY DISEASE OR DISEASE EXTENT.

Nine of the 13 studies excluded patients with previous coronary artery bypass surgery or prior percutaneous transluminal coronary angioplasty (PTCA) and in the remaining 4 studies, exclusions were unclear. The definition of significant angiographic disease percentage stenosis ranged from 50% to 70%. The percentage of patients with one vessel, two vessels and three vessels was described in 10 of the 13 studies. The definition of severe disease or disease extent (multivessel vs. three-vessel or left main artery disease) also differed. In 5 of the 13 studies disease extent was defined as multivessel disease (i.e., more than one vessel involved). In the remaining 8 studies, it was defined as three-vessel or left main disease and in one of them as only left main artery disease and in another the impact of disease in the right coronary artery disease on left main disease was considered. The prevalence of severe disease ranged from 16% to 48% in the studies defining disease extent as multivessel disease and from 10% to 28% in the studies using the more strict criterion of three-vessel or left main disease.

Statistical Techniques

Multivariable analysis is a statistical technique that seeks to separate subjects into different groups on the basis of measured variables.[12] Clinical investigators have commonly used two types of analysis: discriminate function and logistic regression analysis. Logistic regression has been preferred since it models the relationship to a sigmoid curve (which often is the mathematical relationship between a risk variable and an outcome) and it's output is between zero and one (i.e., from zero to 100% probability of the predicted outcome). Thus, the output of a discriminate function is a unit-less numerical score while a logistic regression provides an actual probability.

Not all of the publications of the reviewed studies included the equations derived from the multivariable analyses they performed which would be critical to the validation of their findings.[13] The equations developed in the studies were available for only 4 of the 13 studies predicting disease extent or severity.

Predictors of Disease Severity in 13 Studies (14 Equations)

Variables	Significant Predictor	
Gender	7/9	78%
Chest Pain Symptoms	8/11	73%
Diabetes Mellitus	6/10	60%
Age	8/14	57%
Abnormal Resting ECG	4/8	50%
Elevated Cholesterol	4/10	40%
Family History of CAD	1/4	25%
Smoking History	2/8	25%
Hypertension	1/6	17%
ST-Segment Depression	11/14	79%
ST-Segment Slope	6/8	75%
Double Product	4/7	57%
Delta Systolic BP	5/11	45%
Exercise Capacity	4/13	31%
Exercise Induced Angina	4/13	31%
Maximal HR	1/10	10%
Maximal Systolic BP	0/4	0%

The discriminating power of the variables listed above that appear in more than 50% of the equations above can be assumed. However, the predictive power of other variables remains undecided. Note also the difference in the variables chosen for predicting presence and severity of coronary disease. The reasons why the variables had different results in many of studies remains uncertain but the following sections discuss possible explanations.

Difference of Variable Definition

The way in which many of the clinical risk predictors were defined or classified differed in many of the studies. For example, smoking history was classified as current smoking, history of smoking or both. In all 4 studies where smoking was classified by history, it was not a good predictor. Furthermore, the classification of current smoking was not shown in detail, for instance, how many packs per day, how many years has a person smoked or which type of smoking (pipe, cigar, cigarette) and so on.

Differences in the Degree of Work-up Bias

A problem with these exercise test-angiographic correlation studies has been the failure to remove work up bias. Patients in studies were selected for angiography by their physician while others were excluded. This selection process results in patients with abnormal tests (i.e., with exercise-induced chest pain or ST-depression) being more likely to be chosen while patients with high exercise capacities would be excluded from such studies resulting in a relatively higher prevalence of disease than seen in a clinic population. Prior prediction equations, scores and heart rate adjustment schema were derived from populations with extensive work up bias and probably are not applicable to patients who present to their physician with chest pain.

The Effect of Characteristic (or Variable) Frequency (or Prevalence)

Prevalence in this discussion relates to the difference of frequency in the clinical variables and their impact on prediction. Diabetes was classified by history in 7 studies. All 3 studies, in which the prevalence of diabetes was greater than 19%, demonstrated that diabetes was a good predictor. In contrast diabetes was not a good predictor in 4 studies, where the frequency of diabetes was less than 16%. The same phenomena occurred with hypercholesterolemia. In all 4 studies in which the mean serum cholesterol concentration was more than 240 mg/dl, hypercholesterolemia was a good predictor.

Interactions Between Variables

Morise and colleagues demonstrated that when serum cholesterol concentration was included into the model, smoking lost its significance as a predictor of disease presence and extent. In 4 of the 9 studies where smoking was not a significant predictor, serum cholesterol was included into the model.

The Effect of Drug Administration

In most of the studies that considered maximal heart rate for the presence of disease, patients taking beta-blockers were included. Patients receiving digoxin were usually excluded.

Overfitting

The risk estimates may be unreliable if the multivariable data contain too few outcome events relative to the number of independent variables. In general, the results of models having fewer than 10 outcome events per independent variable are thought to have questionable accuracy.

Missing data

In several studies reviewed, the investigators included patients who had missing data. If a complete data set cannot be included for all patients in a training population, the model will not be generated including the entire population. This can greatly reduce the population size therefore, some investigators designed their models to handle missing data.

Gender Differences

In the extent of disease, the number of equations developed for females was less than 3. Age, chest pain symptoms, ST-segment depression and ST-segment slope were good predictors. In comparison, smoking history, hypertension, family history of CAD, exercise induced angina, maximal heart rate, maximal systolic blood pressure and exercise capacity were not good predictors.

Summary of the Multi-Variable Prediction Studies

While the studies demonstrate that the multi-variable equations out perform simple ST diagnostic criteria this may not be the case for disease severity. These equations generally provide a predictive accuracy of 80% (ROC area of 0.80). That they will function accurately in a clinic or office practice is uncertain since work up bias will never be totally removed. The selection process results in patients with abnormal ST responses and/or chest pain being more likely chosen while patients with high exercise capacities would be excluded from such studies resulting in a relatively higher prevalence of disease than seen in a clinic population. Thus, the coefficients for METs and ST-depression are probably not totally appropriate. In addition, while the discriminating power of the equations may persist when they are applied to another population, the calibration can be off.[14] For instance, the equation may predict a 50% chance of coronary disease given a set of variables in one population when a 70% chance is more appropriate in another population with the same variables.

CONSENSUS OR AGREEMENT

A hypothetical way to make these equations more portable and self-calibrating would be to require a consensus between a number of equations for patient classification as low or high risk. The consensus approach has been used by NASA to calculate the trajectories of spacecraft but has not been applied in health care. Majority would only classify patients as low or high risk if at least 2 of 3 equations agreed; i.e., consensus. In order to evaluate this approach, a probability score was calculated for each patient with a logistic regression equation that was developed in the VA and two other validated equations developed in different populations by Morise and Detrano, calculating probability for angiographic disease with each equation independently for each patient. The population was then partitioned repetitively using probability scores from 20 to 90 in increments of 5 for each equation separately. Using a consensus strategy that required at least two of the three logistic equations to agree at each probability score level, a training set was separated into groups using all equations at each probability score, calculating the prevalence of coronary artery disease in each group below or above the chosen probability score (< 30% or >75%). [15] Two thresholds or probability scores were chosen from results in the training set that separated the population into three groups: low risk (prevalence coronary artery disease < 5%), intermediate risk (5-70%), and high risk (> 70% prevalence for coronary artery disease).

This demonstrated that by using simple clinical and exercise test variables, we could improve on the standard use of ECG criteria during exercise testing for diagnosing coronary artery disease. Using the consensus approach divided the test set into populations with low, intermediate and high risk for coronary artery disease. Since the patients in the intermediate group would be sent for further testing and would eventually be correctly classified, the sensitivity of the consensus approach was 94% and the specificity was 92%. This consensus approach controls for varying disease prevalence, missing data, inconsistency in variable definition, and varying angiographic criterion for stenosis severity. The percent of correct diagnoses increased from the 70% for standard exercise ECG analysis and the 80% for multi-variable predictive equations to greater than 90% correct diagnoses for the consensus approach.

The consensus approach has made population-specific logistic regression equations portable to other populations. Excellent diagnostic characteristics can be obtained using simple data and measurements. The consensus approach is best applied utilizing a programmable calculator or a computer program (such as EXTRA) to simplify the process of calculating the probability of coronary artery disease using the three equations.

REFERENCES

1. Gibbons RJ; Balady GJ; Beasley JW; Bricker JT; Duvernoy WF; Froelicher VF; Mark DB; Marwick TH; McCallister BD; Thompson PD Jr; Winters WL; Yanowitz FG ACC/AHA Guidelines for Exercise Testing. A report of the American College of Cardiology/American Heart Association Task Force on Practice Guidelines (Committee on Exercise Testing).; J Am Coll Cardiol 1997 Jul;30(1):260-311

2. Chassin MR, Kosecoff J, Solomon DH, Brook RH. How coronary angiography is used. Clinical determinants of appropriateness. JAMA 1987; 258:2543-2547.

3. Morris CK, Morrow K, Froelicher VF, Hideg A, Hunter D, Kawaguchi T, Ribisl PM, Ueshima K, Wallis J. Prediction of cardiovascular death by means of clinical and exercise test variables in patients selected for cardiac catheterization. Am Heart J 1993; 125 (6):1717-1726.

4. Marks DB, Hlatky MA, Harrell FE, Lee KL, Califf RM, Pryor DB. Exercise treadmill score for predicting prognosis in coronary artery disease. Ann Int Med 1987;106:793-800.

5. Marks D, Shaw L, Harrell FE, Jr, Hlatky MA, Lee KL, Bengtson JR, McCants CB, Califf RM, Pryor DB. Prognostic value of a treadmill exercise score in outpatients with suspected coronary artery disease. N Engl J Med 1991;325:849-853.

6. Froelicher VF, Morrow K, Brown M, Atwood E, Morris C. Prediction of artherosclerotic cardiovascular death in men using a prognostic score. Am J Cardiol 1994; 73(2):133-138.

7. Detrano R, Gianrossi R, Mulvihill D, Lehmann K, Dubach P, Colombo A, Froelicher VF. Exercise-induced ST segment depression in the diagnosis of multivessel coronary disease: A meta analysis. J Am Coll Cardiol 1989;14:1501-1508.

8. Hartz A, Gammaitoni C, Young M. Quantitative analysis of the exercise tolerance test for determining the severity of coronary artery disease. Int J Cardiol 1989;24:63-71.

9. Ellestad MH, Savitz S, Bergdall D, Teske J. The false positive stress test. Multivariate analysis of 215 subjects with hemodynamic, angiographic and clinical data. Am J Cardiol 1977; 40: 681-687.

10. Braitman LE; Davidoff F. Predicting clinical states in individual patients. Ann Intern Med 1996 Sep 1;125(5):406-12

11. Yamada H, Do D, Morise A, Froelicher V. Review of Studies Utilizing Multi-variable Analysis of Clinical and Exercise Test Data to Predict Angiographic Coronary Artery Disease. Progress in CV Disease, 1997; 39:457-481.

12. Concato J, Feinstein AR, Holford TR. The risk of determining risk with multivariate models. Ann Intern Med 1993; 118: 201-210.

13. Diamond GA. Future imperfect: The limitations of clinical prediction models and the limits of clinical prediction. J Am Coll Cardiol 1989; 14: 12A-22A.

14. Harrell FE Jr; Lee KL; Mark DB. Multivariable prognostic models: issues in developing models, evaluating assumptions and adequacy, and measuring and reducing errors. Stat Med 1996 Feb 28;15(4):361-87

15. Dat Do, Jeffrey A. West, Anthony Morise, and Victor Froelicher. Agreement In Predicting Severe Angiographic Coronary Artery Disease Using Clinical and Exercise Test Data, Am Heart J 1997 Oct; 134:672-9.

32. CARDIOPULMONARY EXERCISE TESTING: CARDIOVASCULAR AND RESPIRATORY LIMITATIONS DETECTED BY EXERCISE GAS EXCHANGE

KARLMAN WASSERMAN

The basic requirement to sustain muscular exercise is an increase in cellular respiration for regeneration of adenosine triphosphate (ATP). The primary role of the cardiovascular system is to supply O_2 to the cells to support aerobic regeneration of adenosine triphosphate (ATP). This requires that O_2 consumption by the mitochondria be increased at a rate proportional to the increase in rate of ATP utilization. Each mole of ATP used to perform exercise requires approximately 1/6 of a mole of O_2 or 3.7 liters. The major function of the cardiovascular system is to supply the tissues with the O_2 needed by the metabolically active tissues. Cardiopulmonary exercise tests (CPET) in which gas exchange in response to exercise is measured breath-by-breath can be used to evaluate the dynamic efficiency with which the cardiovascular system couples respiration at the cells (O_2 consumed and CO_2 produced) to respiration at the airway (O_2 uptake and CO_2 output). This coupling is depicted in the scheme shown in figure 1.

To support the increase in cellular respiration, O_2 and CO_2 transport between the cells and the external airway must match the rate of cellular respiration except for transient lags allowed by the capacitances within the transport system. These include O_2 stores on the venous side of the circulation and small stores of high energy phosphate in the form of creatine phosphate in the myocytes. The increases in O_2 and CO_2 transport require the interaction of the peripheral circulation, heart, pulmonary circulation, blood, lungs and respiratory muscles, all controlled to couple their function to the cellular

331

H.-H. Osterhues et al. (eds.),
Advances in Noninvasive Electrocardiographic Monitoring Techniques, 331–339.
© 2000 *Kluwer Academic Publishers. Printed in the Netherlands.*

Questions Addressed by Cardiopulmonary Exercise Testing*

Question	Example of Disorder	Markers for Abnormality
1. Is exercise capacity reduced?	Any disorder	Maximal $\dot{V}O_2$ - panel 3
2. Is the metabolic requirement for exercise increased?	Obesity	$\dot{V}O_2$-WR relationship – panel 3
3. Is exercise limited by impaired O_2 flow?	Due to ischemic, myopathic, valvular, congenital heart disease?	ECG; LAT; $\Delta\dot{V}O_2 /\Delta WR$; $\dot{V}O_2 /HR$ – panels 2,3,5
	Due to pulmonary vascular disease?	$\Delta\dot{V}O_2/\Delta WR$; LAT; $\dot{V}O_2/HR$; $\dot{V}E/\dot{V}CO_2$ – panels 2,3,5,6
	Due to peripheral arterial disease?	BP; $\Delta\dot{V}O_2/\Delta WR$; LAT – panels 3,5
	Due to anemia, hypoxemia, or COHb?	LAT; $\dot{V}O_2/HR$ – panels 2,3,5
4. Is exercise limited by reduced ventilatory capicity?	Lung; chest wall	BR; ventilatory response – panel 1,7,9
5. Is there an abnormal degree of V/Q mismatching?	Lung; pulmonary circulation; heart failure	$P(A-a)O_2$; $P(a-ET)CO_2$; V_D/V_T; $\dot{V}E/\dot{V}CO_2$ - panels 4,6,9
6. Is there a defect in muscle utilization of O_2 or substrate?	Muscle glycolytic or mitochondrial enzyme defect	LAT, R, $\dot{V}CO_2$; HR vs $\dot{V}O_2$; lactate; lactate/pyruvate ratio – panels 3,8
7. Is exercise limited by a behaviorial problem?	Neurosis	Breathing pattern – panels 7,8
8. Is work output reduced because of poor effort?	Poor effort with secondary gain.	HRR; BR; peak R; $P(A-a)O_2$; $P(a-ET)CO_2$ - panels 2,5,7,8

* Maximum $\dot{V}O_2$ = highest O_2 uptake measured; WR=work rate; BR (breathing reserve)=maximum voluntary ventilation-ventilation at maximum exercise; $\Delta\dot{V}O_2/\Delta WR$ = increase in $\dot{V}O_2$, relative to increase in work rate; V_D/V_T=physiologic dead space/tidal volume ratio; $P(A-a)O_2$=alveolar-arterial PO_2 difference; COHb=carboxyhemoglobin; $P(a-ET)CO_2$ =arterial-end tidal PCO_2 difference; HRR (heart rate reserve)=predicted maximum heart rate-maximum exercise heart rate; $\dot{V}E/\dot{V}CO_2$=ventilatory equivalent for CO_2; Peak R=peak gas exchange ratio. Reproduced from reference 1.

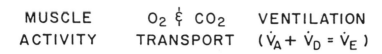

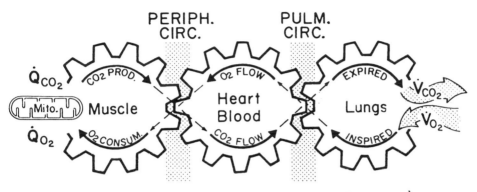

Figure 1. Scheme depicting the coupling of external to cellular respiration $\dot{V}_A$ = Ideal alveolar ventilation / time; $\dot{V}_D$ = physiological dead space ventilation / time; $\dot{V}_E$ = total ventilation measured during expiration / time; $\dot{Q}_{O_2}$ = O_2 consumption; $\dot{Q}_{CO_2}$ = CO_2 production; $\dot{V}_{O_2}$ = O_2 uptake; $\dot{V}_{CO_2}$ = CO_2 output; creat-PO4 = creatine phosphate; Pyr = pyruvate; Lac = lactate; Mito = mitochondria. See text for description of pathophysiological states which interfere with the normal coupling of external to cellular respiration. From ref.1.

respiratory requirement (Fig. 1). Any defect in this interactive system can cause exercise limitation.

Questions addressed by CPET.

Pathophysiological questions appropriate for a physician to ask when caring for a patient with exercise intolerance are shown in Table 1 (1). Using current techniques for making measurements and imposing an exercise stress, CPET provides an efficient way of addressing the questions posed. Examples of disease states which answer "yes" to the posed questions are also listed in Table 1. By identifying the pathophysiology of exercise limitation, a correct clinical diagnosis accounting for the patient's symptom(s) is possible.

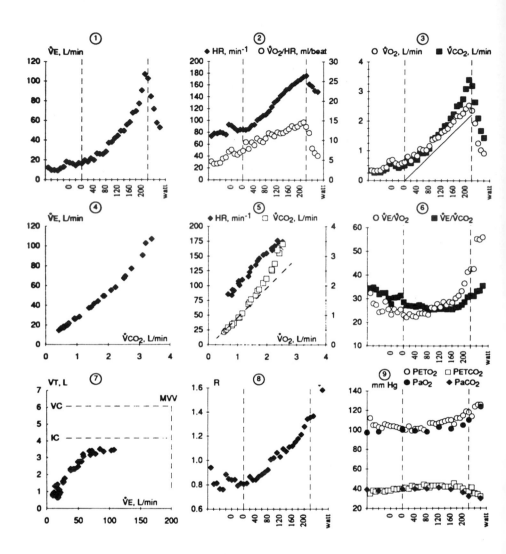

Figure 2. Nine panel graphical array used to describe the cardiovascular, ventilatory, ventilation-perfusion matching and metabolic responses to exercise in the medical record. Study is from a 55 y.o.m. patient (Modified from case 1 of reference 6). The responses are normal. The diagonal line drawn on panel 3 is the normal rate of increase in $\dot{V}O_2$ for the work rate increase (10 ml/min/watt). $\dot{V}E$ = minute ventilation; HR = heart rate; R = respiratory exchange ratio ($\dot{V}CO_2/\dot{V}O_2$); $PETO_2$ = end tidal PO_2 ; $PETCO_2$ = end tidal PCO_2 ; PaO_2 = arterial PO_2 ; $PaCO_2$ = arterial PCO_2 ;MVV = maximal voluntary ventilation; IC = Inspiratory capacity; VC = Vital capacity; watt = unit of power output (work rate). From ref.1.

Testing Protocol.

The testing protocol which has been shown to be very useful in diagnosing defects in the cardiovascular coupling of external (airway) to cellular (muscle) respiration is a progressive incremental exercise protocol in which work rate is increased at a uniform rate (preferably on a cycle ergometer) from unloaded cycling to the level of exercise at which fatigue, dyspnea or pain forces the patient to stop exercise. The cycle is preferable because it provides a true measure of work output to which the gas exchange and metabolic measurements can be related.

Evaluation of Cardiovascular Function from Cardiopulmonary Exercise Testing.

Figure 2 shows the data display that we use to determine the simultaneous performance of the heart, peripheral and pulmonary circulations, the ventilatory system and cellular metabolism. 15 graphs are displayed in 9 panels on a single page for ease of viewing and from which the patterns of change for many different diseases can be easily recognized. Each graph describes the physiological response to exercise of a specific function or organ system. The physiological information revealed by each panel and its graphs follow:

Panel 1- $\dot{V}E$ vs work rate. Normally becomes curvilinear as work rate is increased above the anaerobic threshold (*AT*) except when ventilatory work is excessive, e.g., patients with obesity or lung disease.

Panel 2 - Heart rate (HR) and $\dot{V}O_2$ /HR (equal to stroke volume x arteriovenous O_2 difference) vs work rate. HR is high and $\dot{V}O_2$ /HR is low for a given work rate in patients with certain cardiovascular defects except when under rate control or β-adrenergic blockade.

Panel 3 - $\dot{V}O_2$ and $\dot{V}CO_2$ vs work rate and slope showing predicted rate of increase in $\dot{V}O_2$ for the work rate increase (diagonal line). This is the first panel to address because it gives global assessment of the presence of exercise limitation. $\Delta\dot{V}O_2$ /ΔWR is commonly abnormal in patients with cardiovascular disease, the pattern varying with the defect as previously described (1). $\dot{V}CO_2$ increases above $\dot{V}O_2$ after a lactic acidosis develops and continues to increase steeply despite flattening of $\dot{V}O_2$.

Panel 4 - $\dot{V}E$ vs $\dot{V}CO_2$. A linear relationship until ventilatory compensation for metabolic acidosis (becomes steeper) or CO_2 retention (becomes more shallow) develop. The slope of the linear part increases when the physiological dead space/tidal volume (VD/VT) ratio is increased. Because VD/VT increases in proportion to exercise limitation in patients with chronic heart failure (2), the slope of the linear part is steeper than normal in this disorder (3,4)

Panel 5 - HR vs $\dot{V}O_2$ and $\dot{V}CO_2$ vs $\dot{V}O_2$. HR increases linearly with $\dot{V}O_2$ to the predicted maximums in normal subjects. In patients with heart failure or pulmonary vascular disease, the increase is steep and the relationship may lose its linearity with HR increasing progressively more rapidly than $\dot{V}O_2$. Up to the *AT*, $\dot{V}CO_2$ increases linearly with $\dot{V}O_2$ with a slope of one, or slightly less than one. Then $\dot{V}CO_2$ increases more rapidly, the steepening of the slope depending on the rate of buffering of lactic acid. The breakpoint describes the *AT*. This is the V-slope method for determining *AT* (5). It will be low in patients with poor cardiovascular function.

Panel 6 - Ventilatory equivalent for O_2 and CO_2 ($\dot{V}E$ /$\dot{V}O_2$ and $\dot{V}E$ /$\dot{V}CO_2$) vs work rate. $\dot{V}E/\dot{V}O_2$ decreases to a nadir at the *AT*. $\dot{V}E$ /$\dot{V}CO_2$ decreases to a nadir at the ventilatory compensation point. Both values are high in diseases in which pulmonary blood flow is abnormally reduced to ventilated lung.

Panel 7 - Tidal volume (VT) vs $\dot{V}E$. The patient's vital capacity (VC) and inspiratory capacity (IC) are shown on the VT axis and actually measured maximum voluntary ventilation or FEV$_1$ times 40 are shown on the $\dot{V}E$ axis (MVV). With airflow limitation, maximal exercise $\dot{V}E$ approximates the MVV. Thus the breathing reserve (MVV-$\dot{V}E$ at maximal exercise) is approximately zero. The breathing reserve can not be predicted from resting pulmonary function measurements, alone. With restrictive lung disease, VT may approximate the IC at low work rates and respiratory rate may ultimately increase above 50 or 60.

Panel 8 - Respiratory exchange ratio ($\dot{V}CO_2$ /$\dot{V}O_2$ or R) vs work rate. Usually starts at approximately 0.8 and increases to above 1.0 above the *AT*. Inability or failure to produce an exercise lactic acidosis mitigates increases to values above 1.0. R greater than 1.0 at rest indicates acute hyperventilation. This is reflected by a decreasing PETCO$_2$ in panel 9.

Panel 9 - PETCO$_2$ and PETO$_2$ vs work rate. Low PETCO$_2$ signals either hyperventilation or high VA/Q mismatching. An "R" value above 1 at rest (panel 8) reveals that hyperventilation is acute. Arterial blood gases or knowledge of plasma HCO_3^- differentiates chronic hyperventilation from VA/Q abnormality in patients with a low $PETCO_2$. Arterial blood gases are plotted on this graph to detect abnormal $P(A-a)O_2$ and $P(a-ET)CO_2$ to document low and high VA/Q mismatching, respectively.

The questions that can be addressed by cardiopulmonary exercise testing with respect to pathophysiological diagnosis of various disease processes that limit exercise are shown in Table 1. The relevant panel(s) of data supporting the diagnosis are given in the right column. The answer to the first question relating to exercise capacity is addressed in panel 3 from the measurement of maximum (peak) VO_2 . If it is reduced, we ask if the reduction is due to a cardiovascular limitation (panels 2,3 and 5), ventilatory limitation (panels 1,3,4,7), ventilation-perfusion mismatching (panels 3,6,9) or abnormality in use of metabolic substrate (panels 3, 8).

Poor effort is likely to be revealed by a high heart rate reserve (panel 2), high breathing reserve (panel 7), and a low R (panel 8) at end exercise. In addition, the patient may elicit a chaotic breathing pattern (panel 7) which may cause end-tidal PCO_2 and PO_2 to be quite variable (panel 9), the latter most evident during breath-by-breath monitoring.

Predicted Normal values.

The only parameters which require predicted normal values are the peak or maximal VO_2 and heart rate. The former is normalized by height, age and gender (ref. 6). The latter is scaled to age (220-age). All other measurements have predicted maximal and submaximal values which interrelate to VO_2 or the predicted VO_2 . Predicted normal values for VO_2 max, AT , VCO_2, $\Delta VO_2 / \Delta$ work rate, VE / VO_2, VE / VCO_2, $PETCO_2$, $PETO_2$, VT vs VE, Respiratory Exchange Ratio and Breathing Reserve are provided in reference 6.

Factors Confounding Interpretation of CPET.

Three physiological derangements, not usually considered as diseases of the cardiorespiratory system, may contribute significantly to exercise intolerance due to common cardiorespiratory disorders. These physiological derangements are 1) obesity, 2) anemia and 3) carboxyhemoglobinemia secondary to cigarette smoking.

Obesity adds to the O_2 and cardiac output cost of exercise. It also restricts the ventilatory system and increases the work of breathing. The restriction on ventilatory capacity and the work of breathing become more marked as the $\dot{V}E$ requirement increases.

Anemia reduces the arterial O_2 content and the maximal arteriovenous O_2 difference. Therefore, to achieve a given $\dot{V}O_2$, a greater cardiac output is required than if anemia were not present. Also because the O_2 content of the arterial blood is reduced, the capillary PO_2 decreases to its critical value, inducing anaerobic metabolism and lactic acidosis to take place at a reduced work rate and $\dot{V}O_2$.

The increased carboxyhemoglobin of the heavy cigarette smoker is about 10-12%. This not only reduces the arterial O_2 content to a level which would be found in patients with an arterial PO_2 of about 50-55 mm Hg, but also shifts the oxyhemoglobin dissociation curve to the left making it more difficult for O_2 to dissociate from hemoglobin at a given PO_2 . Thus the capillary PO_2 would fall more rapidly to its critical value, resulting in a lactic acidosis at a reduced level of work (7).

The net effect of these complicating factors is that the amount of external work that the patient can perform is reduced. However, in obesity, the maximal $\dot{V}O_2$ and AT are normal or high when referenced to their ideal body weight. In contrast, the maximal $\dot{V}O_2$, AT and peak work rate are reduced in patients with anemia and increased carboxyhemoglobinemia.

SUMMARY

Diseases of the cardiovascular system translate into abnormal gas exchange during exercise. The peak $\dot{V}O_2$ and the anaerobic threshold may provide the best quantification of the degree of impairment in cardiovascular function and at the least cost. Therefore CPET, with measurements of gas exchange, should play a major role in the evaluation of patients with cardiovascular diseases, particularly when the cause of exercise intolerance is uncertain. Also, it is likely to be especially valuable in determining the severity of the exercise impairment. CPET is a powerful diagnostic tool with great decision-making potential in guiding the management of patients with cardiovascular diseases.

REFERENCES

1. Wasserman, K. Diagnosing cardiovascular and lung pathophysiology from exercise gas exchange. CHEST 112:1091-1101, 1997.

2. Wasserman, K., Y-Y Zhang, A. Gitt, R. Belardinelli, A. Koike, L. Lubarsky, P. Agostoni. Lung function and exercise gas exchange in chronic heart failure. Circulation 96:2221-2227, 1997.

3. Metra, M. D. Raccagni, G. Carini, et.al. Ventilatory and arterial blood gas changes during exercise in heart failure. In: Wasserman K, ed. Exercise gas exchange in heart disease. Arrmonk, NY: Futura, 1996; 125-143.

4. Reindl, I and F. X. Kleber. Exertional hyperpnea in patients with chronic heart failure is a reversible cause of exercise intolerance. Basic Res. Cardiol. 91: Suppl. 1, 37-43, 1996.

5. Beaver, W.L., K. Wasserman and B.J. Whipp. A new method for detecting the anaerobic threshold by gas exchange. J. Appl. Physiol. 60:2020-2027, 1986.

6. Wasserman, K., J. Hansen, D.Y. Sue, B.J. Whipp, R. Casaburi. Principles of Exercise Testing and Interpretation, 2nd Edition. Chapter 6. Baltimore: Williams and Wilkins. 112-131.

7. Koike, A., D. Weiler-Ravell, D.K. Mckenzie, S. Zanconato and K. Wasserman. Evidence that the metabolic acidosis threshold is the anaerobic threshold. J.Appl.Physiol. 68:2521-2526, 1990.

CHAPTER FOUR: METHODS

SECTION THREE: AMBULATORY BLOOD PRESSURE MONITORING

33. WHITE-COAT HYPERTENSION: STATE OF THE ART

PAOLO VERDECCHIA, GIUSEPPE SCHILLACI,
CLAUDIA BORGIONI, ANTONELLA CIUCCI AND
CARLO PORCELLATI

Scipione Riva-Rocci first observed that the standard measurement of blood pressure (BP) triggered an alerting reaction and a pressor rise (1). These observations were subsequently confirmed (2). Mancia *et al.* demonstrated that the average rise in intra-arterial BP during clinical visit is of 27/14 mmHg, that the rise is maximal during the first 4 minutes of the visit, disappears within about 10 minutes and persists over several visits (3-5). The transient pressor rise during clinical visit is referred to as 'white-coat effect' or 'white-coat phenomenon' (6), while the coexistence of persistently high office BP with normal BP outside the medical setting is often referred to as 'white-coat' (7) or 'office' (8) hypertension. The white-coat effect is usually calculated as the difference between clinic BP and average daytime ambulatory BP (9-10).

In a recent study from our laboratory (11) white-coat hypertension was defined by an average daytime ambulatory BP < 131/86 mmHg in women and > 136/87 mmHg in men and its prevalence was 18.9%. The white-coat effect was calculated for systolic and diastolic BP as the difference between clinic BP and average daytime ambulatory BP. Echocardiographic LV mass was slightly but not significantly greater in the group with white-coat hypertension than in the normotensive group (93 *vs* 87 g/m^2, p = n.s.), and increased in the group with ambulatory hypertension (112 g/m^2, p < 0.01). The prevalence of white-coat hypertension markedly decreased from the first to the fourth Joint National Committee V (JNC V) stage of severity of hypertension (33% in I; 11% in II; 3% in III; 0% in IV; p < 0.001). The magnitude of the white-coat effect, which was greater (all p < 0.01) in the group with white-coat

H.-H. Osterhues et al. (eds.),
Advances in Noninvasive Electrocardiographic Monitoring Techniques, 343–349.
© 2000 *Kluwer Academic Publishers. Printed in the Netherlands.*

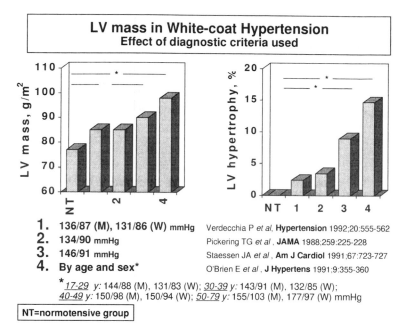

Figure 1. Target organ damage, exemplificated by LV hypertrophy, in white-coat hypertension. Adapted from (15).

hypertension (19.7/12.5 mmHg) than in that with ambulatory hypertension (12.5/4.2 mmHg), increased with the JNC V stage (7/4 mmHg in I, 16/6 mmHg in II, 23/8 mmHg in III, 29/12 mmHg in IV). Furthermore, the magnitude of the white-coat effect did not show any association with echocardiographic LV mass. Also Gosse et al. did not show any association between LV mass at echocardiography and white-coat effect (12). These data suggest that the the difference between clinical BP and awake ambulatory BP (white-coat effect, or phenomenon) may not be a clinically relevant finding, failing to reflect normal state of ambulatory standard BP and LV mass among subjects with standard clinical diagnosis of hypertension. The actual levels of ambulatory BP, not the magnitude of the white-coat effect, should therefore be used to identify the subjects with normal BP outside the clinic and potentially low cardiovascular risk.

White-coat hypertension is usually defined by persistent clinic hypertension with concomitant normal BP levels during usual daily life (6-8). This condition may lead to misclassification of hypertension in some actually normotensive individuals (6-8). Ambulatory BP (7) and self-measured BP (13) have been used to investigate prevalence and clinical characteristics of white-coat hypertension (14). The prevalence of white-coat hypertension varied from less than 20% (15) to more than 60% (13,16), with intermediate values (14,17-21). Frequency of target organ damage in white-coat hypertension is a controversial topic since, for example, echocardiographic LV mass in white-coat hypertension was normal in some studies (8,15) and increased in other studies (18-19). Different definitions of white-coat hypertension and different selection criteria for the normotensive control group may well contribute to explain these discrepancies. In our experience (figure 1), LV mass was not dissimilar between subjects with white-coat hypertension and healthy normotensive controls for cut-off values < 134/90 mmHg in both genders, or < 131/86 mmHg in women and 136/87 mmHg in men (15).

White *et al.* used an even more restrictive definition of white-coat hypertension (i.e., average daytime ambulatory BP < 130/80 mmHg) and found normal values of LV mass in white-coat hypertension (8). Kuwajima *et al.* used a more liberal definition of white-coat hypertension (i.e., average 24-hour systolic BP < 140 mmHg, irrespective of values of diastolic BP) and found a greater LV mass in 20 subjects with white-coat hypertension than in a control normotensive group of 13 subjects (19). Cardillo *et al.* (18) found a greater LV mass in a group of 20 subjects with white-coat hypertension than in a control normotensive group of 18 subjects, but the average daytime ambulatory BP was 12/13% higher in the group with white-coat hypertension than in the normotensive group (126/88 vs 113/78 mmHg, both p < 0.05), hence the different LV mass in the two groups might reflect the association between ambulatory BP and LV mass in the normotensive range (22). Overall, *the normal state of ambulatory BP and LV mass in the subjects with white-coat hypertension suggests that their risk of future cardiovascular complications is potentially low.*

In the setting of the PIUMA study (23), we prospectively followed for up to 7.5 years 1.187 subjects with essential hypertension and 205 healthy normotensive controls who had baseline off-therapy 24-hour non invasive ambulatory blood pressure monitoring. Prevalence of white-coat hypertension was 19.2%. Cardiovascular morbidity, expressed as the number of combined fatal and nonfatal cardiovascular events per 100 patient-years, was 0.47 in the normotensive group, 0.49 in the group with white-coat hypertension, 1.79 in dippers with ambulatory hypertension and 4.99 in non dippers with ambulatory hypertension. After adjustment for traditional risk markers, morbidity did not differ between the normotensive group and the group with white-coat hypertension (p = 0.83).

As compared with the group with white-coat hypertension, cardiovascular morbidity increased in ambulatory hypertension in dippers (relative risk: 3.70, 95% confidence interval: 1.13 to 12.5), with a further increase of morbidity in non dippers (relative risk: 6.26, 95% confidence interval: 1.92 to 20.32). **These**

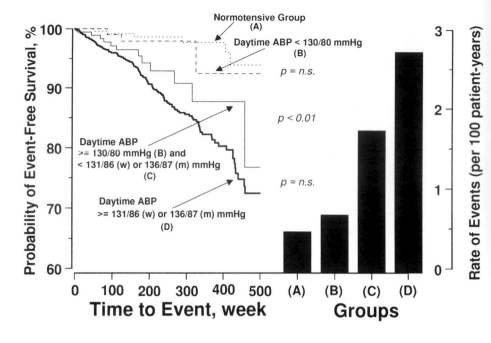

Figure 2. Cardiovascular morbidity in white-coat and ambulatory hypertension. Effects of definition criteria. Adapted from (25).

data show that cardiovascular morbidity is low in white-coat hypertension, and exceedingly high in women with ambulatory hypertension and absent or blunted blood pressure reduction from day to night. Preliminary prospective data from the Cornell group showed a less cardiovascular morbidity in subjects with white-coat hypertension than in those with ambulatory hypertension (9).

In a more recent analysis of the PIUMA database, including about 1.500 hypertensive subjects followed for an average of 4 years and 157 major cardiovascular morbid events, the subgroup with white-coat hypertension was divided up into two subsets with average daytime ambulatory BP < 130/80 mmHg or with intermediate values between 130/80 mmHg and 131/86 mmHg in women or 136/87 mmHg in men.

Figure 2 shows that the rate of major cardiovascular morbid events, expressed per 100 persons per year, was 0.46 in a control group composed by healthy normotensive subjects, 0.67 in the white-coat hypertension group defined more restrictively, 1.72 in the white-coat hypertension group defined more liberally, and 2.71 in the group with ambulatory hypertension. These differences were not significant between the normotensive group and the white-coat hypertension group defined more restrictively, but were significant between the normotensive group and the white-coat hypertension group defined more liberally (24). These data strongly indicate that *we should use a restrictive definition of white-coat hypertension (for example, average daytime BP < 130/80 mmHg), in order to identify a minority of subjects at low probability of developing a major cardiovascular event in the subsequent years.* Also a recent document by the American Society of Hypertension (25) suggests to use restrictive upper limits to define normalcy of ambulatory BP (i.e., average daytime BP < 135 mmHg systolic <u>and</u> 85 mmHg diastolic).

Antihypertensive drug treatment might be withhold in subjects with white-coat hypertension, particularly when two conditions coexist:: low values of daytime ambulatory BP (i.e., < 130/80 mmHg) and absence of organ lesions or other risk factors. The good prognosis in our subjects with white-coat hypertension defined using restrictive criteria supports this possibility, but a final answer will come from larger surveys of the natural history of this condition in the very long-term. Ideally, these longitudinal studies should also compare the response to drug treatment with that to life-style measures in these subjects.

REFERENCES

1. Riva Rocci S. La tecnica della sfigmomanometria. *Gazzetta Medica di Torino* 1897; 10: 181-191.
2. Ayman D, Goldshine AD. Blood pressure determinations by patients with essential hypertension: the difference between clinic and home readings before treatment. *Am J Med Sci* 1940; 200: 465-474.
3. Mancia G, Bertineri G, Grassi G, Parati G, Pomidossi G, Ferrari A, Gregorini L, Zanchetti A. Effects of blood pressure measured by the doctor on patient's blood pressure and heart rate. *Lancet* 1983; 2: 695-698.
4. Mancia G. Parati G, Pomidossi G, Grassi G, Casadei R, Zanchetti A. Alerting reaction and rise in blood pressure during measurement by physician and nurse. *Hypertension* 1987; 9: 209-215.
5. Omboni S, Parati G, Santucciu C, Mutti E, Groppelli A, Trazzi S, Mancia G. "White-coat" effect and patient's response to antihypertensive treatment (abstract n. 50). *J Hypertens* 1994; 12 (Suppl. 3): S10.
6. Mancia G, Parati G. Clinical significance of "white coat" hypertension. *Hypertension* 1990; 16: 624-625.
7. Pickering TG, James GD, Boddie C, Harshfield GA, Blank S, Laragh JH. How common is white-coat hypertension ? *JAMA* 1988; 259: 225-228.

8. White WB, Schulman P, McCabe EJ, Dey HM. Average daily blood pressure, not office pressure, determines cardiac function in patients with hypertension. *JAMA* 1989; 261:873-877.

9. Pickering TG. The ninth Sir George Pickering memorial lecture. Ambulatory monitoring and the definition of hypertension. *J Hypertens* 1992; 10: 401-409.

10. Pickering TG. Blood pressure measurement and detection of hypertension. *Lancet* 1994; 344: 31-35.

11. Verdecchia P, Schillaci G, Borgioni C, Ciucci A, Zampi I, Gattobigio R, Sacchi N, Porcellati C. White coat hypertension and white coat effect. Similarities and differences. *Am J Hypertens* 1995; 8: 790-798.

12. Gosse P, Promax H, Durandet P, Clementy J. "White-coat Hypertension": no harm for the heart. *Hypertension* 1993; 22: 766-770.

13. Julius S, Mejis A, Kones K, Krause L, Schork N, van de Ven C, Johnson E, Petrin J, Sekkarie A, Kjeldsen SE, Schmouder R, Gupta R, Ferraro J, Nazzaro P, Weissfeld J. "White Coat" versus "Sustained" borderline hypertension in Tecumseh, Michigan. *Hypertension* 1990; 16: 617-623.

14. Staessen JA, O'Brien ET, Atkins N and Amery AK on behalf of the Ad-Hoc Working Group. Short Report: ambulatory blood pressure in normotensive compared with hypertensive subjects. *J Hypertens* 1993; 11: 1289-1297.

15. Verdecchia P, Schillaci G, Boldrini F, Zampi I, Porcellati C. Variability between current definitions of 'normal' ambulatory blood pressure. Implications in the assessment of white-coat hypertension. *Hypertension* 1992; 20: 555-562.

16. Spence JD, Bass M, Robinson HC, Cheung H, Melendez LJ, Arnold JMO, Mannuck SB. Prospective study of ambulatory monitoring and echocardiography in borderline hypertension. *Clin Invest Med* 1991; 14: 241-250.

17. Hoegholm A, Kristensen KS, Bang LE, Nielsen JW, Nielsen WB, Madsen NH. Left ventricular mass and geometry in patients with established hypertension and white-coat hypertension. *Am J Hypertens* 1993; 6: 282-286.

18. Cardillo C, De Felice F, Campia U, Folli G. Psychophysiological reactivity and cardiac end-organ changes in white-coat hypertension. *Hypertension* 1993; 21: 836-844.

19. Kuwajima I, Miyao M, Uno A, Suzuki Y, Matsushita S, Kuramoto K. Diagnostic value of elettrocardiography and echocardiography for white-coat hypertension in the elderly. *Am J Cardiol* 1994; 73: 1232-1234.

20. Krakoff LR, Eison H, Phillips RH, Leiman SJ, Lev S. Effects of ambulatory blood pressure monitoring on the diagnosis and cost of treatment for mild hypertension. *Am Heart J* 1988; 116: 1152-1154.

21. Siegel WC, Blumenthal JA, Divine GW. Physiological, psycological and behavioural factors and white-coat hypertension. *Hypertension* 1990; 16: 140-146.

22. Porcellati C, Schillaci G, Verdecchia P, Battistelli M, Bartoccini C, Zampi I, Guerrieri M, Comparato E. Diurnal blood pressure changes and left ventricular mass: Influence of daytime blood pressure. *High Blood Press* 1993; 2: 249-258.

23. Verdecchia P, Porcellati C, Schillaci G, Borgioni C, Ciucci A, Battistelli M, Guerrieri M, Gatteschi C, Zampi I, Santucci A, Santucci C, Reboldi G. Ambualtory blood pressure: an independent predictor of prognosis in essential hypertension. *Hypertension* 1994; 24:793-801.

24. Verdecchia P, Schillaci G, Borgioni C, Ciucci A, Porcellati C. White-coat hypertension. *Lancet* 1996; 348:1444-1445.

25. Pickering T, for an American Society of Hypertension Ad Hoc Panel. Recommendations for the use of home (Self) and ambulatory Blood Pressure Monitoring. *Am J Hypertens* 1996; 9: 1-11.

34. SHOULD ANTIHYPERTENSIVE TREATMENT BE GUIDED BY CASUAL MEASUREMENT OR TROUGH ABPM ?

MARC DE BUYZERE, DENIS L. CLEMENT

INTRODUCTION

Several reliable, convenient, easy to use, validated commercial ambulatory blood pressure (ABP) monitors are now currently available on the market. However, most recommendations, such as those from the Ad Hoc panel of the American Society of Hypertension, the National High Blood Pressure Education Program Coordinating Committee and the Joint National Committee on Prevention, Detection, Evaluation and Treatment of High Blood Pressure restrict ABP to specific conditions. They advise that ABP should not be used indiscriminately for the routine evaluation and management of the hypertensive patient. Most important conditions in which ABP was thought to be helpful included suspected white coat hypertension (WCH), apparent drug resistance, hypotensive symptoms while on antihypertensive drugs, episodic hypertension and autonomic dysfunction (1,2). Individual authors sometimes have more extended lists of clinical indications such as borderline hypertension with target organ damage, orthostatic hypotension and so on (3). All of them agree that ABP is an excellent technique to monitor clinical drug trials, strongly reducing the placebo effect (Table 1).Nevertheless, many investigators in the field have the strong feeling that these are not the final indications and that the answer to the question whether or not the management of the hypertensive patient should be guided by ABP is now turning into a new direction. Next to a number of theoretical advantages of ABP over casual or

H.-H. Osterhues et al. (eds.),
Advances in Noninvasive Electrocardiographic Monitoring Techniques, 351–358.
© 2000 Kluwer Academic Publishers. Printed in the Netherlands.

Table 1 . Ambulatory blood pressure recordings: indications

- patients with apparent drug "resistance"
- suspected white coat hypertension (WCH)
- hypotensive symptoms while on antihypertensive drugs
- episodic hypertension
- autonomic dysfunction
- conflicting data between BP and target organ damage
- (orthostatic) hypotension
- as a research tool for clinical drug trials and studies on the mechanisms of BP-variability

office BP (OBP), two kinds of clinical evidence have been provided by the literature during the last years: cross-sectional studies with target organ damage (particularly left ventricular hypertrophy, LVH) and well-designed prognostic trials.

THEORETICAL ADVANTAGES OF ABP

ABP recordings have been introduced during the past 2 decades to define BP and its shifts better. ABP recorded over a longer period of time may have a number of theoretical advantages and overcome many problems associated with casual or office BP measurements (4). First, the single fact that more measurements are made should provide a better approach to the definition of the mean BP (or BP load) of a subject during a certain observation period (better estimate of means). Secondly, ABP can inform us about the inherent process of BP-variability (night-time BP, day-night dipping, hourly variability, ...), whereas OBP is derived from only a few measurements during the consultation. During the last decade measures of BP-variability have been associated with target organ damage in hypertension. Thirdly, OBP is influenced much more by the conditions during the consultation than ABP: alerting reactions and white coat phenomenon. However, the clinical meaning of high BP peaks, has not been fully clarified. Fourthly, ABP is a very adequate method to document the time-course of effective BP reduction induced by an antihypertensive drug treatment.

Notwithstanding all these theoretical advantages, clinical use of ABP has for a relatively long-time been hampered by a number of shortcomings or practical disadvantages which had to be coped with. We will shortly mention a number of them. Broad scale application of ABP requires non-invasive methodology. In the past, several studies have been published using intra-arterial (i.a.) beat-to-beat measurements of BP. Although the latter studies are important, general management of a hypertensive patient would be difficult to imagine using i.a. ABP. A number of safety aspects are to be dealt with as well. Another important requirement is the aspect of automatic recordings. Older apparatus working semi-automatic (self-inflation), were limited to daytime BP recordings but are now out of the market. The key point to be addressed before any kind of recommendation, is the validation of the commercially available ABP devices. Many devices are on the market, using different measuring principles: auscultatory, oscillometric, combined. Even within the oscillometric devices several algorithms are used, which have not been published in detail by the manufacturers. Several validation protocols for accuracy, precision and reproducibility are available. O'Brien et al. summarized the results of accuracy criteria of the British Hypertension Society protocol (BHS) and the Association for the Advancement in Medical Instrumentation (AAMI) protocol (5).

There is still much controversy in literature what are the optimal time intervals between 2 ABP readings of a 24-h recording. Should it be every 15 min, 30 min or is every 60 min enough ? Several investigators have critical remarks on the definition of day and night time; most agree that fixed clock-times should be replaced by effective hours of sleep or activity based on the patients' diaries and that hours with much arousal should be discarded from the statistical analysis.

Another, but also very important issue and prerequisite before ABP can be used as a tool for patient management is the calculation of reference/normal values (6,7). Staessen et al. collected data for a meta-analysis and provided ABP limits for probable hypertension (6). Once reference values been calculated, it becomes much easier to use ABP recordings to define hypertension and to judge efficacy of drug treatment. It should be realised that at present there are still no ABP limits available based on prognostic studies of morbidity and mortality. A last disadvantage that should be remembered concerns the high costs that are related to ABP monitoring (apparatus, technicians, time-consuming, ...). Studies are ongoing to address the cost-benefits analyses.

CROSS-SECTIONAL STUDIES: TARGET ORGAN DAMAGE VERSUS OBP OR ABP

Many cross-sectional studies (4) have suggested that ABP is a better indicator of the severity of target organ damage than OBP. Most data are available for left ventricular hypertrophy, a well-established risk factor for future cardiovascular events. In the earliest studies OBP and ABP have been correlated with electrocardiographic criteria of LVH (Frank leads, standard leads); later on, echocardiographic measures (wall thicknesses, LVM, LVMI) were used. A first important observation is that in general the relationship between LVH and BP in cross-sectional studies is weak. This may be due to several reasons or shortcomings: low sensitivity of ECG criteria, non standardized protocols for echocardiography, inadequate OBP measurements, non-haemodynamic factors codetermining LVH etc. Nonetheless, in most of these correlation studies between LVH and BP, ABP performed somewhat better than OBP (4). Anyway, the work of Fagard et al. (8,9) should be mentioned that when defining Echo measures by a standardized protocol and measuring casual BP also by protocol (over several days, by a nurse instead of a doctor, ...) the correlations between LVH and respectively casual BP and ambulatory BP are converging. A recent important contribution on the prediction of the regression of LVH by ABP comes from a prospective study in a sample of hypertensives from the SAMPLE-study (10). In 184 well-defined hypertensives (LVH > 110 g/m2 for females and > 131 g/m2 for males) clinic, 24-h ABP and LVH and LVMI were measured before and after treatment with 20 mg o.d. lisinopril with or without 12.5/25 mg o.d. hydrochlorothiazide for 12 months. It turned out that the treatment-induced regression of LVH was better predicted by changes in ABP than by changes in clinic BP over the 12 months follow-up. This illustrates the value of ABP in the management of LVH. Also the group of Fagard et al (11) reported additive value of ABP to explain treatment - induced changes of LV mass. Earlier, using non-invasive 24-h BP recordings in 728 subjects, Palatini et al (12) already suggested that a reduced day-night BP difference and an increased day-time BP-variability were associated with a higher degree of hypertensive cardiovascular complications (a target organ score of 0 to 5 based on fundoscopy, electrocardiogram and chest roentgenogram). No relationship was found between degree of cardiovascular complications and peaks of pressure. In another study by Shimada et al (13) a good correlation was obtained between 24-h ABP and non-dipping in an elderly population. Non-dipping was associated with more left ventricular hypertrophy and with more documented (magnetic resonance imaging) cerebrovascular damage. Nevertheless a few words of caution should be added concerning the concept of dipping. First, the reproducibility of dipping is rather poor. Second, the level of night-time BP is in part determined by the level of day-time BP.

PROGNOSTIC STUDIES USING ABP

The first pioneers' study on the relationship between ABP and cardiovascular morbidity and mortality came in the early 80's. Perloff et al. (14) measured day-time ABP in 1076 patients with hypertension (459 of them treated at the time of the ABP recordings) and followed them for a mean of 5 years. For each subject the observed ABP was compared with the predicted ABP (e.g. expected ABP value on the regression line between ABP and OBP); the difference between observed and predicted ABP was defined as the residual blood pressure. If residual ABP exceeded 10 mmHg systolic or 6 mmHg diastolic, more new fatal and non-fatal cardiovascular events were observed than for ABP values below those values. Because OBP was comparable in the two groups, Perloff et al. (15) concluded that ABP is an important determinant of clinical outcome in essential hypertension.

The trends applied to both SBP and DBP, but were most apparent for less-severe hypertension and patients without previous cardiovascular events. Perloff et al. later performed subanalysis of the same data using the Cox proportional hazards model. For patients not initially treated, who did not sustain a previous cardiovascular event, age, left ventricular hypertrophy, observed and residual ABP, female sex and drug treatment independently predicted the development of future cardiovascular events. However, for patients with a previous cardiovascular event, age and residual ABP (negative), female sex and drug treatment (positive) were independent predictors. Thus, the ABP level was not an independent risk factor in this subanalysis, in contrast to the residual ABP.

In the early nineties other aspects of ABP monitoring have been related to outcome and cardiovascular events. Using intra-arterial blood pressure recordings, Frattola et al. (16), calculated 24-h blood pressure variability in 73 patients. Follow-up was between 4–10 years. The individual initial variables most important to predict end-organ damage at follow-up were initial level of target-organ damage and initial BP-variability.

A few years later, Verdecchia et al. were the first who, with renewed interest, described ABP as an independent predictor of prognosis in hypertension (17). In a large sample of the PIUMA registry, they enrolled 1187 patients with essential hypertension and 205 normotensive controls: all underwent clinic and ambulatory BP recordings. Their main study parameter was combined fatal–non-fatal events/100 patient years. For normotensives the rate was 0.47; for white coat hypertension (< 131/86 mmHg ABP for females, < 136/87 mmHg for males) 0.49. There was a large difference between the rates for ambulatory hypertensive dippers (1.79) and non-dippers (4.99).

Events were particularly high for nondipping women. After adjustment for other factors, Verdecchia et al. could define ABP as an independent risk marker. Events were low for white coat hypertension, and highest for non-dipping women. After those preliminary results in the white coat hypertensives and bearing in mind that several investigators were not convinced that white coat hypertension is an innocuous clinical condition, the same authors addressed the prognostic significance of the white coat effect (18). They documented 6371 persons years from 1522 subjects from the PIUMA registry and took the (clinic-ambulatory) blood pressure differences as a surrogate measure for the white coat effect. During follow up there were 32 fatal and 125 non-fatal events. Analysis for quartiles of the BP difference demonstrated that the difference could not predict cardiovascular morbidity and mortality in essential hypertension. The authors concluded that white coat hypertension is a more innocuous condition than some had thought for a long time.

The most recent and largest study on screening blood pressure versus ABP comes from Ohkubo et al (19) in the Ohasama pilot project. Subjects (n=1542, 565 males) from a Japanese general population have been followed up for 5.1 ± 2.0 years. Subjects were over 40 years old and 473 of them took antihypertensive drugs. Mortality was the main outcome variable. Thirty-seven cardiovascular deaths (24 cerebrovascular and 13 from heart disease) and fifty-six non-cardiovascular events had been documented. The study concluded that systolic 24-h ABP had a stronger predictive power than screening BP for both overall and cardiovascular mortality, using a Cox proportional hazard model.

An interesting secondary finding was the association between low night ABP and non-cardiovascular death. Of course, the latter needs to be confirmed in well-designed studies. All of these recently published studies point into the direction that ABP might be a good tool to manage BP in hypertension. However, the final answer to the question has not been given yet. Many prospective surveys and studies using ABP have been set up and are ongoing, in Europe and the USA. Results are to be expected within the next years. Among them we only mention: OvA, the 24-h ABP arm of Syst-Eur, OCTAVE II, SAMPLE, ... (20-22). OvA (Office versus Ambulatory blood pressure: a European study) aims to study the relation between (cardiovascular) mortality, morbidity, target organ damage and blood pressure expressed either as office or as ambulatory blood pressure (23). Events will be documented over at least 10,000 patients years follow-up. Patients should be treated, but treatment is at the discretion of the physician. Left ventricular hypertrophy is followed at yearly intervals by ECG and Echo, as well as office and ambulatory BP. Mid 1997, inclusion in OvA was stopped when more than 2,300 patients had been enrolled. The OvA study has been constructed as close as possible to the daily routine of an outpatient hypertension clinic. By May 98, almost 6,000 patients/years have been included.

CONCLUSIONS

When answering the question whether the management of hypertensive patients should be guided by office or ambulatory blood pressure, first it should be remembered that the present versions of current guidelines for management of hypertension do not recommend ABP recordings for diagnosis and treatment management of each individual patient. On the contrary ABP recordings are limited to certain well-described conditions. However, many investigators and clinicians in the field feel that this will not be the final answer to the question. Indeed there are arguments, theoretical ones and from clinical studies that point into the direction that ABP will be an interesting and rewarding tool for treatment decisions. The available studies (PIUMA, Ohasama, ...) provide prospective evidence in favour of ABP, but more results from forthcoming studies such as OvA, and 24-h ABP arm of Syst-Eur will be needed to convince leading authorities to adapt current recommendations and guidelines.

REFERENCES

1. Pickering T for an American Society of Hypertension ad hoc panel. Recommendations for the use of home (self) and ambulatory blood pressure monitoring. Am J Hypertens 1995; 9: 1-11.
2. The Sixth Report of the Joint National Committee (JNC VI) on Prevention, Detection, Evaluation and Treatment of High Blood Pressure. Arch Intern Med 1997; 157: 2413-2446.
3. Clement DL. Ambulatory blood pressure recordings: quo vadis ? [Editorial] Neth J Med 1992; 40: 165-171.
4. Clement DL, De Buyzere M, Duprez D. Prognostic value of ambulatory blood pressure monitoring. J Hypertens 1994; 12: 857-864.
5. O'Brien E, Beevers DG, Marshall M. ABPM devices that have fulfilled BHS and AAMI accuracy criteria. ABC of Hypertension London: BMJ Publishing Group 1995, 28.
6. Staessen J, O'Brien E, Atkins N et al. Ambulatory blood pressure in normotensive compared to hypertensive subjects. J Hypertens 1993; 11: 1289-1297.
7. Sega R, Cesana G, Milesi C et al. Ambulatory and home blood pressure normality in the elderly. Data from the PAMELA population. Hypertension 1997; 30: 1-6.
8. Fagard R, Staessen J, Thijs L, Amery A. Multiple standardized clinic blood pressure may predict left ventricular mass as well as ambulatory monitoring: a meta-analysis of comparative studies. Am J Hypertension 1995; 8: 533-540.
9. Fagard R, Staessen J, Thijs L. Prediction of cardiac structure and function by repeated clinic and ambulatory blood pressure. Hypertension 1997; 29: 22-29.

10. Mancia G, Zanchetti A, Agebiti-Rosei E et al. Ambulatory blood pressure is superior to clinic blood pressure in predicting treatment-induced regression of left ventricular hypertrophy. Circulation 1997; 95: 1464-1470.

11. Fagard R, Staessen J, Thijs L. Relationships between changes in left ventricular mass and in clinic and ambulatory blood pressure in response to antihypertensive therapy. J Hypertens 1997; 15: 1493-1502.

12. Palatini P, Penzo M, Racioppa A et al. Clinical relevance of night-time blood pressure and of day-time blood pressure variability. Arch Int Med 1992; 152: 1855-1860.

13. Shimada K, Kawamoto A, Matsubayashi K, Ozawa T. Silent cerebrovascular disease in elderly: correlation with ambulatory pressure. Hypertension 1990; 16: 692-699.

14. Perloff D, Sokolow M, Cowan R. The prognostic value of ambulatory blood pressures. JAMA 1983; 249: 2792-2798.

15. Perloff D, Sokolow M, Cowan R. The prognostic value of ambulatory blood pressure monitoring in treated hypertensive patients. J Hypertens 1991; 9 (Suppl 1): S33-S40.

16. Frattola A, Parati G, Cuspidi C, Albini F, Mancia G. Prognostic value of 24-h blood pressure variability. J Hypertens 1993; 11: 1133-1137.

17. Verdecchia P, Porcellati C, Schillaci G et al. Ambulatory blood pressure: an independent predictor of prognosis in essential hypertension. Hypertension 1994; 24: 793-801.

18. Verdecchia P, Schillaci G, Borgioni C et al. Prognostic significance of the white coat effect. Hypertension 1997; 29: 1218-1224.

19. Ohkubo T, Imai Y, Tsuji I et al. Prediction of mortality of ambulatory blood pressure monitoring versus screening blood pressure measurements: a pilot study in Ohasama. J Hypertens 1997; 15: 357-364.

20. Clement DL, De Buyzere M, Duprez D. Ambulatory blood pressure and prognosis: summary of ongoing studies. J Hypertens 1991; 9 (Suppl 8): S51-S53.

21. Staessen J, Amery A, Clement DL et al. Twenty-four hour blood pressure monitoring in the Syst-Eur trial. Aging 1992; 4: 85-91.

22. Mancia G, Zanchetti A, Agebiti-Rosei E et al. Prognostic value of ambulatory blood pressure: the SAMPLE study. High Blood Pressure 1992; 1: 297-301.

23. Clement DL. Office versus Ambulatory recordings of blood pressure (OvA): a European multicenter study. J Hypertens 1990; 8 (Suppl 6): S39-S41.

35. NON-INVASIVE PULSE WAVE VELOCITY AS A METHOD TO EVALUATE PHYSICAL PROPERTIES OF THE LARGE ARTERIES IN AGING AND HYPERTENSION

JOSÉ L. PALMA-GÁMIZ

INTRODUCTION

Physical properties of the large arteries and in particular the aorta play an important role in cardiovascular physiology and pathophysiology (1). Several studies have strongly suggested an association between the reduction in aortic distensibility and compliance, with a parallel increase in cardiovascular morbidity and mortality (2).

In aging and in hypertension (HT), and more specifically inisolated systolic hypertension (a typical hypertensive form of elderly), there is a significant increase in pulse wave velocity (PWV) as a consequence of the loss in two main arterial properties, i.e., distensibility and compliance.Enlarging arteries are stiffer, and subsequently PWV increases (3).

According to the previous statement, the correct clinical diagnosis of these changes in arterial physical properties in aging and in HT, might provide an excellent approach to cardiovascular mortality and morbidity as well, indicate at the same time the beneficial effects of different antihypertensive compounds. This would be so not only in relation with a reduction on blood pressure values, but also with observation of the possible modifications in the physical properties of the arteries previously mentioned.

H.-H. Osterhues et al. (eds.),
Advances in Noninvasive Electrocardiographic Monitoring Techniques, 359–370.
© 2000 *Kluwer Academic Publishers. Printed in the Netherlands.*

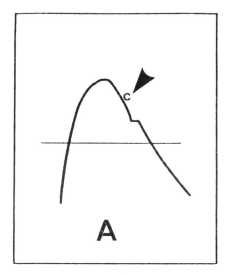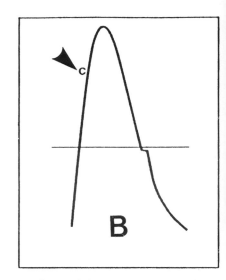

Figure 1. Curve A belongs to a young normotensive subject, while curve B corresponds to an old hypertensive patient. Differences in curve profile, SBP and PP are evident, while MBP remains in both cases at the same level. "C" point represents the counterpulsation effect between incident and reflected waves in both curves.

THE PULSE WAVE VELOCITY

The left ventricular ejection generates a pulse wave into the arterial wall, which travels from the heart to the furthest part of the circulatory system at a speed that varies between 4 to 10 metres per second. This wave is the so-called incident wave. When this incident wave impacts against a stiff vascular structure, for example, the aortic carrefour, or against a significant arterial stenosis, this wave is reflected, travelling in the opposite direction, that is, from the periphery to the heart. Both the incident and the reflected waves crash in some point of the arterial system, generally in the neighbourhood of aortic root, provoking a counterpulsation effect. The point of this crash is important for the mechanics of the left ventricle.

The loss in distensibility and compliance, modifies proportionally blood pressure (BP) curve profile , as shown in figure 1. The higher the loss in distensibility and compliance, the higher the increase in systolic blood pressure (SBP), with no modification on mean (MBP) but slightly reducing diastolic blood presure (DBP) . The inmediate result, is an isolated systolic HT, with a significant increase in pulse pressure (PP). Recent studies have signaled PP as an important marker for cardiovascular mortality and morbidity (4). Also the increase in SBP secondary to a loss of distensibility and compliance, is recognized as the first mechanical factor to induce left ventricular hypertrophy and hcart failure (5).

This form of HT, secondary to the loss on physical properties of the arteries, is common in the elderly, modifying substantially the aortic BP profile as shown in figure 1. The curve on the left corresponds to a young normotensive man, while the aortic curve on the right belongs to an old hypertensive patient in which an exaggerated increase in SBP and PP is observed with small changes in MBP. In this figure 1, we can also observe, in the first case (curve on the left) the reflected wave of the previous cardiac cycle, impacting on the descending slope, when left ventricle is practically at the end of its systolic ejective period, i.e., in the protodiastolic phase. In the other case, (curve on the right) the reflected wave impacts on the ascending part of the aortic curve, that is; in the early systolic phase, provoking a counterpulsation effect, and powerfully increasing cardiac work and myocardial oxygen consumption, leading to left ventricular hypertrophy and heart failure later.

CLINICAL INTEREST

The interest of the scientists on PWV is not new. In 1872, Moens published for the first time in a very interesting paper, the formula to calculate in mammals this PWV. The formula was inexact, but contained all the necessary parameters to calculate properly the PWV in man, such as; wall artery thickness, lateral wall expasion, blood viscosity and the inner diameter of the vessel.

Some years later, in 1922, Bramwell and Hill (6), published a document demonstrating for the first time the ability of the formula for a proper calculation of PWV in a human artery, indicating that velocity on the pulse transmission in man varies from 4 to 10 metres per second. For this experiment, these two scientits, used the common carotid artery of a young man who died from an endocarditis at age of 17. The formula to calculate PWV:

$$PWV = \frac{\Delta\,Pressure}{\Delta Volume} \times \frac{Volumen}{Blood\ viscosity}$$

establishes a relationship, between instantaneous changes in blood volume (delta volume) , blood pressure (delta pressure) and viscosity. From a practical point of view, PWV is the interval time between two arterial pulsations at two different points of the circulatory system, i.e., carotid-femoral, or carotid-radial

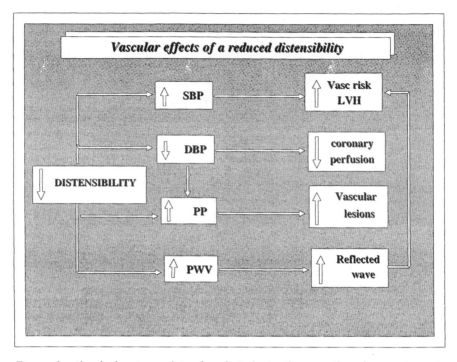

Figure 2. Algorhythm to explain the clinical significance of a decreased aortic compliance in aging and in hypertension. Legend: SBP = systolic blood pressure. DBP = diastolic blood pressure. PP = pulse pressure. PWV = pulse wave velocity.

arteries, or the interval time between the pre-ejection period (QRS) and the arrival of pulse wave to a specific point of the arterial tree.

There are many systems and devices today to calculate PWV in clinical practice. Asmar and co-workers have implemented a system to calculate PWV at rest (7), while Gosse et al. (8), have designed a device to evaluate PWV during a 24-hour out-hospital monitorization combined with simultaneous recording of BP. The Gosse's system, called QKD (Q from QRS, K from Korotkoff 5th sound, and D from diastolic) is based in an algorhythm which permits the automatic calculation of PWV with each measurement of BP during a conventional ambulatory BP monitoring. This QKD expresses the interval time between the pre-systolic period, calculated by the first deflection of the QRS , and the time at which, during the proggresive deflation of the cuff at the arm, the 5th Korotkoff sound is detected, corresponding to the diastolic BP value.

Aortic compliance (C) can be calculated from the data obtained after measuring PWV, and according to the formula previously proposed by Lehmann et al. (9). $PWV^2 = K/r$, where **K** corresponds to the elastic modulus and **r** the blood viscosity. From a practical appraisal, (C) may be calculated as follow:

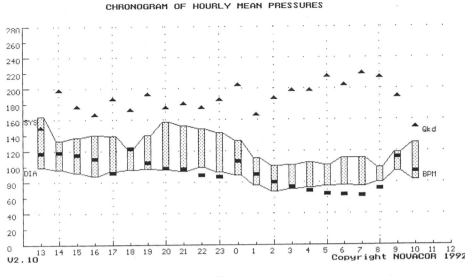

Figure 3

C = 66.7/PWV^2. The same authors have also proposed another formula (10) to calculate a compliance index (CI) independent from the BP values changes as follow: CI = C x (PP x 10.^{3}) / Ln (SBP / DBP) being haemodynamic values measured at brachial artery with the sphygmomanometer.

The clinical significance of a loss in arterial distensibility is summarized in figure 2. An increase in systolic BP is the inmediate result, followed by a decrease of diastolic BP leading in both conditions, to an increase in PP. The distensibility loss also promotes an increase in the transmission of the pulse wave velocity. The increase in SBP is the first mechanical factor to induce LVH increasing cardiovascular risk. The decrease in diastolic BP promotes a reduction in coronary blood perfusion, particularly in those patients with poor coronary reserve increasing the risk for a coronary event. PP correlates highly with vascular lesions, while the acceleration of the reflected waves is also a powerful factor to increase cardiovascular risk.

Figure 3 shows a 24 hour monitoring of a normal subject collecting both systolic and diastolic BP, heart rate and the so-called QKD (black triangles at the upper part) for pulse wave velocity monitoring. There is an indirect relationship between SBP and QKD; the higher the systolic BP, the lower the QKD, expressing an acceleration of PWV, as a consequence of the loss of physical properties of the aorta. The cut-off point for normalcy is currently established at 180 miliseconds, but this cut-off point needs to be reviewed.

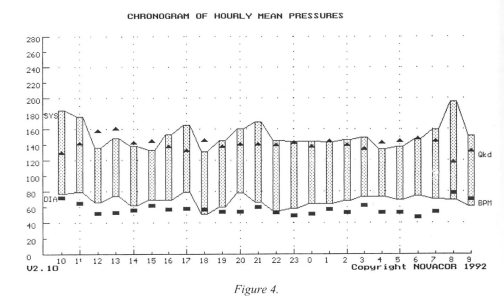

Figure 4.

Figure 4 shows the typical pattern of isolated systolic HT during 24 hours, accompanied by a QKD of a value around 160 miliseconds, indicating a significant loss on aortic distensibility and compliance. QKD as a reflected index of PWV shows an excellent relationship with SBP and PP but not with DBP. It is logical, since DBP depends on peripheral resistances of the arterioles, while SBP is closely related to aortic stiffness.

DISTENSIBILITY AND HYPERTENSION

In our laboratory, 244 hypertensive patients were evaluated during a 24-hour out-hospital period, with simultaneous monitorization of BP and QKD, comparing them to a control group of 30 normotensive subjects. A NOVACOR France system was used in each case. This device permits a peridiocal measurement of SBP, DBP, PP, HR and QKD. For our purposes, measurements were programmed every 15 minutes during the daytime (8 am to 22 pm) and every 20 minutes during nighttime. All the recorded information stored in the automatic ambulatory device was analyzed by means of a standard software.

Table I.

HYPERTENSION & DISTENSIBILITY (QKD)			
	GROUP A HT	GROUP B NT	p
N	244	30	-
Age	61 yrs	51 yrs	0.001
MBP (24 h.)	146/93	121/78	0.001
mQKD (24 h.)	171	189	0.001
% QKD > 180	24%	81%	0.0001
% QKD < 180	76%	19%	0.0001

Table I shows the mean characteristics of both groups. Age was different between normotensives and hypertensives, as was; mean systolic and diastolic BP of 24-hours (p < 0.01) . Mean QKD value was of 171 mseconds for hypertensives, and 189 for normotensives (p < 0.01). Differences were also found in the percentages of QKD below or above the cutt-off point established for this study at 180 msec (p < 0.01). correlating adequaltely these values with mean BP values as well. One hundred and sixty three patients of the previous group, were selected in order to establish the effect of different antihypertensive drugs, not only to evaluate BP values, but also to calculate QKD expressed in miliseconds at basal conditions and on treatment. Table II shows the main results.

All drugs used (diuretics, beta-blockers, alpha-blockers, calcium channel blockers, ACE inhibitors, AT1 receptor blockers, or combined therapy) were effective in lowering mean SBP and DBP during 24-hour of monitorization period, with similar results. Nevertheless, with respect to QKD, only calcium channel blockers, ACE inhibitors and AT1 receptor blockers showed a significant increase in QKD value, indicating a indirect improvement in physical

Table II.

HYPERTENSION & DISTENSIBILITY Effect of drugs				
		BASAL	ON TREATMENT	
DRUG	N	MAP/QKD (24 h)	MAP/QKD (24 h)	p
DIUR	22	148/91 168	136/84 171	NS
BB	21	150/92 170	132/86 170	NS
CCB	30	147/92 171	129/82 181	0.01
AB	11	149/95 173	123/79 173	NS
ACEI	36	151/96 167	130/81 182	0.001
ARB	26	149/89 172	134/81 183	0.001
COMB	17	154/98 168	139/88 176	0.01

properties of the large arteries. Diuretics, alpha-blockers and beta-blockers, were effective in lowering BP, but ineffective in reducing QKD.

A possible explanation for the inability of some antihypertensive compounds to improve large arteries distensibility, even if they have a satisfactory lowering effect on BP values, is the relationship between arterial stiffness and the renin angiotensin system and calcium cellular intake. According to the previous hypothesis, only those drugs able to block calcium influx or renin-angiotensin system, might be effective in reducing not only BP but also improving distensibility by increasing QKD values (11).

This clinical experience permits us to conclude as follows: 1) Arterial distensibility decreases with aging and hypertension. 2) Normalization of SBP and DBP values does not imply a parallel improvement in distensibility, expressed by an increase in QKD values. 3) Only calcium channel blockers, ACE inhibitors and AT1 receptor blockers, are able not only to reduce BP, but also to improve physical properties of the large arteries, and in particular those in the aorta.

But the question to be answered now is: How important are these changes in large arteries in HT. The answer today is clearly quite important; changes in aortic distensibility and compliance in aging and in HT play a major role in cardiovascular morbidity and mortality. In a paper published by Gosse at al. (12), they observed an unfavourable trend in cardiovascular mortality and morbidity during a 36 months follow-up period, in those patients in whom the QKD values were above or below of 187 msec (p < 0.001). Even more, this parameter in the Gosse's study, showed a predicted value more powerful that left ventricular mass index calculated by echocardiography.

ARTERIAL DISTENSIBILITY AND MENOPAUSE

Menopause induces changes in large arteries which become progressively stiffer. Some data have indicated that hormone replacement therapy (HRT) may have a special indication to modify this trend. The indications and contraindications of HRT are currently controversial (13).

Fifty one post-menopausal women aged between 41-60 years (mean 54.2 yrs ±6.5) were compared to a group of 21 women with normal menstruation (14). The age of the control group varies between 45 and 50 years (46.9 yrs ± 3,1). 46,6% of the post-menopausal group, were on HRT. There was more hypertensives among the post-menopausal women (28.6%) than in the control group (19.5%) Table III.

No differences at baseline were observed between post-menopausal women without HRT and control group, in relation to mean QKD values. Nevertheless, in those post-menopausal women, with HRT, normotensives or hypertensives, showed a significant increase in QKD, being even more evident in those patients with HT and HRT.

This study permits us to point out the following conclusions: 1) Arterial distensibility evaluated by QKD decreases after menopause. 2) HRT induces non-significant changes in both systolic and diastolic BP, as recently has been demonstrated in PEPI Study (15). 3) HRT improves both distensibility and compliance in post-menopausal women according to the data observed in our study.

Table III.

DISTENSIBILITY (QKD) & POSTMENOPAUSAL WOMEN			
HRT Evaluation (QKD)			
	GROUP A	**GROUP B**	**P**
Without HRT	184 msec	187 msec	0.039
With HRT / NT	194 msec		
With HRT / HT	209 msec		0.01

Palma-Gámiz JL et al. Am J Hypertens 1998; 11(4):218A

SUMMARY

1.- PWV evaluated by QKD algorhythm and taking into consideration age and systolic BP, may be an excellent tool to evaluate arterial distensibility and compliance of the large arteries and the aorta in particular.

2.- PWV in patients with one or several risk factors, allows the evaluation of their consequences on arterial wall

3.- Changes in PWV is an excellent index of vascular damage, indicating at the same time a clear relationship between HT and wall modificactions of the compliance arteries.

4.- Non-invasive evaluation of arterial distensibility and compliance by QKD, permits an accurate approach to the modification of this parameter when hypertensive patiens are treated with different antihypertensive compounds.

REFERENCES

1.   Safar ME, Laurent S, London GM: The arterial system in essential hypertension. In Clinical research in essential hypertension. Safar M. Ed., Schattauer, Stuttgarrt 1988, pp 115-132.
2.   Riley WA, Freedman DS, Higgs NA et al.: Decreased arterial elasticity associated with cardiovascular disease risk factors in the young. Bogalusa Heart Study. Arterioesclerosis 1986; 6:378-386.
3.   Bouthier JD, De Luca N, Safar M, Simon A. Cardiac hypertrophy and arterial distensibility in essential hypertension.,. Am Heart J 1985; 109:1345-1352
4.   Madhavan S, Lock Ooi W, Cohen H, Alderman MH. Relation of pulse pressure and blood pressure reduction on the incidence of myocardial infarction. Hypertension 1994; 23:395-401.
5.   Ting CT, Chang MS, Wang SP, et al. Regional pulse wave velocities in hypertensive and normotensive human. Cardiovasc Res 1990; 24:865-872
6.   Bramwell JC, Hill AV. The velocity of pulse wave in man. Proc Roy Soc 1922; 93(B):298-306.
7.   Asmar R, Benetos A, Topouchian J., et al. Assessment of arterial distensibility by automatic pulse wave velocity measurement. Validation and clinical application studies. Hypertension 1995; 26:485-490.
8.   Gosse P, Guillo P, Ascher G, Clementy J. Assessment of arterial distensibility by monitoring of the timing of korotkoff sounds. Am J Hypertens 1994;7:228-233.
9.   Lehmann ED, Gosling RG, Fatemi-Langroudi B, Taylor MG: Non-invasive Doppler ultrasound technique for the in vivo assessmentof aortic compliance. J Biomed Eng 1992: 14:250-257.
10. Lehmann ED, Parker JR, Hopkings KD, et al. Validation and reproducibility of pressure-corrected aortic distensibility measurements using pulse-wave-velocity Doppler ultrasound. J Biomed Eng 1993; 15:221-228.
11. Palma-Gámiz JL. Modificaciones anatomofuncionales de las arterias en la hipertensión arterial. Rev Lat Cardiol 1997; 18(4):113-120.
12. Gosse P, Gasparoux P, Ansoborlo P, Lemetayer P, Clementy J. Prognostic value of ambulatory monitoring of the timing of Korotkoff sounds in elderly patients. International Society of Hypertension Proceedings. Glasgow. June 1996.
13. Col N, Eckman M, Karas R, et al. Patient-specific decisions about hormone replacement therapy in postmenopausal women. JAMA 1997; 277:1140-1147
14. Calderón A, Palma-Gámiz JL, Barrios V. Changes on arterial distensibility induced by hormonal replacement therapy in both; hypertensive and normotensive postmenopausal women: Non-invasive ambulatory assessment. Am J Hypertens 1998; 11(4):218A

15. Greendale GA, James MK, Espeland MA, Barret-Connor E. Can we measure prior postmenopausal estrogen/porgestin use. The Postmenopausal Estrogen/Progestin Intervention Trial. The PEPI Investigators. Am J Epidemiol 1997; 146(9):763-770

36. PRONOSTIC IMPLICATIONS OF BLOOD PRESSURE VARIABILITY

JOSÉ RAMÓN GONZÁLEZ-JUANÀTEY AND
CARLOS GONZÁLEZ-JUANATEY

Physiopathologically, systemic arterial hypertension (AH) may be defined as excessive mechanical and neurohormonal cardiovascular stress. It gives rise to a variety of chronic or acute degenerative processes affecting the heart and arteries, and it is these consequences that make it of such importance for public health.

AH AND LEFT VENTRICULAR HYPERTROPHY

Structural and functional cardiac alterations caused by high blood pressure (BP) are collectively known as hypertensive cardiopathy. The myocardium undergoes a series of modifications that constitute the pathogenic nexus between AH and cardiac dysfunction, myocardial ischaemia and alterations of cardiac rhythm (1,2): increased myocyte volume is associated with changes in the composition and mechanical efficiency of contractile protein; increase interstitial volume stiffens the heart and allows infiltration of microvessel walls by conjunctive tissue; and ischaemia is favoured by both structural and functional changes in coronary microcirculation (increased small artery wall thickness due to fibrosis and hypertrophy, hyperplasia of smooth muscle in the tunica media, and unbalanced endothelial production of vasodilators, vasoconstrictors and substances promoting or suppressing cell proliferation and migration).

H.-H. Osterhues et al. (eds.),
Advances in Noninvasive Electrocardiographic Monitoring Techniques, 371–379.
© 2000 *Kluwer Academic Publishers. Printed in the Netherlands.*

These changes at the microstructural or molecular level eventually give rise to left ventricular hypertrophy (LVH). LVH is the first structural change in the hypertensive patient's heart that can be revealed by imaging techniques, and is a powerful predictor of cardiovascular morbidity and mortality: although ECG-detected LVH cases make up only 38% of the LVH cases detected by what is now the standard technique, echocardiography (3), 45% of all deaths due to cardiovascular accidents in the Framinghan study were preceded by ECG-detected LVH, and the 5-year mortality rate among males with and without ECG-detected LVH were 35% and 10-15% respectively (4-6). The more severe the AH of a particular study group, the greater is the prevalence of LVH: whereas only about 12% of randomly selected patients with borderline AH exhibit echocardiographically detected LVH , the prevalence rises to about 20% among patients with sustained AH (7).

Current data suggest that target organ damage due to AH correlates better with ambulatory BP than with in-clinic BP, and that among patients with a given in-clinic BP, target organ damage correlates positively with both mean ambulatory BP and the variability of ambulatory BP (8). Table 1 lists the coefficients of correlation between left ventricular mass and in-clinic and ambulatory BPs, as reported in the four main studies that have addressed this topic. Rowlands *et al.* (9) found significant correlation of LV mass with both in-clinic and intra-arterially monitored ambulatory BP among 50 patients with mild or moderate AH. Similar coefficients of correlation were found by Verdecchia *et al.* (10), not only among 137 randomly selected hypertensives who had received no prior treatment but also among 98 healthy, normotensive subjects. However, correlations were poorer in Devereux *et al.*'s study (11) and higher in Drayer *et al.*'s (12). Studies also differ as regards which is the better correlate of LVH, daytime or night-time BP: in Drayer's and Devereux's studies, daytime BP was the better, especially when recorded during physical or emotional stress (11,12), whereas there was little difference between the two in Rowlands' study (9). Smith *et al.* (13) have reported that left ventricular mass correlates better with night-time than with daytime BP. By contrast, it seems clear that systolic BP correlates with measures of LVH better than diastolic BP: for example in Dayer's study (12) the coefficient of correlation of LV mass index with systolic and diastolic 24-hour mean BP were 0.81 and 0.56 respectively, and the same trend was shown by both the daytime and night-time mean BPs. In view of this, and bearing in mind that in most cases of failure to control BP with an antihypertensive drug it is systolic BP that is uncontrolled (14), it is clear that therapies must be sought that not only control mean BP but also achieve particularly strict control of systolic BP.

WHITE COAT AH

Patients who persistently exhibit high BPs in the clinic but otherwise have normal BPs are said to have "white coat AH". It is thought that their high in-clinic BPs may be a reaction associated with anxiety or alertness in response to the in-clinic situation, and it has been suggested that they should not be classified as hypertensives (15). The prevalence and characteristics of white coat have been investigated using both ambulatory BP monitoring and self-measurement of BP (16), and it has been rigorously defined on the basis of data from transverse studies carried out in various populations to determine the normal ranges of such measures (16,17).

The echocardiographically determined LV mass index of subjects with white coat AH is in most studies significantly smaller than that of patients with hypertensive ambulatory BP; in fact, it is usually found to be similar to that of healthy subjects with normal in-clinic BP (18-20), although some researchers have reported finding significantly greater LV mass index among individuals with white coat AH than among controls with normal in-clinic BP (8,21).

In a recent prospective study of in-clinic hypertensives Verdecchia *et al.* (22) found that white coat AH (defined as the coexistence of hypertensive in-clinic BP with a daytime mean ambulatory BP less than 131/86 mm Hg for women or 136/87 mm Hg for men) is a sign of low cardiovascular risk that is independent of other markers (age, absence of diabetes, absence of previous cardiovascular accidents, in-clinic pulse pressure, serum cholesterol, absence of echocardiographically detected LVH, and in-clinic BP - lower in white coat AH cases than in patients with hypertensive ambulatory BP). Their normotensive group suffered four cardiovascular accidents in the course of the study (0.47 per 100 patient-years) and their white coat AH group three (0.49 per 100 patient-years). These findings are in keeping with the preliminary results of a study by Pickering (23), which showed a smaller incidence of cardiovascular complications among in-clinic hypertensives with white coat AH than among those with higher ambulatory BPs. Pickering's finding that in-clinic pulse pressure is of independent prognostic value (23) has also been corroborated, by a recent prospective study (24). Since AH is generally treated on the basis of in-clinic BP measurements, white coat hypertensives usually receive medication in excess of what would be prescribed on the basis of their ambulatory BP, and it may be the resulting exceptionally strict control of BP that is largely responsible for their better prognosis.

The lesser degree of target organ damage suffered by white coat hypertensives in comparison with hypertensives with both high in-clinic and high ambulatory BP is a direct consequence of their lower vascular stress and more balanced neurohormone production. In addition, Marchesi *et al.* (25) have found that white coat AH and sustained AH are associated with different metabolic patterns, insulin resistance being exhibited by patients with recently diagnosed sustained AH but not by white coat hypertensives. Insulin resistance may well contribute to cardiovascular morbidity and mortality in the former group.

The majority of the data currently available thus suggest that white coat AH is a relatively benign condition that requires no treatment. Because of this, differential diagnosis distinguishing between sustained and white coat AH is now one of the main motives for recording ambulatory BP: Grin *et al.* (26) have reported that screening for white coat AH accounts for 22% of the ambulatory BP determinations performed by health care professionals working in hospitals.

REFRACTORY AH

Another group of patients for whom ambulatory BP measurements would seem to have a significant role to play is composed of hypertensives whose hypertension is refractory to pharmacological treatment. Redón *et al.* (27) have recently shown that for these patients ambulatory BP measurements are of considerable prognostic relevance. In a prospective study in which they monitored patients for between 6 and 96 month (mean 49 months), 86 hypertensives who had persistent in-clinic diastolic BPs > 100 mm Hg in spite of taking three or more antihypertensive drugs were divided in three groups by ambulatory diastolic BP: < 88 mm Hg, 88-97 mm Hg and > 97 mm Hg. Although the groups did not differ as regards in-clinic BP either at the beginning or at the end of the study period, during which in-clinic BP did not change, by the end of the study target organ damage had progressed only in the > 97 mm Hg group, and the incidence of cardiovascular accidents per 100 patient-years was 2.2 in the < 88 mm Hg group, 9.5 in the 88-97 mm Hg group, and 13.6 in the > 97 mm Hg group. Maximum ambulatory diastolic BP was an independent risk factor for cardiovascular accident during the study (relative risk 6.2, 95% confidence interval 1.38-28.1 with $p < 0.02$). Redón *et al.* conclude that in patients with refractory hypertension, high ambulatory BP implies poor prognosis, and recommend that such patients be subjected to ambulatory BP monitoring for semiquantitative risk evaluation.

NIGHT-TIME BP AND CARDIOVASCULAR RISK

The circadian rhythms of normotensive individuals include a drop in BP, by up to 10% of daytime figures, during sleep (28,29). This low-BP phase terminates with a rapid rise in BP upon waking and, in particular, upon getting up and commencing daytime activity (30). A proportion of hypertensives, known as "non-dippers" (31), fail with certain consistency to exhibit the night BP drop: in a recent study in which ambulatory BP was recorded during two 24 h periods separated by 3-5 days, 73% of the hypertensive subjects exhibited the same nocturnal pattern (dipping or non-dipping) on both occasions (32).

It is well documented that left ventricular mass index (33,34), silent cerebrovascular damage (35) and the frequency of ictus (36) are all greater in non-dipping than in dipping hypertensive patients. In the PIUMA study of patients with hypertensive ambulatory BP (22,37), Verdecchia *et al.* found that for any daytime BP value, non-dipping accelerated the impact of AH on target organs; and that for women there was an association between non-dipping and cardiovascular morbidity that was statistically significant even after adjustment for differences in 24 hour mean diastolic and systolic BP (22). The precise mechanisms mediating this association are not known, but it is no doubt relevant that among the women in one of these studies (22) echocardiographically determined LV mass was significantly greater in non-dippers than in dippers even after allowance for differences as regards the independent risk factors LV mass index, diabetes, age and history of cardiovascular accidents (all of which likewise indicated greater risk for non-dipping women). Although larger studies of non-dipping are desirable because of the limitations of the PIUMA study (only 30% of the subjects were followed-up at frequent intervals, and there were only 89 cardiovascular accidents in all), it at least seems clear from the results of Verdecchia *et al.* (22) and Perloff and coworkers (38,39) that for the purposes of assessing the cardiovascular risk of hypertensive patients the determination of night-time BP behaviour by ambulatory BP monitoring is an aid allowing better classification than can be effected only on the basis of in-clinic BP and other classical risk factors.

THE MORNING BP SURGE AND CARDIOVASCULAR RISK

As noted above, following the night-time BP dip, normotensive individuals and most hypertensive patients suffer a rapid increase in BP upon rising in the morning. This "morning BP surge" is accompanied by a large number of other haemodynamic and biochemical events (40,41). Of particular relevance here are an increase in heart rate and systemic resistance, a fall in coronary flow, the peaking of adrenergic activation, an increase in the activity of the renin-angiotensin system and in platelet aggregation, and the alteration of the balance between coagulating and anti-coagulating factors due to an increase in plasminogen inhibitor activity and a fall in plasminogen activator activity (42-44). These physiopathological events are clearly closely inter-related, and together would appear to explain why more cardiovascular accidents occur during the early morning than at other times of day (it is well known that the hourly incidence of stroke, arrhythmia and ischaemic heart disease – silent and symptomatic myocardial ischaemia, acute myocardial infarct and sudden death of ischaemic origin – exhibits a periodicity similar to that of BP (45)).

In view of the above, it seems reasonable to time BP control measures so that their maximum effect coincides with and limits the morning surge, even though no study has yet shown cardiovascular morbidity and mortality to be correlated with the magnitude of the latter. However, this strategy is not effectively implemented by most current antihypertensive therapies: since in practice most patients take the first daily dose of their antihypertensive medication some considerable time after getting up in the morning, the surge generally coincides with the time of *minimum* drug effectiveness, ambulatory BP studies having found that most antihypertensive drugs have little effect at the end of the recommended period between doses. Failure to control the morning BP surge may help explain why meta-analyses (46,47) have found the patients with ischaemic cardiopathy have a higher risk of death from cardiovascular accident when treated with calcium antagonist of short half-life than when treated with other kinds of drug.

Therapeutic regimens that reduce the morning BP surge do exist. They include the use of drugs with long half-lives, and late-night administration of the chronotherapeutic calcium antagonist formulation Verapamil COER (48-51). The results of research on whether such regimens do indeed reduce the cardiovascular risk of hypertensive patients will be greeted with great interest.

REFERENCES

1. Leenen FHH. Increased risk attributed to left ventricular hypertrophy in hypertension. Curr Op Cardiol 1996; 11: 464-470.
2. Weber KT, Anversa P, Amstrong PW, Brilla CG, Brunett JC, et al. Remodeling and reparation of the cardiovascular system: An international perspective. J Am Coll Cardiol 1992; 20: 3-16.
3. Woythaler JN, Singer SL, Kawn OL, Melzer RS, Reulner B, et al. Accuracy of echocardiography versus electrocardiography in detecting left ventricular hypertrophy: Comparison with postmortem mass measurements. J Am Coll Cardiol 1983; 2: 305-311.

4. Kannel WB, Gordon T, Castelli WP, Margoli JR. Electrocardiographic left ventricular hypertrophy and risk of coronary heart disease: The Framingham Study. Ann Intern Med 1970; 72: 813-822.
5. Kannel WB, Gordon T, Offut D. Left ventricular hypertrophy by electrocardiogram. Prevalence, incidence and mortality in the Framingham Study. Ann Intern Med 1969; 71: 89-105.
6. Kannel WB. Prevalence and natural history of electrocardiographic left ventricular hypertrophy. Am J Med 1983; 75 (Suppl 3A): 4-11.
7. Carr AA, Prisant M, Watkins LO. Detection of hypertensive left ventricular hypertrophy. Hypertension 1985; 7: 948-954.
8. Pose A, González-Juanatey JR, Pastor C, Mendez I, Estevez J, Alvarez D, et al. Clinical implications of white coat hypertension. Blood Press 1996; 5: 264-273.
9. Rowlands DB, Glover DR, Ireland MA, McLeay RAB, Stallard TJ, Watson RDS, et al. Assessment of left ventricular mass and its response to antihypertensive treatment. Lancet 1982; 1: 467-470.
10. Verdecchia P, Schillaci G, Guerrieri M, Gatteschi C, Benemio G, Boldrini F, Porcellati C. Circadian blood pressure changes and left ventricular hypertrophy in essential hypertension. Circulation 1990; 81: 528-536.
11. Devereux RB, Pickering TG, Harshfield GA, Kleinert HD, Denby L, Clark L, et al. Left ventricular hypertrophy in patients with hypertension: Importance of blood pressure response to regularly recurring stress. Circulation 1983; 68: 470-476.
12. Drayer JIM, Weber MA, DeYoung JL. BP as a determinant of cardiac left ventricular muscle mass. Arch Intern Med 1983; 143: 90-92.
13. Smith VE, White WB, Karimeddini MK, McCabe EJ, Katz AM. Lowest not highest blood pressure may determine left ventricular filling. Circulation 1986; 74(Suppl II): II-290A.
14. Hammond IW, Devereux RB, Aldemar MH, Lutas EM, Spitzer MC, et al. The prevalence and correlates of echocardiographic left ventricular hypertrophy among employed patients with uncomplicated hypertension. J Am Coll Cardiol 1986; 7: 639-650.
15. Mancia G, Parati G. Clinical significance of "white coat" hypertension. Hypertension 1990; 16: 624-625.
16. Pickering TG, James GD, Boddie C, Harshfield GA, Blank S, Laragh JH. How common is white-coat hypertension? JAMA 1988; 259: 225-228.
17. Julius S, Mejis A, Kones K, Krause L, Schork N, Van der Ven C, et al. "White coat" versus "sustained" bordeline hypertension in Tecumseh, Michingan. Hypertension 1990; 16: 617-623.
18. Hoegholm A, Kristensen KS, Bang LE, Nielsen JW, Madsen NH. Left ventricular mass and geometry in patients with established hypertension and white coat hypertension. Am J Hypertens 1993; 6: 282-286.
19. White WB, Schulman P, McCabe EJ, Dey HM. Average daily blood pressure, not office pressure, determines cardiac function in patients with hypertension. JAMA 1989; 261: 873-877.
20. Cardillo C, De Felice F, Campia U, Folli G. Psychophysiological reactivity and cardiac end-organ changes in white-coat hypertension. Hypertension 1993; 21: 836-844.

21. Verdecchia P, Schillaci G, Boldrini F, Zampi I, Porcellati C. Variability between current definitions of "normal" ambulatory blood pressure: implications in the assessment of white coat hypertension. Hypertension 1992; 20: 555-562.

22. Verdecchia P, Porcellati C, Schillaci G, Borgioni C, Ciucci A, Batistelli M, et al. Ambulatory blood pressure. An independent predictor of prognosis in essential hypertension. Hypertension 1994; 24: 793-801.

23. Pickering TG. Clinic measurement of blood pressure and white-coat hypertension. In: Pickering TG (ed.). Ambulatory Monitoring and Blood Pressure Variability. London, UK: Science Press Ltd, 1991: 7.1-7.14.

24. Coca A. Actual blood pressure control: are we doing things right? J Hypertens 1996; 16(Suppl 1): S45-S51.

25. Marchesi E, Perani G, Falaschi F, Negro C, Catalano O, Ravetta V, et al. Metabolic risk factors in white coat hypertensives. J Hum Hypertens 1994; 8: 475-479.

26. Grin JM, McCabe EJ, White WB. Management of hypertension after ambulatory blood pressure monitoring. Ann Intern Med 1993; 118: 833-837.

27. Redon J, Campos C, Narciso ML, Rodicio JL, Pascual JM, Ruilope LM. Prognostic value of ambulatory blood pressure monitoring in refractory hypertension. A prospective study. Hypertension 1998; 31:712-718.

28. Litter WA, West MJ, Honour AJ, Sleight P. The variability of arterial pressure. Am Heart J 1978; 95: 180-186.

29. Pickering TG, Harshfield GA, Kleinert HD, Blank S, Laragh JH. Blood pressure during normal daily activities, sleep and exercise. JAMA 1982; 24: 992-996.

30. Khoury A, Sunderajan P, Kaplan N. The early morning rise in blood pressure is related mainly to ambulation. Am J Hypertens 1992; 5: 339-344.

31. Kleinert HD, Harshfield GA, Pickering TG, Devereux RB, Sullivan PA, Marion RM, et al: What is the value of home blood pressure measurement in patients with mild hypertension? Hypertension 1984; 6: 574-578.

32. Verdecchia P, Schillaci G, Boldrini F, Guerrieri M, Zampi Y, Porcellati C. Quantitative assessment of day-to-day spontaneous variability in non-invasive ambulatory blood pressure measurements in essential hypertension. J Hypertens 1991; 9 (Suppl 6): S322-S323.

33. Rizzoni D, Muiesan ML, Montani G, Zulli R, Calebich S, Agabiti-Rosei E. Relationship between initial cardiovascular structural changes and daytime and nighttime blood pressure monitoring. Am J Hypertens 1992; 1992; 5: 180-186.

34. Kumar A, Ventura HO, Messerli FH, Frohlich DE, et al. Diurnal variation of blood pressure in elderly patients with essential hypertension. J Am Geriart Soc 1984; 32: 896-992.

35. Shimada K, Kawamoto A, Matsubayashi K, Nishinaga M, Kimura S, Ozawa T. Diurnal blood pressure variations and silent cerebrovascular damage in elderly patients with hypertension. J Hypertens 1992; 10: 875-878.

36. O'Brien E, Sheridan J, O'Malley K. Dippers and non-dippers. Lancet 1988; 2: 397.

37. Verdecchia P, Schillaci G, Gatteschi C, Zampi I, Battisteli M, Bartoccini C, et al. Blunted nocturnal fall in blood pressure in hypertensive women with future cardiovascular morbid events. Circulation 1993; 88: 986-992.

38. Kobrin Y, Oigman Perloff D, Sokolow M, Cowan R. The prognostic value of ambulatory blood pressure. JAMA 1983; 249: 2792-2798.

39. Perloff D, Sokolow M, Cowan R, Juster RP. Prognostic value of ambulatory blood pressure measurements: further analysis. J Hypertens 1989; 7(Suppl 3): S3-S10.

40. Johnstone MT, Mittleman M, Tofler G, Muller JE. The pathophysiology of the onset of morning cardiovascular events. Am J Hypertens 1996; 9: 22S-28S.

41. Touitou Y, Haus E (eds.). Biologic rhythms in clinical and laboratory medicine. Springer Verlag, New York, 1992.

42. Brezinski DA, Tofler GH, Pahjola-Sintonen S, Willich SN, Schafer AI, Czeisler C, William GH. Morning increase in platelet aggregability: association with assumption of the upright posture. Circulation 1988; 78: 35-40.

43. Tofler GH, Brezinski D, Schafer AI, Czeisler CA, Rutherford JD, Willich SN, Glearson RE, Williams GH, Muller JE. Concurrent morning increase in platelet aggregability and the risk of myocardial infarction and sudden cardiac death. N Engl J Med 1987; 316: 1514-1518.

44. Petralito A, Mangiafico RA, Gibilino S, Cuffari MA, Miano MF, Fiore CE. Daily modifications of plasma fibrinogen, platelet aggregation, Howell's time, PTT, TT, and anti-thrombin III in normal subjects and in patients with vascular disease. Chronobiologica 1982; 9: 195-201.

45. White WB. A chronotherapeutic approach to the management of hypertension. Am J Hypertens 1992; 9: 29S-33S.

46. Pahor M, Guralnik JM, Corti C, Foley DJ, Carbonin PU, Havlik RJ. Long-term survival and use of antihypertensive medications in older persons. J Am Geriatr Soc 1995; 43: 1191-1197.

47. Furberg CD, Psaty BM, Meyer JV. Nifedipine. Dose-related increase in mortality in patients with coronary heart disease. Circulation 1995; 92: 1326-1331.

48. Pickering TG, Levenstein M, Walmsley P, for the Hypertension and Lipid Trial Study Group. Nighttime dosing of doxazosin has peak effect on morning ambulatory blood pressure: results of the HALT study. Am J. Hypertens 1994; 7: 844-847.

49. Sundberg S, Luurila OJ, Kohvakka A, Gordin A. The circadian heart rate but not blood pressure profile is influenced by the timing of beta-blocker administration in hypertensives. Eur J Clin Pharmacol 1991; 40: 435-436.

50. Palatini P, Racioppa A, Raule G, et al. Effect of timing of administration on the plasma ACE inhibitory activity and the antihypertensive effect of quinapril. Clin Pharmacol Ther 1992; 52: 378-383.

51. White WB, Black HR, Weber MA, Elliot WS, Bryzinski B, Fakonhi TD. Comparision of effects of controlled onset extended release verapamil at bedtime and nifedipine gastrointestinal therapeutic system on arising on early morning blood pressure, heart rate, and heart rate-blood pressure product. Am J Cardiol 1998; 81: 424-431.

CHAPTER FOUR: METHODS

SECTION FOUR: MAGNETOCARDIOGRAPHY

37. MAGNETOCARDIOGRAPHIC TECHNOLOGY: STATE OF THE ART

S.N. ERNÉ AND H.-P. MÜLLER

ABSTRACT

The non-invasive detection of high resolution magnetocardiographic signals generated by the electrical activation of the heart requires the development of high-resolution magnetic field sensors (superconducting quantum interference devices (SQUIDs)). The ability of multichannel recording and adequate computational power allows an application of this technique suitable for clinical use. The magnetic shielding of the detection chamber is a necessity for a high signal to noise ratio. The basic technical performances, an overview of large MCG systems and as an example for a clinical MCG system a description of the performance of Argos 55 - the new MCG system in Ulm - is presented.

INTRODUCTION

Biomagnetism is the study of magnetic fields that originate in biological systems. Since the first report of a magnetic field of the human body in the 1960s, the advance of this discipline was hampered by the fact that magnetic fields produced by biological activity are extremely weak, and conventional instruments had difficulty in resolving all but the strongest of the biomagnetic fields. The breakthrough came in the 1970s with the development in low temperature physics laboratories of a field sensor of dramatically improved

383

H.-H. Osterhues et al. (eds.),
Advances in Noninvasive Electrocardiographic Monitoring Techniques, 383–392.
© 2000 *Kluwer Academic Publishers. Printed in the Netherlands.*

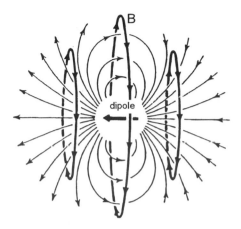

Figure 1. Electric and magnetic field caused by a current dipole.

sensitivity, known as the Superconducting Quantum Interference Device (SQUID). This instrument provides the possibility to discover magnetic fields of many organs of the body. As the fields are much weaker than the magnetic noise of the environment, the earliest applications were limited to measurements that could be recorded in either a remote location or an elaborately shielded chamber. The first magnetically shielded room consisted of two layers of ferromagnetic shielding and one layer of aluminium. Nowadays, highly sensitive multi-channel SQUID-magnetogradiometers inside magnetically shielded rooms with several layers of high permeability material and additional active shielding are the state of the art.

ORIGIN OF BIOMAGNETIC SIGNALS

Moving charge produces a magnetic field in the surrounding space. A further connection between the electric and the magnetic field is that a changing magnetic field produces an electric field. This is called Lenz law. Biomagnetism is primarily an exercise in magnetostatics, meaning that the currents and fields change slowly enough that electromagnetic radiation can be ignored. Under this condition the magnetic field at each position in space is determined exactly by the pattern of the electrical current. This association of a magnetic field with an electrical current is demonstrated in fig. 1. The magnetic field vector is perpendicular to the electric potential caused by a current dipole. Thus, having the same origin, the magnetic as well as the electric field of a biomagnetic source in principle carry the identical information, but they are measured in different ways. Thus, due to different detection techniques, the magnetic signal can carry more information than the electrical signal.

SIGNAL DETECTION - SQULD-TECHNOLOGY

The magnetic field can be detected in several ways: Fluxgate magnetometer, induction-coil magnetometer, magnetic resonance magnetometer, etc. Those magnetometers are appropriate for certain limited applications, but for all-around versatility and ultimate sensitivity the SQUID offers significant advantages. Despite the inconvenience and cost of the liquid helium that is presently needed for cooling, the most effective and sensitive way to detect very low changes in the magnetic field is the use of a SQUID magnetometer. The SQUID technology uses the quantum mechanical properties of defined metal alloys at low temperatures to measure changes in the magnetic field by the Josephson effect.

SHIELDED ROOMS

Historically the development of biomagnetism is strongly connected with magnetically shielded rooms. Presently there are existing three ways of shielding: eddy-current shielding, magnetic shielding and active shielding. Passive magnetic shielding requires ferromagnetic materials with high relative permeability. High permeability materials have a large flux density for a given value of magnetic field strength. That means, if the material is formed in the shape of a container it tends to retain the magnetic flux within the wall rather than outside and thus it shields the interior space. The shielding factor of passive magnetic shielding systems depends on the permeability of the material, the wall thickness and on the shape of the shield. It can be shown that for a given quantity of magnetic material, a more sophisticated construction can produce a better shielding factor as compared with a single, thick-walled shield.

Eddy current shielding is based on the use of conducting materials such as copper or aluminium. The principle is very simple: time-varying magnetic fields induce circulating currents in the conducting material in such a way that their magnetic field tends to cancel the changes of the impressed magnetic field inside the conducting material and the enclosed space. The shielding effect is essentially determined by a characteristic parameter of the material, the skin depth. The skin depth is depending on the conductivity of the material and

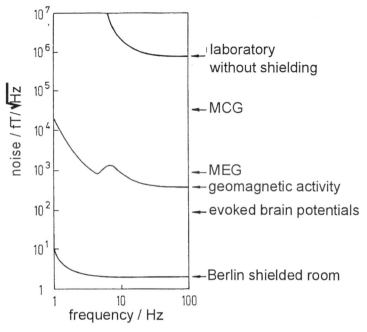

Figure 2. Frequency dependence of magnetic field strengths.

on the frequency of the alternating field. An alternative to the passive shielding techniques is active shielding: This consists in the generation of a suitable magnetic field to compensate the ambient disturbing field. Additional active shielding depends on sensing the local field and providing a corresponding field to stabilise it. Active systems consist of several magnetometers to detect the field to be compensated, an arrangement of field coils to generate the compensating field and a suitable controller to close the feedback loop. A good application of the active shielding is to improve the performance of a passive shield at low frequencies.

For an overview of the frequency dependence of magnetic noise and the shielding performances and the biomagnetic fields to be measured see fig. 2. It should be mentioned that the quality of SQUID based signal detection does not only depend on the surroundings and the environment but also on the quality and the low noise level of the SQUID-sensors, the amplifiers and the whole detection hardware.

EXAMPLE: THE NEW MAGNETIC SHIELDED ROOM IN ULM

To accommodate the biomagnetic instrumentation of the Ulm Biomagnetic Laboratory, a new magnetic shielded room was built in co-operation with Amuneal Co. On the basis of the standard structural set-up and the standard set of three layers of high permeability material with a thickness of 1.57 mm for shielding in the low frequency range. The fourth outer shell, constructed with aluminium plates with a thickness of 0.5", works as an eddy current shield for shielding of AC stray fields. Additionally, an active shielding system was designed and built around the shielded room. It was designed in two parts, a static compensation and a dynamic compensation using each one a dedicated set of three pairs of coils. The static compensation has the task to remove the influence on the external layer of high permeability material of the static earth magnetic field which is with its intensity of about 50µT the larger contribution to the environmental magnetic field. The shielding performance at 0.01 Hz is 42 dB and at 36 Hz is better than 100 dB. The high quality of the new magnetically shielded room in Ulm is shown in fig. 3.

The dynamic compensation is based on a feedback loop technique and compensates the variations of the environmental field measured by a dedicated SQUID triplet which is integrated in the biomagnetic sensor system.

STATE OF THE ART: LARGE MCG SYSTEMS

Nowadays there exist many large MCG systems in the world that have the performance to measure cardiac signals with a sufficient low noise level and thus good signal quality (tab. 1). For practical use the minimum requirements for a clinical MCG system are described in the following:

- The thorax has to be covered by at least 50 measurement sites, i.e. SQUID sensors, to detect the heart signal simultaneously.
- The minimum number of body surface potential mapping (BSPM) channels for simultaneous recording is 90.
- The number of auxiliary monitoring channels (breathing, etc.) should be greater than 8.
- For refilling of the dewar for the liquid helium the minimum maintenance interval is 7 days.
- The shielding at 0.01 Hz should be at least 38 dB and at 50 Hz the shielding should be better than 100 dB.

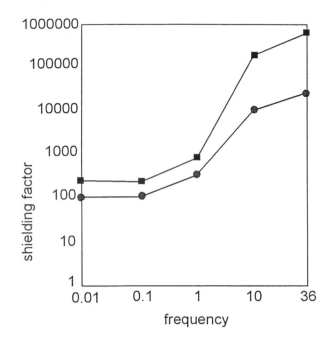

■ Ulm magnetically shielded room
● performances of comparable magnetically shielded rooms

Figure 3. Measured shielding performances.

Table 1. Survey of large MCG systems

Location		Meas. sites		Sensor config.
Berlin-Steglitz	Non commer.	49	7.2x7.2 mm²	magnet.
Bochum	CTF	64	Ø 2 cm	ax. grad.
Chieti	AtB	55	9x9 mm²	magnet.
Erlangen	BTI	2x37	Ø 2 cm	ax. grad.
Helsinki	Neuromag	37	8x8 mm²	grad.
Jena	Philips	2x31	Ø 2 cm	grad.
Ulm	Atb/non commer.	55	8x8 mm²	magnet.

The newest development is Argos 55, a MCG system recently installed at the Ulm University in a new magnetic shielded room.

NEWEST DEVELOPMENT: ARGOS 55 - THE MCG SYSTEM IN ULM

The new MCG system installed at the Ulm University is specifically designed for clinical application and routine use and this implies that a large number of patients are to be investigated. To reach this goal, the system design meets the requirements of reliability and high field sensitivity. The MCG sensor system is operating inside the magnetic shielded room described above. The sensor system consists of a planar dewar, housing a complex architectural structure with sensors distributed over three levels. The maintenance interval of the dewar is 7 days. The first level i.e. the primary measurement plane holds 55 SQUID sensors. The sensing elements are integrated magnetometers with a square shape of 12.7 mm in diagonal. The sensors are uniformly distributed over the inner surface of the dewar, according to a hexagonal geometry,
covering a circular surface of about 23 cm in diameter. The measurement plane is 18 mm from the outer dewar bottom. Nineteen additional SQUIDs are mounted on the second level and are used as reference channels 90 mm from the measurement plane. On the third level there is a magnetometric triplet located 70 mm from the reference plane to control the active shielding system. Operating in the shielded environment the systems show on all channels a white noise level better than 7fT√Hz and 10fT√Hz with and without software noise cancellation, respectively. A software gradiometer set-up is easily performed by subtraction of the background field sensed by selected reference channels from the signal of each primary channel.

The patient handling set-up is made of non magnetic material and is an emulation of the standard set-up for clinical cardiac electrophysiology (fig. 4).

A high speed optical connection transfers the data from the acquisition hardware to the real time pre-processing system, controlled through the operator console. The real time pre-processing is performed on the fly by an array of Digital Signal Processors, carrying out the noise compensation (software gradiameters), the digital bandpass filtering and the requested decimation to 18 bit at a sampling frequency of maximum 10 kHz.

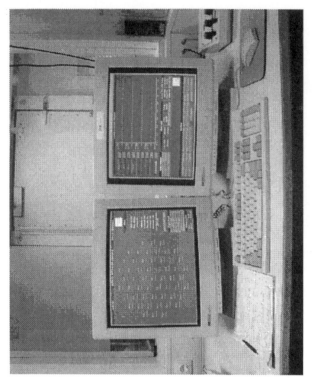

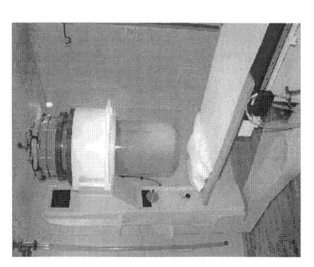

Fig. 4: Left: General view of sensor, system gantry and patient table in the Ulm shielded room. Right: Biomagnetic Operator Console with all signals displayed in real time mode.

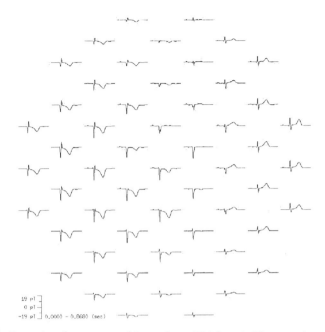

Figure 5. Example of an averaged heart beat (100 beats). The signals were recorded simultaneously at 55 positions.

Fig. 5 shows MCG signals as they are displayed on the analysis console. Additionally 128 BSPM channels can be recorded simultaneously and the number of auxiliary monitoring channels is 16.

DISCUSSION

Nowadays in the world there are several MCG systems with a technical performance that allows for the clinical application of MCG measurements. When clinical measurements are considered there is a need to observe a large number of patients and thus short measurement time, fast data analysis and large storage capability. Up to date it was not possible to validate the results of magnetocardiography at a clinical level, thus not allowing an evaluation of the clinical routine use of MCG in the contest of clinical work in cardiology. A clinical system has to perform a standard MCG measurement within a global time of 15-20 min per patient, leading to a possible throughput of 30 patients per day. First measurement results show that these numbers are realistic for the Argos 55 system.

REFERENCES

1. Williamson SJ, Romani G-L, Kaufman L, Modena I (eds.): Biomagnetism: An Interdisciplinary approach. NATO ASI Series, Plenum Press, New York, 1983.
2. Erné SN et al The Berlin Magnetically shielded Room (BMSR), Section B - Performances. Erné SN, Hahlbohm HD, Lübbig H (eds): Biomagnetism. Berlin, New York: Walter deGruyter 79-88, 1981.
3. Drung D, IEEE Trans. Appl. Supercon. 5 2112-2117, 1995.
4. Pasquarelli A, Kammrath H, Tenner U and Erné SN The new Ulm Magnetic Shielded Room. Proceedings of BIOMAG98, Sendai, Japan, 1998.
5. Pasquarelli A, Tenner U and Erné SN Use of an Additional Active Shielding System to enhance the low-frequency performances of a Magnetic Shielded Room. Proceedings of IWK98, Ilmenau, Germany, 1998 .
6. Pasquarelli A and Rossi R Miniaturized SQUID-electronics for biomagnetic multichannel applications. Proceedings of ISEC97, Berlin, Germany, 3 74-76, 1997.
7. Corby NR Jr, Miller PD, Hogle RA and Pasquarelli A A Realtime, High-Bandwidth, Programmable Digital Signal-Processing System for Monitoring, Acquisition, Filtering and Archival Storage of Biomagnetic Signals. Proceedings of Biomag '96, Santa Fe, 1996.
8. Martin K, Erné SN, Law C, Mallik J and Tatar B Multiple Modality Biomagnetic Analysis System. Proceedings of Biomag '96, Santa Fe, 1996.

38. ISCHEMIA AND HIBERNATION IN MAGNETOCARDIOGRAPHY

MARKKU MÄKIJÄRVI

INTRODUCTION

Detection, quantification and localization of ischemia is clinically important. New therapeutic interventions for revascularization enable treatment of new and larger patient groups. These techniques include coronary angioplasty and stenting, debulking methods like rotablation, mini-invasive surgery as well as surgical or percutaneous transmyocardial laser revascularization. Several noninvasive technologies for ischemia detection already exist: radionuclide methods, magnetic resonance imaging, stress echocardiography and positron emission tomography. However, many of these methods are either expensive or not available for most clinical centers. Therefore, new techniques for detection of myocardial ischemia are still warranted.

ELECTROMAGNETIC CHANGES CAUSED BY ISCHEMIA

Myocardial ischemia and necrosis cause clearcut changes in the electrophysiological properties of the myocardium. The resting transmembrane potential decreases and the upstroke amplitude of the action potential and its velocity is lowered (Janse 1981). The conduction velocity decreases markedly and unhomogenously in the ischemic areas resulting in the dispersion of the activation front. Ischemic and infarcted regions should therefore have different electromagnetic properties reflecting e.g. changes in the amplitudes and

H.-H. Osterhues et al. (eds.),
Advances in Noninvasive Electrocardiographic Monitoring Techniques, 393–400.

current densities of the recorded signals. The ST-segment changes have been experimentally shown to be a secondary result of a primary injury current that is interrupted during the ST-interval (Cohen 1975).

The magnetic field generated by the heart is produced by the same ionic currents in the volume conductor, which produce the ECG (Cohen 1972). Since the MCG and ECG are produced by the same class of currents, the MCG has the same morphological features as the ECG, such as QRS-complex and T, P and U-waves. However, there are some fundamental differences: the MCG is sensitive to closed loop currents (so called vortex currents) and the magnetic signals do not depend on the skin resistivity and other troublesome fields unlike the ECG (Plonsey 1972). Observed differences in the patterns of repolarization in the epicardium and endocardium could also be caused by ischemia and thus support a current distribution with possible loop (vortex) character (Antzelewich 1990, Wikswo 1982). These experimental findings are supported by the study of Brockmeier et al. producing stress by pharmacological agents in normal subjects and recording multichannel magnetocardiography and electrocardiography simultaneously (Brockmeier 1997). During peak stress and maximum heart rates, comparison of the repolarization showed substantial changes in the MCG up to T-wave inversions. In the ECG only junctional ST-segment shifts were present. In detailed analysis of the electromagnetic fields, it was found that when the current dipole moment change at the onset of the T-wave were marginal, the magnetic dipole moment changed drastically. The authors hypothesized the changes in the intensity and the orientation of the magnetic dipole to reflect the so called vortex currents as the biophysical basis of these differences of nonpathological origin between MCG and ECG.

ISCHEMIA IN MAGNETOCARDIOGRAM

Basicly, detection of all different types of ischemia by MCG has been reported in the literature. MCG has been shown to be able to detect and localize acute ischemia caused by acute myocardial infarction (Seese 1995) or induced by exercise (Seese 1995, Hänninen1998). Changes on magnetocardiograms in chronic ischemic heart disease have also been reported (Saarinen 1989, Leder 1996 and 1998, Hailer 1998, Van Leeuwen 1998). In these studies, acute and chronic ischemia have caused both morhological and spatio-temporal changes in MCG map patterns. QRS changes, ST-segment shifts and T-wave inversions have been seen resembling the alterations in the ECG recordings. In addition, the orientation of the magnetic field maps seems to change drastically during acute or silent ischemia (Van Leeuwen 1998, Hänninen 1998).

On the contrary, chronic ischemia is typically characterized by reduced amplitude and decreased current densities reconstructed by the minimum norm estimation (Saarinen 1989, Seese 1995, Leder 1996 and 1998). Qualitative identification of ischemia by MCG can be easily done by comparing normals and ischemic patients during resting state and exercise, but reliable quantification and localization of ischemic myocardial areas requires still high-quality 3-D imaging (i.e. magnetic resonance imaging) and preferably sophisticated individualized torso models (Leder 1998).

EXERCISE INDUCED ISCHEMIA IN MCG

Already in the 1970's ischemic ST-segment depressions similar to ECG has been reported after an exercise test of coronary heart disease patients (Saarinen 1974, Cohen 1976). Saarinen et al. showed that the ratio of ST-segment depression to R-wave amplitude after exercise is even greater in the MCG than in the ECG (Saarinen 1974). Cohen et al. reported ST-depression visible in the MCG but not in the standard exercise ECG (Cohen 1976). In the beginning of 1980's Cohen et al. demonstrated exercise induced ischemic ST-segment shifts in the direct current MCG in a patient with coronary artery disease after a step stress test (Cohen 1983).

Many years later Seese et al. investigated 11 patients with coronary heart disease and positive exercise ECG (Seese 1995). They were studied using an amagnetic bicycle ergometer in the magnetically shielded room. MCG was recorded before and immediately after exercise when signs of ischemia were still present in ECG. The minimum norm estimation was used to reconstruct the current density distribution during the ST-segment and the data were combined with X-ray and MRI images. The results were compared with coronary angiography and myocardial scintigraphy. During ischemia there was a significant elevation or depression of the ST-segment both in MCG and ECG in all patients. The injury currents were in most cases directed from the ischemic area to the non-ischemic area. For example, anterior ischemia caused an injury current directed from the apex to the base of the heart. The anatomical location of the injury currents was in topographical agreement with the results of the reference methods.

Very recently Hänninen et al. have shown further evidence of the diagnostic power of MCG to detect ischemia and viability (Hänninen 1998). In this study they investigated 18 patients with single vessel coronary artery disease compared with 18 normals. The subjects performed a symptom limited exercise test pedalling a nonmagnetic ergometer in supine position. The rotation of the magnetic field vector was found to be a good parameter for identification of coronary artery disease. Patients with a stenosis of the left anterior descending artery showed a mean rotation of 94 degrees of the field vector during the ST-segment compared to 49 degrees in patients with right coronary stenosis and 33 degrees in normals. On the other hand, patients with right coronary stenosis had their T-wave field rotated up to 44 degrees 4 minutes post exercise compared to 29 degrees of the left anterior descending stenosis and 8 degrees of the normals. The clinical reference methods were coronary angiography and thallium stress test. This preliminary study shows that exercise MCG can detect and localize ischemia at least in patients with single vessel coronary artery disease.

ACUTE MYOCARDIAL INFARCTION AND MCG

So far there are very few clinical MCG observations from the acute phase of myocardial infarction in man. Seese et al. have reported 5 patients studied during the very first days of acute myocardial infarction (Seese 1995). Patients were examined in the acute phase of myocardial infarction. The minimum norm estimation was used to reconstruct the current density distribution during the ST-segment and the data were combined with X-ray and MRI images. The results were compared with coronary angiography and myocardial scintigraphy. Acute myocardial infarction (ischemia and necrosis) caused a significant elevation or depression of the ST-segment both in MCG and ECG in all patients. The injury currents induced by transient ischemia and infarction of the same anatomical region were found to flow in opposite direction. This change of direction was reflected to either ST-depression or ST-elevation in morphological signals.

MCG changes owing to previous myocardial infarction have earlier been reported by several authors. However, the total number of reported cases is small and does not allow much detailed analysis of the MCG patterns in various infarct locations. Lant et al. have demonstrated the complementary nature of electrocardiographic and magnetocardiographic data also in patients with ischemic heart disease (Lant 1990). In post infarction patients they have shown that the differences between MI patients and normals were greater in ECG mapping especially during Q-wave and in MCG mapping, on the contrary, during the repolarisation. In particular, MCG mapping showed complex, non-dipolar structure in patients with non Q-wave infarction. According to these investigators this could have been caused by prolonged ischemic injury increasing tangential current flow through the spared subendocardial tissue.

Lately, Van Leeuwen and collegues have developed an index for the variability of the QT-interval dispersion called Smoothness Index. With this index they could reliably separate myocardial infarction patients from normals (van Leeuwen 1996).

CHRONIC ISCHEMIA AND MYOCARDIAL VIABILITY

There are still very few clinical studies on chronic myocardial ischemia and viability by MCG. Leder et al. investigated 40 subjects half of them patients with a history of myocardial infarction (Leder 1996). All patients underwent 12-lead-electrocardiogram, stress-test, echocardiography, coronary angiography, and most of them Tl-SPECT. Individual volume conductor properties and physiologically meaningful constraints for current generator reconstructions were extracted from T1-weighted 3D-MR-images. Current density was calculated for myocardial support points using depth normalized minimum norm least square estimates and overlayed with 3D-MR-images. Results show that the current density is increasing from QRS onset to QRS maximum. The majority of healthy myocardial regions has high current densities. Corresponding to the absence of electrical active myocardial tissue, MCI shows reduced current density for regions of infarcted myocardium. Infarcted areas have current densities < 1 $\mu A/mm^2$. The current density distribution correlates with other cardiological investigations (eg. left heart catheterization, scintigraphy, echocardiography). These are promising results for further application of current density reconstruction algorithms. In 55% of 40 patients/normals investigated, MCI had complete correspondence with the other cardiological findings, in 27% they found partly correspondence and 18% MCI failed to provide correct diagnosis.

Recently same authors published a very detailed analysis of two infarction patients (one anterior and one inferior) and two healthy controls using the same methods and confirming the results of the initial series (Leder 1998). The main finding of these studies was the markedly decreased regional current densities in the areas corresponding to the infarcted segments of the heart defined by the clinical reference methods. The authors conclude that the proposed multiple dipole model may in the best case be able to distinguish viable from scarred myocardium. However, further studies are needed in order to define the spatial resolution and the diagnostic performance of this method. In addition, the ability of this method to identify and localize chronic ischemia or hibernation (not scar) remains unknown.

Specific changes during the repolarization phase of the cardiac electric cycle have recently been proposed to be related to coronary heart disease and possible silent chronic ischemia (Van Leeuwen 1998, Hailer 1998). In the study by Van Leeuwen et al. patients with significant coronary stenosis but without myocardial infarction were found to have alterations of the magnetic field map orientation resembling the changes detected in infarction patients although there were no changes in the standard 12-lead ECG (Van Leeuwen 1998). Moreover, the QT-interval of the coronary patients was found to be more dispersed, more variable between neighboring channels and map pattern globally altered (Hailer 1998).

We have recently started a study, which is designed to test the diagnostic performance of MCG mapping to detect and localize areas of hibernating myocardium. The viability of the myocardium is confirmed by a full set of other diagnostic tests: exercise ECG, thallium stress test, dobutamine MRI and positron emission tomography (PET). The preliminary results of the first three patients look promising but there is a clear need for better software and modelling concerning chronic ischemia.

ADVANTAGES AND DISADVANTAGES OF MCG

Magnetocardiography has many advantages for a clinical method. First of all, it is fully noninvasive. There is no real need to attach anything extra to the patient. Current operating multi-channel systems are also very fast. A full measurement is carried out in just a couple of minutes. Both of these features mean highest patient comfort. Magnetocardiography can offer multiple electromagnetic parameters at one shot for complete electromagnetic characterization of the patient's heart. In addition, the spatio-temporal resolution is much higher than in conventional electric methods. Moreover, this novel technology always carries a substantial potential for extracting new physiological and pathophysiological information of the heart's electric acitivity.

There are of course some disadvantages. The equipment is still expensive. The need of a shielded room excludes the wide applicability of the method as a quick bed-side test. The system is sensitive to any metal objects, which is an exclusion criteria for some patients.

CONCLUSIONS

Until now the information content of the electromagnetic signals of the heart is used clinically only in the form of very limited standard 12-lead electrocardiogram. The more extensive electric mapping methods are time consuming to apply clinically and complicated to analyze, the fast technical development during the last years resulting in increased computer performance together with new algorithms and advanced source modelling, magnetocardiography (MCG) is offering now new independent information from normal and pathological cardiac function. Detection and localization of ischemia and viability would concern a large number of cardiac patients, if MCG method proves to be useful. Studies on the prognostic value of MCG after myocardial infarction are currently under way.

In the present state, we can conclude that detection of acute ischemia by MCG is definitely possible and the MCG method might even be more sensitive than the ECG in this task. This is probably related to the special properties of the MCG such as the ability to detect so called tangential injury currents (loop currents, vortex currents). Also the localization of ischemic areas should be possible accurately enough for clinical purposes. This application still needs more development and validation work. For the moment, the identification of chronically ischemic or hibernating myocardium by MCG has to be proven although the initial experience seems to be promising. There is still a clear need for better mathematical models for ischemia and large enough clinically appropriate patient studies. The increasing availability of high performance multichannel MCG systems in clinical environment will strongly contribute to these efforts.

REFERENCES

1. Antzelevitch C, Litowsky SH, Lukas A. Epicardium versus endocardium: Electrophysiology and pharmacology. In Zipes DP, Jalife J, eds.:cardiac Electrophysiology: From Cell to Bedside. WB Saunders, Philadelphia, 1990, pp. 386-395.
2. Brockmeier K, Schmitz L, Bobadilla Chavez J, Burghoff M, Koch H, Zimmermann R, Trahms L. Magnetocardiography and 32-lead potential mapping: Repolarization in normal subjects during pharmacologically induced stress. J Cardiovasc Electrophysiol 1997;8:615-626.
3. Cohen D, McCaughan D. Measurements and a simplified interpretation of magnetocardiograms from humans. Circulation 1969;39:395-402.
4. Cohen D, Kaufman LA. Magnetic determination of the relationship between the S-T-segment shift and the injury current produced by coronary artery occlusion. Circ Res 1975;36:414-424.
5. Cohen D, Lepeschkin E, Hosaka H, Massell BF, Myers G. Abnormal patterns and physiological variations in magnetocardiograms. J Electrocardiol 1976;9:398-409.
6. Cohen D. Steady fields of the heart. In: Williamson SJ, Romani G-L, Kaufman L, Modena I, eds. Biomagnetism. An Interdisciplinary Approach. New York, Plenum Press, 1983, pp. 265-274.
7. Hailer B, Van Leeuwen P, Pilath M, Lange S, Gr̄nemeyer D, Wehr M. Changes in the spatial dispersion of QT-interval in patients with coronary artery disease. PACE 1998;21(4 Part II):908.

8. Hänninen H, Takala P, Mäkijärvi M, Montonen J, Nenonen J, Katila T, Toivonen L. Dtection of exercise induced myocardial ischemia by multichannel magnetocardiography in patients with single vessel coronary artery disease. 8th International Congress of Holter and Noninvasive Electrocardiology, Annals of Noninvasive Electrocardiology 1998.

9. Janse MJ, Kl9ber AG. Electrophysiological changes and ventricular arrhythmias in the early phase of regional myocardial ischemia. Circ Res 1981;49:1069-1081.

10. Lant J, Stroink G, ten Voorde B, Horacek BM, Montague TJ. Complementary nature of electrocardiographic and magnetocardiographic data in patients with ischemic heart disease. J Electrocardiol 1990;23:315-322.

11. Leder U, Hemmann A, Eichorn J, Pohl HP, Hoffmann M, Huck MP, Nowak H, Haueisen J, Michaelsen S, Kuhnert H, Muller S. Segmentation of realistically shaped surfaces from 3D MRI for biomagnetic myocardial current imaging. Proceedings of the 10th International Conference on Biomagnetism, Sante Fe, 1996.

12. Leder U, Pohl H-P, Michaelsen S, Fritschi T, Huck M, Eicchorn J, Muller S, Nowak H. Noninvasive biomagnetic imaging in coronary artery disease based on individual current density maps of the heart. Int J Card 1998;64:83-92.

13. Plonsey R. Comparative capabilities of electrocardiography and magnetocardiography. Am J Cardiol 1972;29:735-736.

14. Saarinen M. Magnetocardiogram in coronary artery disease. Ann Clin Res 1989.

15. Saarinen M, Karp PJ, Katila TE, Siltanen P. The magnetocardiogram in cardiac disorders. Cardiovasc Res 1974;8:820-834.

16. Seese B, Moshage W, Achenbach S, Killmann R, Bachmann K. Magnetocardiographic (MCG) analysis of myocardial injury currents. In: Biomagnetism: Fundamental Research and Clinical Applications. Baumgartner C, Deecke L, Stroink G, Williamson SJ (eds). Elsevier Science, IOS Press, Amsterdam, 1995, pp 628-632.

17. Van Leeuwen P, Hailer B, Wehr M. Spatial distribution of QT-intervals: an alternative approach to QT-dispersion. PACE 1996;19:1894-1899.

18. Van Leeuwen P, Hailer B, Donker D, Lange S, Wehr M. Noninvasive diagnosis of coronary artery disease at rest on the basis of multichannel magnetocardiography. PACE 1998;21(4 Part II):908.

19. Wikswo JP Jr, Barach JP. Possible sources of new information in the magnetocardiogram. J Theoret Biol 1982;95:721-729

39. MAGNETOCARDIOGRAPHY AT THE TURN OF THE MILLENIUM

V. HOMBACH AND B. SCHARF

HISTORICAL REMARKS

In 1963 Baule and McFee used an induction coil to measure magnetic signals produced by the human heart (1). The technique of super conducting technology in a specially shielded room was introduced in 1970 by Cohen and co-workers (2) and further described in 1974 by Lepeschkin (3). The next improvement was the development of gradiometric detection coils that allowed MCG recordings in unshielded laboratories (4-8). In 1974 Siltanen (9) described the current MCG lead system, a standard grid and the normal MCG pattern. Recordings of the His-Purkinje-system by magnetocardiography from body surface were first reported by Farrell in 1978 (10), and ventricular late fields as correlates to ventricular late potentials by Erné in 1983 (11). In 1985 the first three-dimensional localization of abnormal cardiac microfields by MCG was described by Erné (12). Since 1983 isofield contour maps for imaging the magnetic field distribution during cardiac de- and repolarisation have been used routinely (12, 13, 14). In general, among the the pioneers of magnetocardiography the names of Katila (15), Awano (8), Cohen (2), Siltanen (9), Fenici (13), Romani (16) and Erné (11, 12) have to be mentioned in particular, because they have contributed significantly to the technical development and clinical application of modern magnetocardiography.

H.-H. Osterhues et al. (eds.),
Advances in Noninvasive Electrocardiographic Monitoring Techniques, 401–411.
© 2000 *Kluwer Academic Publishers. Printed in the Netherlands.*

TECHNICAL ASPECTS

The technology of magnetocardiography is described in more detail in the chapter by Erné and Müller. Principal components of a modern large MCG system are:

- A multi-sensor system, i.e. at least 50 measurement sites by SQUID for simultaneous detection of heart signals.
- A minimum number of 90 channels for body-surface potential mapping.
- A number of greater than 8 of auxiliary monitoring channels (breathing etc.).
- An appropriate shielding room with shielding at 0.01 Hz at least 38 dB and at 50 Hz better than 100 dB.
- A maintenance interval of the dewar of 7 days, i.e. the time interval between refilling of the dewar with liquid helium.

The newest development in magnetocardiography is the Argos 55, an MCG system recently installed at the Ulm University in a new magnetically shielded room with excellent shielding properties. All the investigational programmes in ischemic heart disease patients, as described below, will be performed by the Ulm group using this equipment.

CLINICAL APPLICATIONS OF MAGNETOCARDIOGRAPHY

Since the 1980s a number of widely differing studies in normal individuals and patients with different cardiac diseases have been performed using magnetocardiography, in most of these studies only small numbers of individuals have been investigated. The different fields and aims of these studies can be differentiated and listed as follows:

Fetal heart rate measurements
Recording of atrial repolarisation
Measurement of left-ventricular hypertrophy
Abnormal cardiac depolarisation (arrhythmias)

Localization of accessory pathways (WPW-syndrome)
Localization of foci of ventricular tachycardia
Localization of ventricular late depolarisation as late fields

Ischemic heart disease

stress induced myocardial ischemia
localization and extent of myocardial infarction
hibernating mycardium

FETAL HEART ACTIVITY

In a study of Quinn and co-workers in 1994 (18) 106 low-risk pregnant women at 20th - 42nd week of gestation were studied by magnetocardiography. This technique was acceptable to pregnant women and QRS-complexes were successfully demonstrated in 68/106 (67%) of the unaveraged traces. Using off-line averaging techniques on these 68 cases, P-waves were obtained in 75% and T-waves in 72%. QRS-duration demonstrated a positive linear correlation with increasing gestation. No significant relation was found between measurements of the fetal MCG-wave forms and the pH results from umbilical veins.

In 1995 van Leeuwen et al. (17) described a method for recording the fetal magnetocardiogram, which was not affected by intermediate tissue, in particular by the insulating effect of the vernix caseosa. They also described fetal magnetocardiograms with a good signal-to-noise ratio from the beginning of the second trimester, and examples of the recording and evaluation techniques were given. By identifying all fetal beats an average beat could be calculated, by which signal morphology and cardiac time intervals were determined. Furthermore by producing a beat-to-beat time series heart rate variability could be measured from time and frequency domain technologies. The authors concluded that magnetocardiography holds the promise of improved antenatal surveillance as of the second trimester of pregnancy.

In a later study by Menendez and co-workers in 1998 (19) a total of 104 MCG recordings were performed in 53 pregnant women from the 10th week of gestation onwards. The fetal magnetocardiogram was recorded non-invasively over the mother's abdomen in a magnetically shielded room. Fetal heart beats were generally detected from the 20th / 21st week of gestation onwards, in a few cases fetal beats could be recorded as early as in the 16th week. Time intervals and amplitudes of the fetal magnetocardiogram increased in concordance with fetal growth, whereby P-wave duration, PQ-interval and QRS duration increased significantly with fetal growth. Moreover the group was able to record fetal arrhythmias in 20 cases (26-38th week), including episodes of ventricular and supraventricular arrhythmias or AV-block. The authors concluded that the fetal magnetocardiogram could become a new diagnostic instrument for monitoring fetal well-being during pregnancy.

ATRIAL REPOLARISATION

As to atrial repolarisation only one study describes magnetocardiographic data in four normal subjects at rest and during mild exercise with high spatial correlation, which could be used for removal of atrial components between the PQ segment (20). Whether this technology will be of clinical significance for studying signals during atrio-ventricular conduction, remains to be determined.

LEFT VENTRICULAR HYPERTROPHY

Left ventricular hypertrophy in patients with cardiomyopathy has been studied in 18 patients with arterial hypertension and in 32 healthy males as controls (21). Elements of the magnetocardiogram of normal subjects were analysed morphologically over 36 points of precordial leads, and left ventricular hypertrophy was confirmed by echocardiography in 11/18 (61%) within the magnetocardiogram in 16/18 (84%) and in the conventional ECG in 7/18 (34%) of patients with arterial hypertension. Left atrial hypertrophy was discovered primarily by echocardiography and magnetocardiography. The authors recommend magnetocardiography as an effective tool in the diagnosis of hypertensive heart disease.

ABNORMAL VENTRICULAR DEPOLARIZATION

The broadest clinical application of magnetocardiography has been reported for abnormal cardiac depolarisation either due to accessory pathways or to ectopic or reentrant mechanism (arrhythmia substrate) in patients with ventricular tachycardia. Some groups have reported the localization of accessory pathways in patients with WPW syndrome (22-27). The largest study in this respect has been published by Mäkijärvi et a. 1993 (27), describing the magnetocardiographic localization of the pre-excitation site in 26 WPW patients, in whom an average accuracy of site localization of 2±1 cm in comparison to the results obtained by invasive catheter mapping could be achieved. In our own series of 11 patients with ventricular pre-excitation the localization of the Kent bundle could be compared between catheter mapping and magnetocardiographic mapping (28). In all of these 11 patients magnetocardiography was able to reconstruct the site of pre-excited ventricular myocardium, however, the difference between catheter mapping and magnetocardiographic localization was between 0 cm to 6 cm (in the latter case the accessory pathway was localized over the liver by MCG). In three cases localization was identical, in one case the difference was 1 cm, in three patients 3 cm, and in one patient each the difference was 3,4,5 and 6 cm, respectively. These results are in line with those reported by Fenici and other authors (22,23,26). Therefore, we can conclude that localizing the insertion of the accessory pathway by magnetocardiography is at present limited, further refinements of the computer algorithms have to be expected before the definite value of localization of accessory pathways by MCG may become a firm clinical application.

Data on the localization of VT-foci are much more limited. We studied four patients with sustained ventricular tachycardia, and the reentrant circuit was localized by both catheter mapping and magnetocardiography (28). In one patient the localization was similar to that described by an algorithm of Kuchar 1989 according to the surface 12 lead ECG. In a second patient with inferior aneurysm post infarction the difference of the VT focus was 1 cm between magnetocardiographic and catheter mapping. In the third patient with right ventricular dysplasia the origin was identical as determined by both MCG and catheter mapping. In a fourth patient with arrhythmogenic right ventricular dysplasia a difference of 5 cm was seen between the origin of the VTs determined by MCG (localization of the dipole within the left ventricular apex) and the mean septum on the right ventricular aspect as determined by catheter mapping. Mooshage and co-workers (29) reported better results in 12 patients with ventricular tachycardia, because phantom and pacing studies demonstrated the spatial localization accuracy to be better than 15 mm for a dipole to dewar distance below 15 cm.

In patients in whom sustained ventricular tachycardia is not present in history or cannot be provoked by programmed stimulation a secondary approach to localize the arrhythmogenic substrate might be the detection and localization of ventricular late fields, which may correspond to ventricular late potentials within the signal averaged surface ECG. In our series of eight patients, four with VT and four without VT (28, 30) the localization of ventricular late fields within the MCG was performed with the last 30 ms of the QRS-complex. In all patients MRI imaging was added in order to assign the calculated localization of the magnetic dipole to the corresponding anatomic structure. In all patients with VT its focus was known by catheter mapping. In the four patients with VT the differences between the origin as determined by MCG and catheter mapping was 2,7,5 and 1 cm, respectively, the mean difference was 3.8 cm.

Mäkijärvi and co-workers (31) compared the diagnostic value of ventricular late fields in the MCG with high resolution surface ECG for diagnosing patients with ventricular tachycardia. A total of 30 subjects, 10 with documented VT and old myocardial infarction, 10 patients with old infarction without complex ventricular arrhythmias and 10 normals were studied. The duration of the QRS-complex in the magnetocardiogram was significantly longer in ventricular tachycardia patients compared to those without VT and to the normals. The root mean square field of the last 60 ms of the QRS-complex was significantly smaller in VT patients and also the duration of low amplitude signal less than 700 FT was longer in VT patients than in MI patients without VT. The sensitivity and specificity in identifying VT patients were both 80%, and the positive and negative predictive values were 78% and 86%, respectively. High resolution ECG performed slightly better with a sensitivity of 90%, specificity of 90 % and positive and negative predictive values of 90%. The authors concluded that the new MCG technique seemed helpful in screening patients at risk of VT after myocardial infarction.

ISCHEMIC HEART DISEASE

Theoretically, magnetocardiography could be used for diagnosing myocardial ischemia (acute and chronic) particularly as to the extent and localization of mycardial infarctions and for assessing myocardial viability in chronic myocardial ischemia. There have been several reports showing that acute and chronic ischemia may cause both morphological and spatio-temporal changes in MCG map patterns (32, 33, 34) and the orientation of the magnetic field maps may change drastically during acute or silent ischemia (35, 36). Chronic ischemia is characterized by a reduced amplitude and decreased current density reconstructed by the minimum norm estimation (32,33,36,37).

In patients with acute myocardial infarction the magnetocardiogram may show ST segment depressions and elevations similar to the ECG, and injury currents of the same anatomical region as confirmed by angiography were found to flow in an opposite direction (38). Another approach is the use of the variability of the Q-interval dispersion, called smoothness index, using this index patients with myocardial infarction could be reliably separated from normals (39).

Another exciting area to use magnetocardiography is chronic ischemia and the recognition of myocardial viability in patients with chronic severe stenosis or post myocardial infarction. Some authors could show a reduced current density for regions of infarcted myocardium, and the localization of current density distribution may correlate with the area of interest as documented by left heart catheterization or echocardiography (32). Mäkijärvi and co-workers have recently started a study to detect and localize areas of hibernating myocardium (see chapter of Mäkijärvi).

FUTURE DIRECTIONS OF MAGNETOCARDIOGRAPHY

There are some important advantages of magnetocardiography as compared to other non-invasive electrocardiographic methods. Magnetocardiography is a fully non-invasive tool without need to attach anything extra to the patients (e.g. recording electrodes). It is a multi-channel system and a full measurement of the cardiac excitation can be performed within some minutes with highest patient comfort. For some beats a complete electromagnetic characterization of the patients' hearts can be performed and this spatio-temporal resolution is much higher than with conventional electric methods. Despite the fact that magnetocardiographic equipment is very expensive and needs a shielded room and is sensitive to any metal objects within the patient, at this time it is a must to further test this very promising new method.

In the past magnetocardiography has been mainly used to localize abnormal cardiac excitation in patients with accessory pathways or with ventricular tachycardia. Since the intracardiac mapping and ablation technology has been improved considerably, comparison of magnetocardiographic excitation patterns with intracardiac mapping may only be used to refine and improve the computer algorithms for better spatial resolution of the magnetocardiogram. There are some much more important areas to use and test the clinical significance of magnetocardiography in patients with ischemic heart disease. This relates to three main important groups of patients, patients with stable coronary heart disease and significant stenosis to document the extent and localization of myocardiac ischemia, patients with myocardial infarction to estimate the region and extent of infarcted myocardium, and last but not least the very important group of patients post MI or with chronic severe stenosis and areas of impaired ventricular function, which may be still viable (so called hibernating myocardium). In our own group we will mainly focus on these three patient groups, and we will compare the results of magnetocardiographic "imaging" with changes of myocardial perfusion in MRI and perfusion and viability studies using Positron Emission Tomography (PET). The next five to ten years will be exciting because many groups in Germany and Europe are now going into this very promising field of magnetocardiography.

REFERENCES

1. Baule GM, R McFee. Detection of the magentig field of the heart. Am Heart J 66, 95-96, 1963.

2. Cohen D, EA Edelsack, JE Zimmermann. Magnetocardiograms taken inside a shielded room with a superconducting point-contact magnetometer. Appl Phys Lett 16, 278-280, 1970.

3. Lepeschkin E. Tentative analysis of the normal magnetocardiogram. Adv Cardiol 10, 325-332, 1974.

4. SaarinenM, PJ Karp, TE Katila, P Siltanen. The magnetocardiogram in cardiac disorders. Cardiovasc Res 8, 820-834, 1974

5. Opfer JE, YK Yeo, JM Pierce, LH Rorden. A superconducting second-derivative gradiometer. IEEE Trans Mag MAG 9, 536-539, 1974

6. Karp PJ, TE Katila, M Saarinen, P Siltanen, TT Varpula. Etude Comparative de manétocardiogrammes normaux et pathologiques. Ann Cardiol Angeiol 27 (1), 65-70, 1978.

7. Barbanera S, P Carelli, R Leoni, GL Romani, F Bordoni, I Modena, RR Fenici, P Zepilli. Biomagnetic measurements in unshielded, normally noisy enviroments. In: Biomagnetism: Erné SN, HD Hahlboom and H Lubbig (eds), Berlin-New York, Walter de Gruyter, pp 139-149, 1981.

8. Awano N, K Owada, K Machip, S Kariyone, I Awano. A study on magnetocardiograms of normal subjects. Japan Circulation J 46, 870, 1982

9. Siltanen P, M Saarinen, T Katila, J Ahopelto. Magnetocardiogram in healthy men and women. Proc VIII World Congr Cardiol, Buenos Aires (abtsr), 1974

10. Farrell DE, J Tripp, R Nordgren. Non-invasive information on the PR segment of the cardiac cycle: an assessment of the clinical potential of the electric and magnetic methods. Proc SPIE 167, 173-177, 1978

11. Erné SN, RR Fenici, H-D Halboom, W Jaszcuk, HD Lehmann, M Maselli. High-resolution isofiled mappoing in magnetocardiography. Il Nuovo Cimento 2D, 291-300, 1983

12. Erné SN. High resolution magnetocardiography: modeling and sources localization. Med Biol Eng Comp 23, suppl: 1447-1450, 1985

13. Fenici RR, M Masselli , SN Erné, HD Halbohm. Magnetocardiographic mapping of the PR-interval phenomena in an unshielded laboratory. In: Biomagnetism-Applications and Theory, Weinberg H, G Stroink and TE Katila (eds), New York-Toronto, Pergamon Press, pp 137-141, 1985

14. Gonnelli R, P Galeone, M Sicuro. A biomagnetic approach to the localization of the necrotic area in inferior myocardial infarction. Proc XIV ICMBE and VII ICMP, Espoo, Finland, 1985

15. Katila T, R Maniewski, M Mäkijärvi, J Nenonen, P Siltanen. On the accuracy of source localization in cardiac measurements. Phys Med Biol 32, 125-131, 1987

16. Romani GL. An application of SQUID sensors to medicine and physiol. Physica 126, B:70-81, 1984

17. Van Leeuwen P, M Schussler, H Bettermann, S Lange, W Hatzmann. Magnetocardiography for assessment of fetal heart actions. Geburtshilfe-Frauenheilkd 55, 642-646, 1995

18. QuinnA, A Weir, U Shahani, R Bain, P Maas, G Donaldson. Antenatal fetal magnetocardiography: a new method for fetal surveillance ? Br J Obstet Gynaecol 101 (10), 866-870, 1994

19. Menendez T, S Achenbach, W Moshage, M Flug, E Beinder, A Kollert, A Bittel, K Bachmann. Prenatal recording of fetal heart action with magnetocardiography. Z Kardiol 87, 111-118, 1998
20. Kawaoka PY, SM Yamashiro. Separation of cardiac conduction system and atrial activities by spatial regression. Med Eng Phys 18 (1), 45-50, 1996
21. Nikitin IP, AV Shabalin, EN Ermakova, AV Kytmanov, NV Golyshev, BM Rogachevsky, SV Motorin. Magneto-, electro- and echocardiography in detecting symptoms of the „hypertensive heart". Klein Med Mosk 74 (5), 29-31, 1996
22. Fenici RR, M Masselli, L Lopez, G Melillo. Clinical value of magnetocardiography. In: Electrocardiography and Cardiac Drug Therapy. HombachV, HH Hilger and HL Kennedy (eds), Dordrecht, Boston, London, Kluwer Academic Publishers, pp 239-258, 1989
23. Hombach V, M Kochs, P Weismüller, M Clausen, E Henze, P Richter, M Höher, A Peper, T Eggeling, WE Adam. Localization of ectopic ventricular depolarization by ISPECT radionuclide ventriculography and by magnetocardiography. ISPECT and MCG for ectopic mapping. Int J Card Imag 7 (3-4), 225-235, 1991
24. Weismüller P, K Abraham-Fuchs, S Schneder, P Richter, M Kochs, J Edrich, V Hombach. Biomagnetic non-invasive localization of accessory pathways in Wolff-Parkinso-White syndrome. Pacing Clin Electrophysiol 14, 1961-1965, 1991
25. Weismüller P, K Abraham-Fuchs, S Schneider, P Richter, M Kochs, V Hombach. Magnetocardiographic non-invasive localization of accessory pathways in the Wolff-Parkinson-White syndrome by a multichannel system. Eur Heart J13, 616-622, 1992
26. Nenonen J, M Mäkijärvi, L Toivonen, K Forsman, M Leinio, J Montonen, Jarvinen, P Keto, P Hekali, T Katila. Non-invasive magnetocardiographic localization of ventricular pre-excitation in the Wolff-Parkinson-White syndrome using a realistic torso model. Eur Heart J 14, 168-174, 1993
27. Mäkijärvi M, J Nenonen, L Toivonen, J Montonen, T Katila, P Siltanen. Magnetocardiography: supraventricular arrythmias and preexcitation syndromes. Eur Heart J 14, suppl E, 46-52, 1993
28. Weismüller P. Nichtinvasive Lokalisation des Ursprungs pathologischer Erregungen im ventrikulären Herzmuskel. Habilitationsschrift Ulm 1993
29. Moshage W, S Achenbach, K Gohl, K Bachmann. Evaluation of the non-invasive localization accuracy of cardiac arrhythmias attainable by multichannel magnetocardiography. Int J Card Imaging 12, 47-59, 1996
30. Weismüller P, P Richter, K Abraham-Fuchs, W Haerer, S Schneider, M Höher, M Kochs, J Edrich, V Hombach. Spatial differences of the duration of ventricular late fields in the signal-averaged magnetocardiogram in patients with ventricular late potentials. Pacing Clin Electrophysiol 16, 70-79, 1993
31. Mäkijärvi M, J Montonen, L Toivonen, P Siltanen, MS Nieminen, M Leinio, T Katila. Identification of patients with ventricular ntachycardia after myocardial infarction by high resolution magnetocardiography and electrocardiography. J Electrocardiol 26, 117-124, 1993
32. Leder U, A Hemmann, J Eichhorn, HP Pohl, M Hoffmann, MP Huck, H Nowak, J Haueisen, S Michaelsen, H Kuhnert, S Müller. Segmentation of realistically shaped surfaces from 3D MRI for biomagnetic myocardial current imaging. Proc 10th International Confererence on Biomagnetism, Santa Fé, 1996

33. Leder U, H-P Pohl, S Michaelsen, T Fritschi, M Huck, J Eichhorn, S Müller, H Nowak.. Noninvasive biomagnetic imaging in coronary artery disease based on individual current desnsity maps of the heart. Int J Cardiol 64, 83-92, 1998

34. Hailer B, P Van Leeuwen, M Pilath, S Lange, D Grönemeyer, M Wehr. Changes in the spatial dispersion of the QT-interval in patients with coronary artery disease. PACE 21 (Part II), 908, 1998

35. Van Leeuwen P, B Hailer, D Donker, S Lange, M Wehr. Noninvasive diagnosis of coronary artery disease at rest on the basis of multichannel magnetocardiography. PACE 21 (Part II), 908, 1998

36. Häninen H, P Takala, M Mäkijärvi, J Montonen, J Nenonen, T Katila, L Toivonen. Detection of exercise induced myocardial ischemia by multichannel magnetocardiography in patients with single vessel coronary artery disease. 8th International Congresss of Holter and Non-invasive Electrocardiology 1998 in Ulm. ANE 3 (3), 241, 1998.

37. Saarinen M. Magnetocardiogram in coronary artery disease. Ann Clin Res 1989

38. Seese B, W Moshage, S Achenbach, R Killmann, K Bachmann. Magnetocardiographic (MCG) analysis of myocardial injury currents. In: Biomagnetism: Fundamental Research and Clinical Applications. Baumgartner C, L Deecke, G Stroink, SJ Williamson (eds), Elsevier Science^, IOS Press, Amsterdam, 1995, pp 628-632

39. Van Leeuwen P, B Hailer, M Wehr. Spatial distribution of QT-intervals: an alternative approach to QT-dispersion. PACE 19, 1894-1899, 1996

CHAPTER FIVE: ANALYSIS TECHNIQUES

SECTION ONE: NON-LINEAR DYNAMICS

40. METHODS OF NON-LINEAR DYNAMICS

MALTE MEESMANN, CHRISTIAN BRAUN, ANSGAR FREKING,
MARCUS KOLLER AND PETER KOWALLIK

INTRODUCTION

Noninvasive risk stratification of patients post myocardial infarction has
gained renewed interest, since prophylactic therapy for sudden cardiac death
has primarily to consider the expensive and invasive therapy with the
implantable cardioverter/defibrillator [25]. In addition to left ventricular ejection
fraction and number of ventricular extrasystoles [3], measures of heart rate
variability (HRV) are often used for risk stratification. HRV is usually
analyzed in the time and frequency domain [4,17,22]. These methods describe the
linear correlations in HRV. In addition, *nonlinear components* in HRV have
been demonstrated [20,16,7] and are being explored for improvement of risk
prediction [13,29,32]. In this article, we briefly review methods that have been used
to describe and/or quantify *nonlinear* components in HRV. Methods using
symbolic dynamics are presented elsewhere in this book.

1/F- FLUCTUATIONS

HRV analysis in the frequency domain is well established in the HF ($0.15 - 0.4$
Hz) and LF ($0.04 - 0.15$ Hz) frequency bands. However, most of the spectral
power is contained in the very low and ultra low frequency bands. These have
been used as integrated measures (VLF, ULF) and as such have a high
correlation to the standard deviation as a global measure [5]. Plotting the

H.-H. Osterhues et al. (eds.),
Advances in Noninvasive Electrocardiographic Monitoring Techniques, 413–420.
© 2000 *Kluwer Academic Publishers. Printed in the Netherlands.*

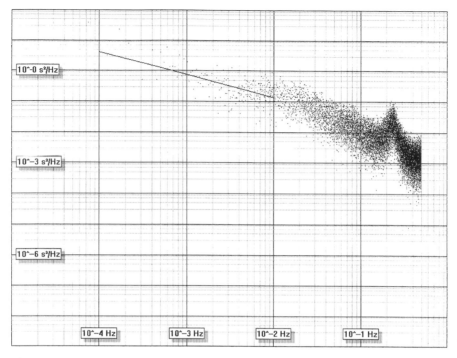

Figure 1. Log-log plot of the periodogram from a 24 hour Holter recording of a normal person. Four power values of neighboring frequencies are averaged. Note the increase in power at lower frequencies which can be fitted by a straight line, indicating a power law with the spectral power density proportional to $f^{-0.9}$.

smoothed periodogram of a 24 hour record in a log-log fashion, one can easily see that the power is proportional to $1/f^\alpha$ which represents a (nonlinear) power law (Figure 1). The slope of the power spectrum at frequencies below 0.01 Hz can be fitted with linear regression using the averaged power values [6]. Alternatively, the unsmoothed spectrum can be fitted by the maximum likelihood method [24]. The latter method accommodates the fact that the error of the unsmoothed spectrum has an exponential non-Gaussian distribution. A simple and intuitive time domain estimate of this power law behavior has been performed using counting statistics [21 23 28].

In patients post myocardial infarction the $1/f$-slope is an independent risk predictor, with greater risk indicated by a steeper slope [6 22]. In a recent study, $1/f$-fluctuations proved to be an important risk predictor in the elderly [14]. It is tempting to speculate that slopes approaching a value of 2 represent integrated white noise of a system which is no longer controlled by specific physiologic mechanisms [33].

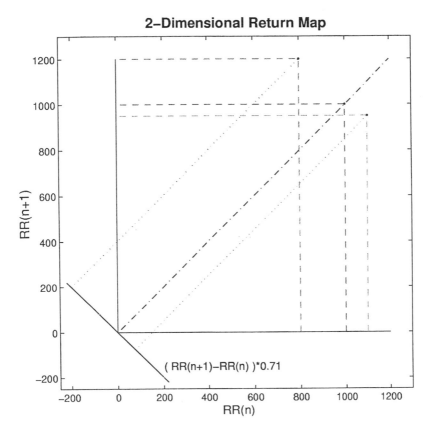

Figure 2. Cartoon of a return map of 3 artificial pairs of consecutive RR-intervals (800-1200, 1000-1000, 1100-950). The first value of each pair is plotted on the x-axis with the corresponding second value on the y-axis. This constitutes a two-dimensional embedding with a delay of 1. As is evident from geometry, the projection of points on the oblique line (vertical to the line of identity) represents the distribution of consecutive differences. Thus, the more the points are away from the line of identity, the larger the beat-to-beat variability.

RETURN MAP

In the usual depiction of a Holter recording the RR-intervals are presented consecutively over time. In the return map, however, each interval is plotted on the y-axis with the previous RR-interval as x-coordinate. As can be seen from Fig. 2, this plot indirectly depicts the differences of successive RR-intervals. Thus, the beat-to-beat dynamics in HRV, i.e. the *change* in RR-intervals, are presented as a function of the previous RR-interval.

Early applications of this method were performed by Anan[1] and Babloyantz[2]. Visual inspection of these plots has lead to a delineation of different patterns

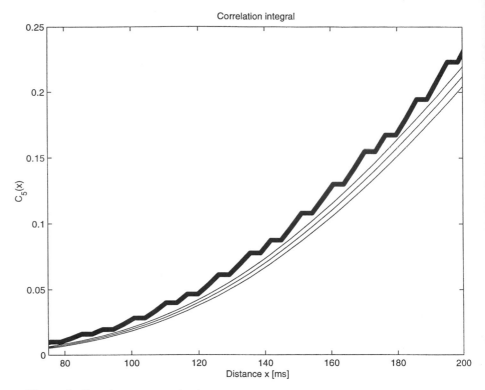

Figure 3. Correlation integral of a stationary segment of 16384 RR-intervals after embedding in 5 dimensions using delay coordinates. The thick line represents the values of the original time series. The thin lines represent the mean (± 2 standard deviations) of the correlations integrals of 25 corresponding surrogate data sets. For more details the reader is referred to Ref. 7.

such as "torpedo" or "complex" [37]. The latter has been associated with an adverse prognosis in patients post myocardial infarction [15]. The return map is a graphical representation of a two-dimensional embedding. This embedding uses delay coordinates to generate a multidimensional phase space from only one observable.

CORRELATION INTEGRAL

The correlation integral quantitatively describes the distribution of consecutive RR-intervals, embedded in a high-dimensional phase space in similar fashion as explained before. It can be used to detect differences between time series of RR-intervals and corresponding time series with identical linear properties but without any nonlinear components, so called *surrogate data* [30]. Figure 3 shows the mean of correlation integrals and the mean ± 2 standard deviations for these linear time series (thin lines). The correlation integral of the original time series of RR-intervals (thick line) lies outside this 2σ-range of therefore significantly differs from the linear surrogate data sets. This demonstrates that the time series of RR-intervals can not completely be described by linear methods[7].

CORRELATION DIMENSION

The dynamics of "chaotic systems" are drawn towards attractors that have, in most cases, a non-integer dimension, a so called fractal dimension [12]. The dimension of the attractor can in principle be estimated by the slope of the regression line fitting the correlation integrals of increasing embeddings. The requirements for estimating the correlation dimension from embeddings have been delineated by Takens [31] and Sauer [27]. Basic assumption for the detection of an attractor is the deterministic coupling of the variables involved. Embedding data in a meaningful way basically requires a high time and amplitude resolution, stationarity, and a data range of several orders of magnitude. These conditions are rarely encountered in biological data.

A widely used algorithm to estimate the correlation dimension was developed by Grassberger and Procaccia [11]. It works nicely for low-dimensional chaotic systems but its application to biological data, including HRV has remained problematic. Early skepticism was put forth by Ruelle[26] and Grassberger himself who said about the correlation dimension (D_2): „If a system is low-dimensional you don't need it. If it is high-dimensional it will not work" [10].

NONLINEAR PHENOMENA IN MYOCARDIAL REPOLARIZATION

Rate-dependent fluctuations in cardiac action potential duration and refractoriness are important determinants of cardiac tachyarrhythmias. The dependence of action potential duration on heart rate can be described using a nonlinear unidimensional map [9], where action potential duration is a function of the preceding diastolic interval. Iteration of this map reproduces the dynamics of action potential duration found in driven preparations, including period doubling bifurcations and chaos [8,35]. Certain features of this map, e.g. a region of a steep slope (>1), may also determine whether single spiral waves of electrical activity may splinter into multiple spirals, which has been proposed as a mechanism for the transition of ventricular tachycardia to ventricular fibrillation [36]. It has been shown recently that a steep slope in this map produces alternans of action potential duration [19], which may pertain to T-wave alternans which is a well established harbinger of malignant ventricular arrhythmias.

The dynamics of this one-dimensional map may also be used for *controlling* the dynamics of action potential duration. In a computer model [34] as well as in real-time experiments [18] complex ("chaotic") dynamics in action potential duration have been reduced to simpler oscillations. This has been achieved by delivering single, appropriately timed extrastimuli that drive the system to its fixed point.

SUMMARY

1/f-fluctuations are frequently encountered within a rather narrow scaling region. In „healthy" situations, the slope is close to 1. A steeper slope (approaching 2) may indicate loss of control in the system considered and can be used as an independent risk predictor.

Methods of nonlinear dynamics are a powerful tool in descriptive data analysis of biological time series. Nonlinear components can be demonstrated in these time series which can not be assessed by linear methods (i.e. conventional spectral analysis). The physiological and clinical importance of these nonlinear components remains to be established in large scale studies.

Demonstration of low-dimensional chaos in complex signals (e.g. RR-intervals) should be considered with great caution.

ACKNOWLEDGMENT
We would like to thank Dante R. Chialvo, MD, Robert F. Gilmour, PhD, Klaus-D. Kniffki, PhD, and Rainer Scharf, PhD, for continuing discussions. This work is being supported by a grant from the "Bundesministerium für Forschung und Technologie (BMBF)".

REFERENCES

1. Anan T, Nakagaki O, Nakamaru M: An application of Lorenz and multi-Lorenz plot to computerized to computerized analysis of arrhythmia. *Jpn.Heart J.* 1982;23:694-696
2. Babloyantz A, Destexhe A: Is the normal heart a periodic oscillator? *Biol.Cybern.* 1988;58:203-211

3. Bigger JTJr, Fleiss JL, Kleiger RE, Miller P, Rolnitzky LM, Multicenter Post-infarction research group: The relationships among ventricular arrhythmias, left ventricular dysfunction, and mortality in the 2 years after myocardial infarction. *Circulation* 1984;69:250-258

4. Bigger JTJr, Fleiss JL, Rolnitzky LM, Steinman RC: Frequency domain measures of heart period variability to assess risk late after myocardial infarction. *J.Am.Coll.Cardiol.* 1993;21:729-736

5. Bigger JTJr, Fleiss JL, Steinman RC, Rolnitzky LM, Kleiger RE, Rottman JN: Correlations among time and frequency domain measures of heart period variability two weeks after acute myocardial infarction. *Am.J.Cardiol.* 1992;69:891-898

6. Bigger JTJr, Steinman RC, Rolnitzky LM, Fleiss JL, Albrecht P, Cohen RJ: Power law behavior of RR-interval variability in healthy middle-aged persons, patients with recent acute myocardial infarction, and patients with heart transplants. *Circulation* 1996;93:2142-2151

7. Braun C, Kowallik P, Freking A, Hadeler D, Kniffki K-D, Meesmann M: Evidence for nonlinear components in heart rate variability of healthy persons. *Am.J.Physiol.* 1998;in press

8. Chialvo DR, Gilmour RFJr, Jalife J: Low dimensional chaos in cardiac tissue. *Nature* 1990;343:653-657

9. Glass L, DT Kaplan: *Understanding nonlinear dynamics.* New York, Springer, 1995, pp 1-420

10. Grassberger, P. 1994, personal communication

11. Grassberger P, Procaccia I: Measuring the strangeness of strange attractors. *Physica* 1983;9D:189-208

12. Grassberger P, Schreiber T, Schaffrath C: Nonlinear time sequence analysis. *Int.J.Bif.Chaos* 1991;1:521-547

13. Ho KKL, Moody GB, Peng C-K, Mietus JE, Larson MG, Levy D, Goldberger AL: Predicting survival in heart failure case and control subjects by use of fully automated methods for deriving nonlinear and conventional indices of heart rate dynamics. *Circulation* 1997;842-848

14. Huikuri HV, Mäkikallio TH, Airaksinen J, Seppänen, T, Puukka P, Räihä J, Sourander LB: Power-law relationship of heart rate variability as a predictor of mortality in the elderly. *Circulation* 1998;97:2031-2036

15. Huikuri HV, Seppänen T, Koistinen MJ, Airaksinen KEJ, Ikäheimo MJ, Castellanos A, Myerburg RJ: Abnormalities in beat-to-beat dynamics of heart rate before the onset of life threatening ventricular tachyarrhythmias in patients with prior myocardial infarction. *Circulation* 1996;93:1836-1844

16. Kanters JK, Holstein-Rathlou N-H, Agner E: Lack of evidence for low-dimensional chaos in heart rate variability. *J.Cardiovasc.Electrophysiol.* 1994;5:591601-601

17. Kleiger RE, Miller JP, Bigger JTJr, Moss AJ: Decreased heart rate variability and its association with increased mortality after acute myocardial infarction. *Am.J.Cardiol.* 1987;59:256-262

18. Koller ML, Riccio ML, Gilmour RFJr: Control of local dynamics in ventricular tissues. *Proceedings of the Upstate New York Electrophysiological Society 10/97* 1998 (Abstract)

19. Koller ML, Riccio ML, Gilmour RFJr: Dynamic restitution of action potential duration during electrical alternans and ventricular fibrillation. *Am.J.Physiol.* 1998, in press

20. Kurths J, Voss A, Witt A, Saparin P, Kleiner HJ, Wessel N: Quantitative analysis of heart rate variability. *CHAOS* 1995;

21. Meesmann M, Boese J, Chialvo DR, Kowallik P, Bauer WR, Peters W, Grüneis F, Kniffki K-D: Demonstration of 1/f fluctuations and white noise in the human heart rate by the variance-time-curve: Implications for self- similarity. *Fractals* 1993;1(3):312-320

22. Meesmann M, Brüggemann T, Wegscheider K, Kowallik P, Kniffki K-D, Andresen D: The slope of 1/f-fluctuations of the heart period power spectrum is a powerful risk predictor in patients following myocardial infarction. *PACE* 1996;19:606(Abstract)

23. Meesmann M, Grüneis F, Flachenecker P, Kniffki K-D: A new method for analysis of heart rate variability: Counting statistics of 1/f fluctuations. *Biol.Cybern.* 1993;68:299-306

24. Meesmann M, Schmidt G: Technical advances in heart rate variability processing. *Cardiac Electrophysiology Review* 1998;3:340-344

25. Moss AJ, Hall J, Cannom DS, Daubert SL, Higgins SL, Klein H, Levine JS, Saksena S, Waldo AL, Wilber D, Brown MW, Heo MftMADITI: Improved survival with an implanted defibrillator in patients with coronary disease at hihg risk for ventricular arrhythmia. *N.Engl.J.Med.* 1996;335:1933-1940

26. Ruelle D: *Zufall und Chaos*. Berlin, Springer, 1992, pp 1-207

27. Sauer T, Yorke JA, Casdagli M: Embedology. *J.Stat.Phys.* 1991;65:579-616

28. Scharf R, Meesmann M, Boese J, Chialvo DR, Kniffki K-D: General relation between variance-time curve and power spectral density for point processes exhibiting $1/f^\beta$-fluctuations with special reference to heart rate variability. *Biol.Cybern.* 1995;73:255-263

29. Schmidt G, Morfill GE, Barthel P, Hadamitzky M, Kreuzberg H, Demmel V, Schneider R, Ulm K, Schömig A: Variability of ventricular premature complexes and mortality risk. *PACE* 1996;19:976-980

30. Schreiber T, Schmitz A: Improved surrogate data for nonlinearity tests. *Phys Rev Lett* 1996;77:635-638

31. Takens F: Detecting strange attractors in turbulence. In: Dynamical systems and turbulence. *Lect.Notes Math.* 1981;898:

32. Voss A, Hnatkova K, Wessel N, Kurths J, Sander A, Schirdewan A, Camm AJ, Malik M: Multiparametric analysis of heart rate variability used for risk stratification among survivors of acute myocardial infarction. *PACE* 1998;21:186-192

33. Wagner CD, Persson PB: Two ranges of blood pressure power spectrum with different 1/f characteristics. *Am.J.Physiol.* 1994;Heart Circ.Physiol36:H449-H454

34. Watanabe M, Gilmour RFJr: Strategy for control of complex low dimensional dynamics in cardiac tissue. *J.Math.Biol.* 1996;35:73-87

35. Watanabe M, Otani NF, Gilmour RFJr: Biphasic restitution of action potential duration and complex dynamics in ventricular myocardium. *Circ.Res.* 1995;76:915-921

36. Winfree AT: How does ventricular tachycardia decay into ventricular fibrillation?, in Shenasa M, Borggrefe M, Breithardt G (eds): *Cardiac Mapping*. 1993,

37. Woo MA, Stevenson WG, Moser DK, Trelease RB, Harper RM: Patterns of beat-to-beat heart rate variability in advanced heart failure. *Am.Heart J.* 1992;123:704-710

41. HEART RATE VARIABILITY AND NON-LINEAR DYNAMICS

ALBERTO MALLIANI, ALBERTO PORTA, NICOLA MONTANO
AND STEFANO GUZZETTI

Heart rate variability (HRV) is in part the result of numerous and complex rhythmical oscillations that can be extracted from time series with spectral methodology (1,2,3). This approach in the frequency domain has made it possible to indirectly explore the neural regulation of cardiovascular function and in particular to assess the changes in sympathovagal balance (2,3).

However, the harmonic components describe only part of HRV. Recently, some studies (4,5,6) have provided evidence that non-linear and non-harmonic dynamics are present in heart rate. In fact, the system seems to display a behavior ranging from a regular periodicity to an erratic pattern which, from the geometrical and dynamical point of view, might have a deterministic rather than a stochastic nature. Hence, what may be often interpreted as a noise effect could be hypothesized to pertain to a non-linear deterministic system, extremely sensitive to initial conditions, a pattern generally assumed as defining a chaotic system (7,8).

The sinus rhythm system consists of the sino-atrial node activity controlled by multiple and complex neural mechanisms which constitute a near-perfect theoretical substrate for the generation of chaos (7).

A few mathematical theorems suggest that a chaotic process might be studied by looking at a realization of a time series, sufficiently long and adequately sampled, which may provide the invariant information that quantifies the chaotic dynamics of the system. Consequently, it is possible to make quantitative inferences about the dynamic structure of the entire system from the behavior of a single variable.

H.-H. Osterhues et al. (eds.),
Advances in Noninvasive Electrocardiographic Monitoring Techniques, 421–428.
© 2000 *Kluwer Academic Publishers. Printed in the Netherlands.*

In a previous study (6) we used parameters that quantify non-linear dynamics (D2 correlation dimension, K2 Kolmogorov entropy, self-similarity exponent and Lyapunov exponents) in order to compare the behavior of a normal sinus rhythm to that of heart-transplanted patients. It was found not only that non-linear dynamics are likely to be present in HRV, but that system complexity decreases in transplanted patients (a finding that was attributed to the loss of neural modulation of heart rate).

One of the limitations of this approach was, however, that large time series were needed, a fact that is often incompatible with physiological and clinical studies.

Moreover the finding of a non-integer correlation dimension or a positive Lyapunov exponent is not a sufficient condition to demonstrate the existence of a chaotic process.

An alternative approach based on the change of a control parameter in the experimental protocol and on the classification of the evoked non-linear dynamics can be followed. This approach allows to construct a bifurcation diagram indicating the parameter value determining a change in the behavior of the experimental preparation. If a standard "route to chaos" is found, such as a period doubling cascade (9), the claim for chaos is more robust. This approach appears closer to physiology than a mere application of signal processing methods and can be performed over short data sequences (classification methods do not imply the use of large amount of samples).

For example, Guevara et al (10) classified the non-linear interactions between periodic trains of current pulses and the spontaneous rhythmical activity of aggregates of chick ventricular heart cells when the stimulation frequency was changed. In this way he was able to observe a period doubling route to chaos.

In the field of cardiovascular variability Porta et al (11), on the basis of recordings of efferent preganglionic cardiac sympathetic discharge and ventilation in decerebrate artificially ventilated cats, classified the non-linear interferences between the low frequency (LF, around 0.1 Hz) and the high frequency (HF, synchronous with respiratory activity) oscillations and the ventilatory cycles. In this experimental protocol (12) the control parameter was the mean sympathetic firing rate that was changed by means of experimental maneuvers such as the inferior vena cava occlusion (IVCO) or aortic constriction (AC) while keeping constant the ventilatory frequency at 0.3 Hz. While IVCO, by reducing the arterial pressure, determined a reflex sympathetic activation, AC, by increasing the arterial pressure, caused a sympathetic inhibition. At control a prevalence of 1:1 dynamics is more frequently observed, the sympathetic discharge oscillates with each ventilatory cycle (Fig.1a). The frequency tracking locus (FTL) is used to characterize these non linear interactions (3,11). Each sympathetic response to ventilatory cycles is represented by a vector, its

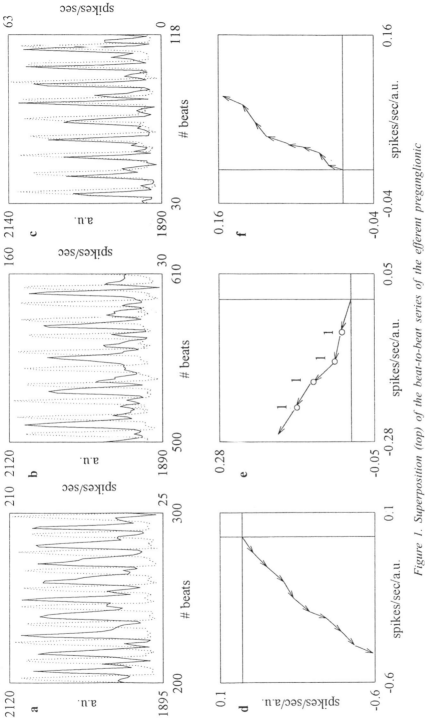

Figure 1. Superposition (top) of the beat-to-beat series of the efferent preganglionic cardiac sympathetic activity (solid line) and ventilation (dotted line) (upper panels) and relevant frequency tracking locus (FTL) (lower panels) at control (a,d) during inferior vena cava occlusion (b,e) and aortic occlusion (c,f) (from Ref. 11).

magnitude being proportional to the amplitude of the sympathetic burst. As to the vector phase it is related to the time occurrence of the sympathetic burst inside the ventilatory cycle. A missed response is represented in the FTL as an open circle labeled by the number 1. The 1:1 dynamics is represented by the FTL as a sequence of vectors with almost fixed length and phase (Fig.1d). Sympathetic activation produced by IVCO induces a 1:2 dynamics with peaks of sympathetic discharge every two ventilatory cycles (Fig.1b). Its FTL appears as a regular sequence of vectors and open circles (Fig.1e). It was observed that, during IVCO, the sympathetic discharge was locked to a subharmonic of ventilation and various locking ratios were found (mainly 1:2; 1:4; 1:6; 1:8 dynamics). Therefore, while in the so-called control conditions ventilation interfered more with HF central rhythm generators, during IVCO the interaction between ventilation and spontaneous LF sympathetic oscillations were privileged. During AC the sympathetic discharge was more frequently coupled in 1:1 fashion with ventilation (Fig.1c,f), thus evidencing that ventilation mainly entrained the HF oscillator.

This is an example of non-linear analysis performed on short segment of data: a rich set of dynamics is evoked by changing an adequate control parameter and the classification of the non-linear interferences is performed by a simple graphical tool. Other control parameters can be changed in order to explore the system (e.g. the frequency of the ventilation) and other tools can be used to perform classification of the interferences.

Another recent approach to the analysis of non-linear dynamics of short data sequences is based on the quantification of regularity of the time series. The regularity is measured by means of functions quantifying the entropy rate of a process (i.e. the amount of information carried by a sample of the series when a certain amount of previous samples are known). These functions exploit the conditional probability to understand if the series is more or less predictable from its own past. If the series is strictly periodic (i.e. it is completely predictable) the entropy rate is zero. If the series is a white noise (i.e. it is completely unpredictable) the entropy rate is high. The entropy rate of a series with some level of regularity is between these two extremes. Several functions were proposed to approximate the entropy rate of short segments of data and to derive indexes of regularity. The most widely utilized index is the approximated entropy proposed by Pincus (14). More recently, Porta et al (15) proposed a new function, referred to as corrected conditional entropy (CCE). The main advantage of this function is that the derived index of regularity is obtained without setting a priori the embedding dimension of the reconstructed phase space (i.e., the number of previous samples used to predict). When applied to short data sequence (around 250-300 samples) the CCE exhibits a minimum and the smaller is its value the more regular is the series.

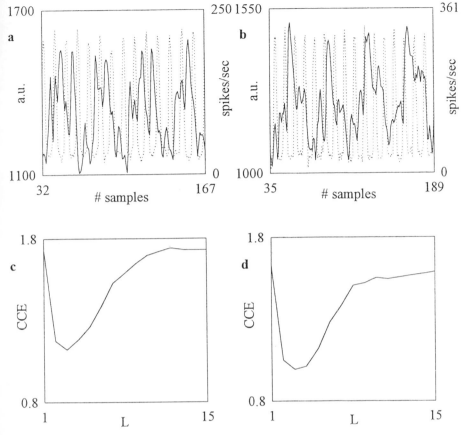

Figure 2. Beat-to-beat variability of sympathetic discharge (solid line) superposed to ventilation (dotted line) (upper records) in the same animal during control (a) and during inferior vena cava occlusion (b). The corrected conditional entropy (CCE) functions exhibit a well defined minimum which was at L=3 smaller during inferior vena cava occlusion (d) than during control conditions (c) (from Ref. 15).

An example of regularity analysis performed by using the CCE is shown in Fig.2. The analysis was also in this case performed on the beat-to-beat variability series of the sympathetic discharge in relation to ventilatory cycles. During IVCO (15) the LF oscillation was locked to ventilation with a 1:4 pattern and strong regularity (the minimum of the CCE decreases, Fig.2d). During AC the sympathetic discharge, although characterized by a dominant HF rhythm, was not so regular (15). Hence the sympathetic activation produced by IVCO determines a more synchronous firing than the sympathetic inhibition induced by AC. After spinalization at C1 level the preganglionic efferent cardiac sympathetic activity was decreased and phase-locked periodic dynamics could not be

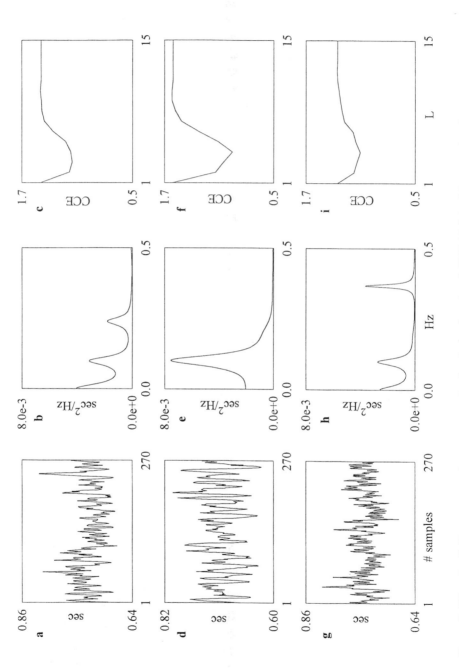

Figure 3. RR series (left), autoregressive power spectra (central column) and CCE (right) of the considered experimental conditions on the same subject: rest (a,b,c), head-up tilt (d,e,f) and controlled respiration at 20 breaths per minute (g,h,i). (from Ref. 16).

found. In these conditions although the sympathetic activity still exhibited LF and HF oscillations they were unlocked to ventilation. As a result the minimum of the CCE increased thus quantifying the loss of the regularity of the sympathetic discharge variability (15). It is likely that the spinal section reduced the ability of the supraspinal centers to entrain and synchronize the spinal sympathetic outflow. The pattern generators were still able to exhibit a rhythmic activity but less coordinated and organized.

A similar analysis was performed on the beat-to-beat variability series of heart period (16). Experimental conditions of sympathetic excitation (90 degree head-up tilt, T) and sympathetic inhibition (controlled respiration at 20 breaths per minute, CR) were analyzed. While T is able to increase the LF oscillation and the regularity of the heart period series (the minimum of the CCE is smaller in respect to resting conditions), CR determines the increase the HF component but the minimum of the CCE remains unchanged. This suggests that a sympathetic activation is more important in increasing the regularity of the heart period variability than an external input like respiration.

In our current research we are trying to combine in different experimental conditions these approaches to the study of rhythmical and non rhythmical components of HRV.

REFERENCES

1. Akselrod S, Gordon D, Ubel FA, Shannon DC, Cohen RJ: Power spectrum analysis of heart rate fluctuation: a quantitative probe of beat-to-beat cardiovascular control. *Science* 1981;213:220-222

2. Pagani M, Lombardi F, Guzzetti S, Rimoldi O, Furlan R, Pizzinelli P, Sandrone G, Malfatto G, Dell'Orto S, Piccaluga E, Turiel M, Baselli G, Cerutti S, Malliani A. Power spectral analysis of heart rate and arterial pressure variabilities as a marker of sympathovagal interaction in man and conscious dog. *Circ Res* 1986;58:178-193

3. Malliani A, Pagani M, Lombardi F, Cerutti S. Cardiovascular neural regulation explored in the frequency domain. Research Advances Series, *Circulation* 1991;84:482-492

4. Goldberger AL, West BJ. Applications of non linear dynamics to clinical cardiology. *Ann NY Acad Sci* 1987;504:195-213.

5. Sugihara G, Allan W, Sobel D, Allan KD. Non-linear control of heart rate variability in human infants. *Proc Natl Acad Sci* 1996;93:2608-2613.

6. Guzzetti S, Signorini MG, Cogliati C, Mezzetti S, Porta A, Cerutti S, Malliani A: Non-linear dynamics and chaotic indices in heart rate variability of normal subjects and heart-transplanted patients. *Cardiovasc Res* 1996;31:441-446.

7. Denton TA, Diamond GA, Helfant RH, Khan S, Karagueuzian H: Fascinating rhythm: A primer on chaos theory and its application to cardiology. *Am Heart J* 1990;120:1419-1440

8. Glass L, Mackey MC. From clock to chaos: the rhythms of life. Princeton University Press. Princeton, 1998.

9. May RM. Simple mathematical models with very complicated dynamics. *Nature* 1976;261:459-467.

10. Guevara MR, Shrier A, Glass L. Phase-locked rhythms in periodically stimulated heart cell aggregates. *Am J Physiol* 1988;254:H1-H10.

11. Porta A, Baselli G, Montano N, Gnecchi-Ruscone T, Lombardi F, Malliani A, Cerutti S. Classification of coupling patterns among spontaneous rhythms and ventilation in the sympathetic discharge of decerebrate cats. *Biol Cyber* 1996;75:163-172.

12. Montano N, Lombardi F, Gnecchi-Ruscone T, Contini M, Finocchiaro ML, Baselli G, Porta A, Cerutti S, Malliani A. Spectral analysis of sympathetic discharge, R-R-interval and systolic arterial pressure in decerebrate cats. *J Autonom Nerv Syst* 1992;40:21-32

13. Kitney RI, Bignall S. Techniques for studying short-term changes in cardio-respiratory data. In: Di Rienzo et al. (eds) Blood pressure and heart rate variability. IOS Press, Amsterdam, 1992 pp 1-23.

14. Pincus SM. Approximated entropy as a measure of system complexity. *Proc Natl Acad Sci USA* 1991;88:2297-2311

15. Porta A, Baselli G, Liberati D, Montano N, Cogliati C, Gnecchi-Ruscone T, Malliani A, Cerutti S. Measuring regularity by means of a corrected conditional entropy in sympathetic outflow. *Biol Cybern* 1998;78:71-78

16. Porta A, Baselli G, Guzzetti S, Magatelli R, Montano N, Cogliati C, Malliani A, Cerutti S. Synchronisation analysis of heart rate period variability signal based on corrected conditional entropy. *Computers in Cardiology*, IEEE Computer Society Press, Los Alamitos, California, 1997:24;121-124

42. SYMBOLIC DYNAMICS

A. VOSS, N. WESSEL, J. KURTHS, A. WITT, A. SCHIRDEWAN,

K.J. OSTERZIEL, M. MALIK AND R. DIETZ

INTRODUCTION

Symbolic dynamics did start with Hadamard [1] ideas to more complicated systems in 1898. The most important point of this work is the simple description of the possible sequences that can arise in geodesic flows on surfaces of negative curvature. He introduced a finite set of forbidden symbol pairs and defined possible sequences as those that do not contain any forbidden symbol pair. Later on, Hedlund and Morse [2, 3] used this method to prove the existence of periodic and other dynamics in different classical dynamical systems. They showed that in many circumstances such a finite description of a system's dynamics is possible and performed their investigations by finding interesting sequences satisfying the constraints defined by the corresponding symbolic dynamical system.

Now we understand symbolic dynamics as a rapidly growing part of dynamical systems. Although it was originally developed as a method to study basic structures and behavior of dynamical systems, the methods and the technology have found significant applications in various fields of sciences. Some of the major fields for applications of symbolic dynamics are linear algebra, data storage (coding), data transmission (information theory), data analysis and processing as well as life sciences. Paulus et al. [4] applied symbolic dynamics in animal experiments. Studies of the dynamics in heart rate generation with symbolic dynamics started 1993 with Voss et al. [5] and were followed by other investigations [6, 7]. Several studies in EEG processing [8-10] emphasize

H.-H. Osterhues et al. (eds.),
Advances in Noninvasive Electrocardiographic Monitoring Techniques, 429–437.
© 2000 *Kluwer Academic Publishers. Printed in the Netherlands.*

Two different tachograms

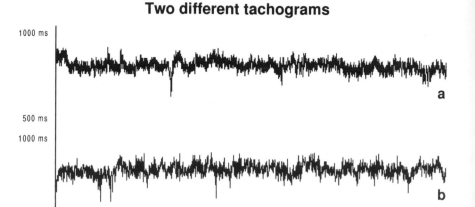

Spectra of the tachograms

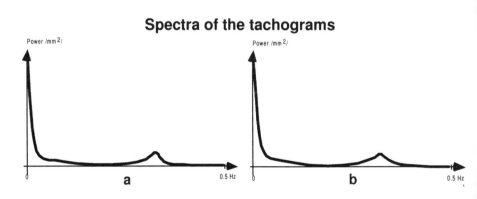

Word distributions of the tachograms

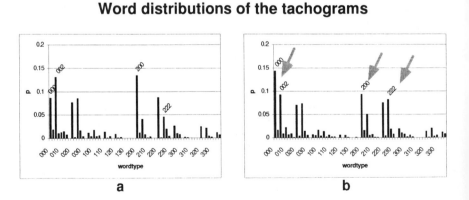

Figure 1. Application of symbolic dynamics in HRV analysis. From two tachograms (upper traces) with identical mean and standard deviation the related spectra (middle traces) show a high degree of congruence. The resulting word distributions (lower part) show impressive differences highlighted with arrows.

the increased importance of symbolic dynamics in characterizing biological systems.

Heart rate variability reflects the complex interactions of many different control loops of the cardiovascular system. In relation to the complexity of the sinus node activity modulation system, a more predominantly non-linear behavior has to be assumed. In this way the detailed description and classification of dynamic changes using time and frequency measures is often not sufficient. Therefore we have introduced new methods of non-linear dynamics derived from the symbolic dynamics to distinguish between different states of the autonomic interactions.

METHOD

The motivation for applying methods from nonlinear dynamics in heart rate variability is drawn in figure 1. Two different short time tachograms (represented by the beat-to-beat interval length as a function of time) produce identical values of the heart rate variability (HRV) time domain measures (mean: 831/831 ms, standard deviation: 29/29 ms). The spectra derived from these tachograms show a rather similar behavior and the frequency domain measures (total power 'P': 0.000120/0.000115, high frequency component in normalized units 'HFn': 0.707/0.645) do not differ sufficiently (4.2% resp. 8.8% difference). However, the nonlinear measures from symbolic dynamics extracted from the displayed word distributions show high significant differences between both time series (number of forbidden words 'forbword': 24/19 that are 21%, intermittent high variability phvar20: 0.0132/0.0304 that is related to about 130% difference!).

Symbolic dynamics

Symbolic dynamics is based on a coarse-graining of the dynamics of a signal. The time series are transformed into symbol sequences with symbols from a given alphabet (figure 2). Some detailed information is lost but the coarse dynamic behavior remains and can be analyzed. Depending on the time series we have to define the type and number of symbols. Long time series allow a higher number of symbols (a higher resolution of the analysis) than short time series. Symbolic dynamics, as an approach to investigate complex systems facilitates the analysis of dynamic aspects of the HRV.

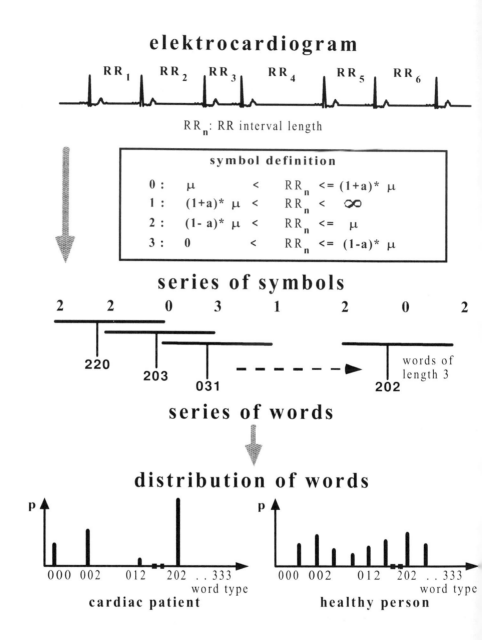

Figure 2. Basic principle of symbolic dynamics with 4 symbols and words of length 3. First, symbols were extracted from the ECG depending on the relation of an actual beat-to-beat interval to the weighted mean following the rules within the box. Then, words of length 3 are formed, counted and displayed as word distributions.

There are several procedures to characterize symbol strings. In studies of short term HRV records we did use the probability distribution of length 3 words (words which consist of 3 symbols of a four letter alphabet). In this way, one obtains 64 different types of words (bins). A 30 minutes ECG corresponds to about 1800 RR-intervals in the tachogram, so that there are about 28 words in each bin. Too few words per bin reduce the accuracy of the word distribution estimation. We recommend to use at least 12 words per bin. For a 24 hour analysis the number of symbols can be increased to 6 (word of length 5).

The Shannon and Renyi entropies calculated from the distributions of words are suitable measures for the complexity in the time series. A high percentage of words consisting only of the symbols '0' and '2' is a measure for decreased HRV, conversely a measure of increased HRV would consist of a high percentage of all words that contain the symbols '1' and '3'. Higher values of these entropies refer to higher complexities in the corresponding tachograms and lower values to lower ones. The Shannon entropy is the classical measure of information theory. It extracts the information contents of a symbol sequence. The concept of Renyi entropy was introduced as a generalization of Shannon's concept. Both types of entropy are described more in detail in [11].

A further method is to count the so called 'forbidden words' in the distribution of words, that is the number of words which seldom or never occur. A high number of forbidden words reflects a reduced dynamics in the time series.

The parameter 'wsdvar' is a measure of the time series variability depending on a word sequence. The resulting word sequence $\{w_1, w_2, w_3...\}$ is transformed into a sequence $\{\bar{s}_1, \bar{s}_2, \bar{s}_3...\}$ in the following way:

$$
\bar{s}(w_i) = \begin{cases}
3 & \text{if} & n_{13}(w_i)=3 & \wedge & s_{13}(w_i)='1' \\
2 & \text{if} & n_{13}(w_i)=2 & \wedge & s_{13}(w_i)='1' \\
1 & \text{if} & n_{13}(w_i)=1 & \wedge & s_{13}(w_i)='1' \\
0 & \text{if} & n_{13}(w_i)=0 & & \\
-1 & \text{if} & n_{13}(w_i)=1 & \wedge & s_{13}(w_i)='3' \\
-2 & \text{if} & n_{13}(w_i)=2 & \wedge & s_{13}(w_i)='3' \\
-3 & \text{if} & n_{13}(w_i)=3 & \wedge & s_{13}(w_i)='3'
\end{cases} \qquad i=1,2,3,...
$$

where $n_{13}(w_i)$ represents the number of symbols '1' or '3' in the word w_i and $s_{13}(w_i)$ is that symbol '1' or '3' that occurs first in the word w_i. The word dynamics parameter 'wsdvar' is defined as the standard deviation of this sequence $\bar{s}_i$.

An additional mode of symbolic dynamics for low or high variability analysis was developed. In this way we observed 6 successive symbols of a simplified alphabet, consisting only of symbols '0' or '1'. Here the symbol '0' stands for a difference between two successive beats lower than a special limit (5, 10,

20, 50, 100 ms) whereas '1' represent those cases where the difference between two successive beats exceeds this special limit:

'1': $|t_n-t_{n-1}| \geq$ limit

'0': $|t_n-t_{n-1}| <$ limit

Words consisting only of an unique type of symbols (either all '0' or all '1')
were counted. These measures were called 'plvar5', 'plvar10', 'plvar20' (word
type '000000'), 'phvar20', 'phvar50' and 'phvar100' (word type '111111'). As
an example 'plvar10' represents the probability of the word type '000000'
occurrence with the special limit of 10 ms. In opposition 'phvar100' represents
the probability of the word type '111111' occurrence with the special limit of
100 ms.

APPLICATIONS OF SYMBOLIC DYNAMICS

Test of independence

700 long-term tachograms from patients after myocardial infarction were analyzed [12]. We calculated heart rate variability parameters from time (5 parameters) and frequency domain (4) as well as from non-linear dynamics (10).
Then the correlations between non-linear, time and frequency measures were
estimated. Heart rate variability analysis based on non-linear parameters presents an independent assessment and shows only low correlations with time
(r<0.4) and frequency (r=0.3) domain parameters.

The capability of symbolic dynamics to detect nonlinearities in time series was
proved with amplitude adjustmented surrogates [13].

High risk stratification

A multiparametric heart rate variability analysis was performed [11, 14] to
prove if combined heart rate variability (HRV) measures of different domains
improve the result of risk stratification in patients after myocardial infarction.
Standard time domain, frequency domain and non-linear dynamics (symbolic
dynamics) measures of HRV assessment were applied to 572 survivors of
acute myocardial infarction. The discriminant analysis shows a separation of
patients suffered by all cause mortality in 80% (best single parameter 74%)
and sudden arrhythmic death in 86% (73%). All parameters show a high significant difference (p<0.001) between survivors and non-survivors based on
two-tailed t-test. The specificity level of the multivariate parameter sets is at
the 70% sensitivity level (ROC) about 85-90%, whereas HRVi as the standard
measurement of global heart rate variability shows maximum levels of 70%.
The PPA in the all cause mortality group is at the 70% sensitivity level twice

as high as the univariate HRV measure and increases to more than fourfold as high within the VT/VF group. In this population, the multiparametric approach with the combination of four parameters from all domains especially from symbolic dynamics seems to be a better predictor of high arrhythmia risk than the standard measurement of global heart rate variability.

Twin studies

We tested the hypothesis of a genetic influence on heart rate variability. This genetic influence was assessed in 62 twin pairs (30 monozygotic, 32 dizygotic). From all twins long term ECG records were obtained, edited and analyzed. Heart rate variability analysis was performed on the basis of parameters from time domain, frequency domain and non-linear dynamics.

Twin pairs show a significant lower difference in the parameter values than other randomly selected and age matched couples ($p<0.001$). This reflects a considerable familial influence. Most parameters of time domain, non of the frequency domain at all and half of the non-linear dynamics show significant differences between twin pairs and non-twin pairs. As a result of the comparison between monozygotic and dizygotic twin pairs we find a significant lower parameter difference in the monozygotic pairs ($p<0.05$). These results [15] suggest that there is a clear genetic component in heart rate generation and HRV besides family environmental influences. Therefore, analysis of HRV might become a useful method in phenotyping severe genetic changes in cardiovascular diseases.

CONCLUSIONS

Symbolic dynamics is a useful tool in several fields of complexity analysis in science. We have applied symbolic dynamics mainly to characterize the dynamics of heart rate variability. Symbols represent now levels of time differences between successive beats. Symbolic dynamics is an independent method (correlation to standard time and frequency measures) and increases within a multiparametric approach the predictive accuracy in high risk stratification. Complexity measures based on non-linear dynamics separate best between different patient groups because of the partly non-linear behavior of the heart rate generation. Parameters of time domain alone are less efficient in high risk stratification. Measures of frequency domain lead to an improved discrimination between different patient groups probably due to their strong correlation with physiological phenomena. The combination of parameters of time and frequency domain and non-linear dynamics leads to an optimal detection rate of patients after myocardial infarction with high risk for sudden cardiac death.

The results from the twin studies show that there is a genetic component in heart rate generation and HRV besides family environmental influences. Therefore, the analysis of HRV might become a useful method in phenotyping different genetic changes in cardiovascular diseases.

The primary results of these studies show the effectiveness of symbolic dynamics in the HRV analysis. It also shows the advantage of combining symbolic dynamics with conventional methods from time and frequency domain. This leads to an improved precision in the diagnosis of cardiovascular diseases.

REFERENCES

1. Hadamard J. Les surfaces à courbures opposées et leurs lignes geodésiques. J. Math. pures appl., pages 27-73, 1898.
2. Morse M. Recurrent geodesics on a surface of negative curvature. Trans. Amer. Math. Soc., 22:84-110, 1921.
3. Morse M and Hedlund GA. Symbolic dynamics. American J Math., 60:815-866, 1938.
4. Paulus MP, Geyer MA, Gold LH, Mandell AJ. Application of entropy measures derived from the ergodic theory of dynamical systems to rat locomotor behavior. Proc Natl Acad Sci U S A, 87(2):723-727, 1990.
5. Voss A, Dietz R, Fiehring H, Kleiner HJ, Kurths J, Saparin P, Vossing HJ, Witt A. High Resolution ECG, Heart Rate Variability and Nonlinear Dynamics: Tools for High Risk Stratification. Computers in Cardiology, IEEE Computer Society Press, Los Alamitos, 261-264, 1993
6. Kurths J, Voss A, Witt A, Saparin P, Kleiner HJ, Wessel N. Quantitative analysis of heart rate variability. Chaos, 5: 88-94, 1995.
7. Palazzolo JA, Estafanous FG, Murray PA. Entropy measures of heart rate variation in conscious dogs, Am J Physiol Heart Circul Physiol, 43(4) : H1099-H1105, 1998
8. Xu JH, Liu ZR, Liu R. The measures of sequence complexity for EEG studies, Chaos 4(11):2111-2119, 1994
9. Rapp PE, Schmah T. Complexity measures in molecular psychiatry, Molec Psychiatry 1 (5): 408-416, 1996
10. Engbert R; Schiek M, Scheffczyk C, Kurths J, Krampe R, Kliegl R, Drepper F. Symbolic dynamics of physiological synchronization: Examples from bimanual movements and cardiorespiratory interaction, Nonlinear Analysis Theory Methods And Applcations. 30(2): 973-984, 1997
11. Voss A, Kurths J, Kleiner HJ, Witt A, Wessel N, Saparin P, Osterziel KJ, Schurath R, Dietz R. The application of methods of non-linear dynamics for the improved and predictive recognition of patients threatened by sudden cardiac death. Cardiovascular Research, 3: 419-433, 1996

12. Voss A, Hnatkova K, Wessel N, Dietz R, Malik M. Non-Linear Parameters Contribute to Heart Rate Variability Analysis Independently from Time and Frequency Measures. Proceedings of Europace97, Monduzzi Editore, 191-195, 1997

13. Theiler J, Eubank S, Longtin A, Galdrikian B, Farmer JD. Testing for nonlinearity in time series: the method of surrogate data. Physica D 58: 77-94, 1992

14. Voss A, Hnatkova K, Wessel N, Kurths J, Sander A, Schirdewan A, Camm AJ, Malik M. Multiparametric analysis of heart rate variability used for risk stratification among survivors of acute myocardial infarction. Pace 21(1 Pt 2):186-192, 1998

15. Busjahn A, Voss A, Knoblauch H, Knoblauch M, Jeschke E, Wessel N, Bohländer J, McCarron J, Faulhaber HD, Schuster H, Dietz R, Luft FC. Angiotensin-Converting Enzyme and Angiotensinogen Gene Polymorphisms and Heart Rate Variability in Twins. Am J Cardiol 8: 755-760, 1998

CHAPTER FIVE: ANALYSIS TECHNIQUES

SECTION TWO: NEWER SIGNAL DETECTION AND ANALYSIS TECHNIQUES

43. NEURAL CLASSIFICATION IN HIGH-RESOLUTION ECG SIGNAL PROCESSING

HANS A. KESTLER, FRIEDHELM SCHWENKER, GÜNTHER PALM, JOCHEN WÖHRLE and MARTIN HÖHER

INTRODUCTION

The incidence of sudden cardiac death (SCD) in the area of the Federal Republic of Germany is about 100.000 to 120.000 cases per year. Apart from cases of ventricular fibrillation (VF) related to myocardial ischaemia, e.g. acute myocardial infarction, the main reason for SCD is the occurrence of ventricular tachyarrhythmiaslike ventricular fibrillation with functional cardiac arrest and sustained ventricular tachcardias (VT) as a cause of a chronic arrhythmogenic substrate. The latter group exhibits, in comparison to individuals who survive a life-threatening acute myocardial infarction, a high risk of a recurrent cardiac arrest. Sudden cardiac death most often occurs in the presence of coronary artery disease (CAD) (90% of SCD patients). In a significant number of patients (13%–20%) it is the initial symptom of CAD. VF emerges in most cases (70%) secondarily from a VT and only in 10% primarily from a premature beat [7, 12].

In postinfarction studies with animals it has been shown that the substrate for singular or repeated ventricular arrhythmias is a localized damaged myocardium with abnormal conduction characteristics. This can cause reentrant activation. Such regions have been explored with microelectrodes and have been found to contain nonconducting cells with no evidence of depolarization, poorly conducting cells with poor action potential upstrokes, as well as normal-appearing action potentials [1]. This causes slow or irregular propagation of activation. It is possible to detect these delayed signals with the high-resolution electrocardiogram.

In this study multilayer perceptron and prototype based artificial neural network models are used to classify data from the high-resolution electrocardiogram. Two studies, capturing different aspects of conduction defects are exemplarily reported. The first is based on established features [3] derived from signal averaged QRS-complexes and mainly describes a prolongation of cardiac exitation

441

H.-H. Osterhues et al. (eds.),
Advances in Noninvasive Electrocardiographic Monitoring Techniques, 441–452.
© 2000 *Kluwer Academic Publishers. Printed in the Netherlands.*

that extends beyond the normal QRS (*late potentials*). The second study centers on capturing morphology changes of the T-wave [18] in beat-to-beat recordings (*T-wave alternans*).

METHODS

High-Resolution ECG

The high-resolution ECG (HRECG) provides information about low-level signal sources (μV range) from within the heart not obtainable with standard ECG (mV range) techniques. The standard ECG is usually recorded from 12 leads with an analog device. The HRECG is recorded from three bipolar, orthogonal leads (X, Y, Z).

All registrations are done with a low noise amplifying system inside a Faraday cage in order to minimize the influence of external noise sources. The analog signal bandwidth of the system (Corasonix, Oklahoma, U.S.A.) is 0.05–300 Hz. The ECGs were digitized with 16 bit analog/digital resolution at a sampling rate of 2.000 Hz for signal averaged recordings and 1000 Hz for beat-to-beat recordings.

Signal Averaging and Late Potential Assessment

Signal-averaged HRECGs were recorded from three bipolar orthogonal leads X, Y and Z within a Faraday cage on the day of the electrophysiological (EP) study. Averaging of 128-500 cardiac cycles resulted in a residual noise level of <0.9 μV. Standard ventricular late potential (VLP) analysis was performed using the Simson method [3, 20]. The averaged X,Y,Z signals were filtered between 40–250Hz with a four-pole Butterworth filter and afterwards summed into a vector magnitude $V = \sqrt{(x^2 + y^2 + z^2)}$, cf. Fig. 1. Onset and offset of the vector QRS were automatically determined and visually checked. Three time-domain variables were calculated: total duration of the filtered QRS (QRSD), root mean square voltage of the last 40 ms of the QRS (RMS), and duration of the low amplitude signal below 40 μV (LAS). In patients without intraventricular conduction defects the following limits were used to define abnormal findings: QRSD > 114 ms, LAS > 38 ms, and RMS <20 μV [2]. Recordings were defined as VLP positive if two out of the three criteria were met.

T-Wave Variability Assessment

T-wave microvariation measurement utilizes the vector of standard deviations of the amplitude of corresponding points of the T-wave, cf. Fig. 2. As on- and off-points of the T-wave are difficult to localize, 400 ms of signal after the QRS-off point – this included the T-wave – were used. Prior to the quantification of

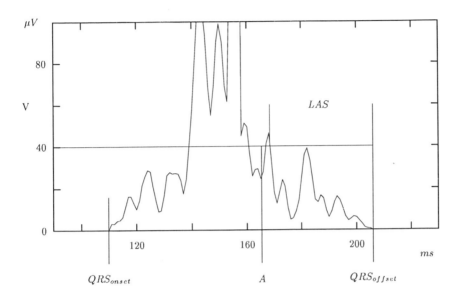

- QRSD (QRS-Duration):
$$QRSD := QRS_{offset} - QRS_{onset}$$

- RMS (Time A: $A := QRS_{offset} - 40ms$):
$$RMS := \sqrt{\frac{1}{QRS_{offset} - A} \sum_{i=A}^{QRS_{offset}} V_i^2}$$

- LAS (Duration of the low amplitude signal below 40 μV):
$$LAS := QRS_{offset} - argmax\{i \mid V_i \geq 40\mu V\}$$

Figure 1: Signal averaged heartbeat (QRS complex) of a highresolution ECG recording. The displayed signal shows late potentials at the end of the QRS complex. The calculation of the three standard features QRSD, RMS and LAS is depicted. The V on the y-axis stands for the so called vector-signal which is calculated from the single lead filtered and averaged signals through: $V = \sqrt{(X^2 + Y^2 + Z^2)}$.

Measurement of T-wave variability:

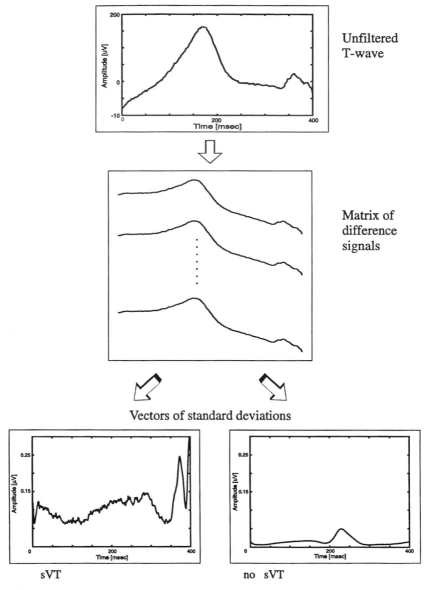

Figure 2: Calculation stages of intra T-wave variability vectors. The individual unfiltered T-wave (400 ms from the QRS-off point) is subtracted from its smoothing spline (difference signal); standard deviations of corresponding points are calculated, resulting in a variability vector.

variability, the beats were preprocessed to suppress the main electrical exitation. Each beat was subtracted from its cubic spline smoothed version (spline filtering). This filter is adapted to the individual beat, a procedure which does not induce any artefacts not present in the original signal. Next, the amplitude of the filtered beat is normalized to zero mean and a standard deviation of 1 μV, cf. Fig. 2. The time alignment of the original beats was achieved by maximizing the cross-correlation function between the first and every other beat for each individual.

Electrophysiological Study

Programmed ventricular stimulation was performed from the right ventricular apex and the right ventricular outflow tract. The stimulation protocol included up to two extrastimuli at sinus rhythm and also during pacing with a basic cycle lengths of 430, 370, and 330 ms, and up to three extrastimuli during pacing with a basic cycle length of 500 ms. Impulse strength was twice the stimulation threshold. A pathological EP-result was defined as an inducible sustained monomorphic ventricular tachycardia (sVT) >30 s in duration or associated with hemodynamic instability requiring immediate defibrillation. Unreproducible VF or ventricular salvos (<30 s) were considered unspecific findings and those patients were declared not inducible.

Neural Classification

Artificial neural networks (ANNs) are effective and versatile computational models originally constructed to the mode of function of neurons. Here, we will briefly describe four pradigms of ANNs: The multilayer perceptron, learning vector quantization (LVQ), radial basis function networks (RBF) and a combination of LVQ and RBF. These feed-forward networks are used for classification of features extracted from time series. ANNs learn from examples, that means they adapt their internal parameters according to some learning algorithm by being presented correctly preclassified data.

Multilayer Perceptron

The multilayer perceptron network (MLP) consisted of one hidden layer of model neurons. The input layer acted as a dummy layer, providing the inputs for the first hidden layer, the output layer was comprised of the same model neurons as those in the hidden layer. The individual neuron realizes a mapping from $\mathbb{R} \rightarrow \mathbb{R}^n$, n denotes the input dimension. This is performed by a weighted summation of the current input vector $x \in \mathbb{R}^n$ and a sigmoid transfer function g:

$$y = g\left(\sum_{k=1}^{n} w_k \cdot x_k \right); \quad g(h) = \tanh(h); \quad w - \text{weight vector.}$$

The net was trained using conjugate gradient descent with line search (Powell's method with restarts, see Press et al. [17] for details). Compared to the popular backpropagation algorithm, in which successive search directions are perpendicular, conjugate optimization methods use as the new search direction a compromise between the gradient direction and the previous search direction [6]:

$$\mathbf{d}^{\text{new}} = -\nabla E^{\text{new}} + \beta \mathbf{d}^{\text{old}},$$

$$E = \text{energy function}, \quad \mathbf{d} - \text{search direction}.$$

Codebook determination with supervised competitive and gradient descent learning

We briefly describe the algorithm used for training the radial basis function network. It consists of two strategies, competitive and gradient descent learning, which are then combined. A more detailed descrpition and analysis can be found in [11].

In supervised competitive learning networks, each prototype vector $c_1, \ldots, c_k$ is labeled with its classmembership $\omega(c_j) \in Y$. This mapping $P : \{1, \ldots, k\} \rightarrow \{1, \ldots, l\}$ is realized by an additional set of fixed connections between the prototype layer and an output layer of l threshold neurons with a threshold value $\theta \in (0, 1)$.

Only neuron j^* – the winning neuron – is active with output $y_{j^*} = 1$ and the others are silent, $y_j = 0, j \neq j^*$, consequently the networks output is the binary vector $z \in \{0, 1\}^l$ with $z_{P(j^*)} = 1$ and $z_p = 0$ for $p \neq P(j^*)$. We assume that the classes $\omega_1, \ldots, \omega_l$ are coded into a set of l binary vector T_p of length l in such a way that $T_{ip} = \delta_{ip}$, here T_{ip} denotes the i-th component of T_p and δ_i is defined by $\delta_{ip} = 1$ if $i = p$ and 0 otherwise. Therefore the binary output $z \in \{0, 1\}^l$ represents $\omega(c_{j^*})$, the classmembership of the winning neuron j^*.

Presenting a vector x^μ in $\mathbb{R}^n$ together with its classmembership ω^μ (encoding ω^μ into T^μ) and using T^μ as a *teaching signal* to the neurons of the output layer, the winning neuron j^* is then adapted according to the learning rule:

$$\Delta c_{ij} = \eta(t)\delta_{j^*j}(x_i^\mu - c_{ij})(2T_{P(j)}^\mu - z_{P(j)}^\mu). \tag{1}$$

$z \in \{0, 1\}^l$ is the activity vector of output layer neurons and $\eta(t)$ is a decreasing learning rate. This competitive learning algorithm has been suggested by Kohonen [13] for vector quantization and classification tasks, it is called *Learning Vector Quantization* (LVQ1) From this algorithm T. Kohonen derived the LVQ2 and LVQ3 network training procedures, these are useful algorithms for the fine-tuning of a pre-trained LVQ1-network.

Gradient Descent Learning in RBF-Networks

In a *radial basis function (RBF)*-network the input vector $x \in \mathbb{R}^n$ is fed into a layer of k hidden neurons, each calculating the distance $d_j = \|x - c_j\|$ between its weight vector $c_j \in \mathbb{R}^n$ (prototype vector) and the currently presented input x. This distance d_j is transformed by a nonlinear transfer function $h : \mathbb{R}_+ \to \mathbb{R}_+$ – the radial basis function – to the neurons output $y_j = h(\|x - c_j\|)$, e.g. the Gaussian density function $h(s) = \exp(-s^2/\sigma^2)$. Each neuron $p \in \{1, \ldots, l\}$ of the output layer receives inputs from all hidden neurons $j \in \{1, \ldots, k\}$ weighted by b_{jp}, such that its activity is given by the weighted sum:

$$z_p = \sum_{j=1}^{k} b_{jp}\, h(\|x - c_j\|). \tag{2}$$

In function interpolation, radial basis functions with fixed prototype vectors have been extensively studied [14]. RBF-networks with free prototype vectors are shown to be universal approximators which are able to approximate continous functions with arbitrary precision [15] – this property implies that RBF-networks with adjustable prototypes are powerful enough for classification tasks [16]. Determining the gradient direction leads to the learning rules: for both types of parameters b_p and c_j. For a single example of the training set (x^μ, T^μ) these weight update rules are:

$$\Delta b_{jp} = \eta_1(t)(T_p^\mu - z_p^\mu)y_j^\mu, \tag{3}$$

$$\Delta c_{ij} = \eta_2(t)(-h'(d_j^\mu))(x_i^\mu - c_{ij}) \sum_p (T_p^\mu - z_p^\mu)b_{jp}. \tag{4}$$

Combined strategy of learning in RBF networks

We will briefly describe the class-specific partitoning algorithm developed in our group [19, 11]. It consists of a strategy for the splitting and merging of prototypes c_j based on their class labels: Given a labeled data set $S := \{(x^\mu, \omega^\mu)|\mu = 1, \ldots, M\}$ with $x^\mu \in \mathbb{R}^n$ and $\omega^\mu \in \{0, \ldots, 1\}$, two thresholds ($\Theta_{\text{outlier}}$ and Θ_{merging} have to be estimated from S.

(1) Start with no prototypes.
(2) Select a training sample.
(3) Detect nearest prototype.
(4) IF prototype insertion condition = TRUE
   - use training sample as new prototype

   ELSE
   - adapt closest prototype

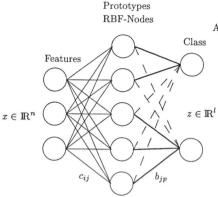

Prototypes
RBF-Nodes

Features

Class

$x \in \mathbb{R}^n$

$z \in \mathbb{R}^l$

c_{ij}

b_{jp}

Algorithm

a) Use the shown network architecture and adapt the prototype vectors c_j according to the supervised competitive learning algorithm (1);

b) Take these c_j as prototypes for the RBF-nodes;

c) Connect each RBF-node to its "class neuron" in the output layer with a strong weight value ($= 1$) as shown in the figure;

d) Introduce additional connections from each RBF-node to the other output neurons and initalize these connections with small random values ($-\epsilon, \epsilon$), $0 < \epsilon \ll 1$;

e) Train this RBF-network according to the learning rules (3) and (4).

Figure 3: The switch of a neural network from competitive to gradient descent learning. The hidden layer consists of k units. After the switch to gradient descent all weights (c_{ij} and b_{jp}) are adapted not only the output layer.

- check merging condition

(5) GOTO (2).

The result of this class-specific partitioning algorithm is a Voronoi tessellation of the input space X, creating larger cells in homogeous regions of X and smaller cells in more complex regions near decision boundaries. The initial kernel widths σ_j for the RBF prototypes are set to $\sigma_j = \gamma d(c_j, c_i)$, e.g. $\gamma = 0.5$, where c_i is the closest prototype to c_j with $w(c_i) \neq w(c_j)$.

The RBF learning procedure starts from this initial setting of prototypes c_j and kernel widths σ_j, see Ref. [19]. After the initialization of the prototypes with the procedure described above the switch to the RBF network follows (cf. Fig. 3).

SELECTED STUDIES

Prototype based Classification of Signal-Averaged High-Resolution Electrograms

Signal-averaged high-resolution ECG's were obtained from 137 subjects separated into two groups: (A) 71 healthy subjects. 15 of these were healthy volunteers without symptoms or history of heart disease. 56 were patients with no history of myocardial infarction, angina, ventricular arrhythmia on resting ECG or by 24 hour Holter monitoring or syncope. All had normal ECG's, normal ejection fraction (cardiac catheterization) and were on no cardiac medication. (B) 66 patients with coronary heart disease in which clinical sustained ventricular tachycardia was inducible at electrophysiologic study. Patients with bundle branch block were not included and no patient was receiving antiarrhythmic medication at the time of the study.

A sequence of classifications was performed using the leaving-one-out method. This procedure utilizes the available samples more effectively compared to a simple sample partition into a training and test set. It is as follows: One sample is taken out, the classifier is designed with the remaining $N - 1$ samples and then tested on the unused sample. This procedure is repeated N times, thus using all samples most effectively. The classification results are counted (four categories as there are two classes) and give an estimate of the classification error [4].

The conventional VLP analysis gave the following results:

Accuracy	Sensitivity	Specificity	Positive predictive value	Negative predictive value
0.759	0.682	0.831	0.790	0.740

Using our algorithm, described in the previous section, several training runs were performed with different numbers of prototyp vectors ($l = 10, ..., 30$), their performance lay in the same order of magnitude. Utilizing the leaving-one-out method a typical RBF-classifier (here 20 prototypes, 3 inputs, 2 outputs) performed as follows:

Accuracy	Sensitivity	Specificity	Positive predictive value	Negative predictive value
0.854	0.803	0.901	0.883	0.831

Multilayer Perceptron based Classification of beat-to-beat Recordings

Unfiltered high-resolution beat-to-beat ECG's (16 bit, 1000 Hz) were recorded in 95 subjects separated into two groups: (A) 51 healthy volunteers (mean±SD, 24±4.2 ys) without any structural heart disease and no cardiac risk factors and (B) 44 patients (61±8.8 ys) with coronary heart disease and a history of myocardial infarction (no bundle branch block). In all patients a sustained ventricular tachy-cardia (>30 s) was inducible twice at electrophysiologic study. Two hundered and fifty consecutive sinus beats per individual were employed for microvariability measurement of the T-wave.

The conventional VLP analysis gave the following results:

Accuracy	Sensitivity	Specificity	Positive predictive value	Negative predictive value
0.789	0.636	0.922	0.875	0.746

The MLP network was utilized as a classifier. It was trained to predict the group membership of the variability vector. Different training runs with variing number of hidden neurons (range: 3-8) were performed. The final net consisted of 400 inputs, 3 hidden neurons and 2 output neurons. Class membership was coded into a "one out of two" vector. The best leaving-one-out result with the least number of hidden neurons was:

Accuracy	Sensitivity	Specificity	Positive predictive value	Negative predictive value
0.811	0.750	0.863	0.825	0.800

CONCLUSION

Our initial application of the backpropagation algorithm for VLP analysis was to use it as an alternative classification tool based on the standard time-domain parameters. Since patient groups with and without malignant arrhythmias are not fully separable by each of the single parameters, the fixed cutoff points sometimes cause borderline results, which are contradictory between subsequent ECG recordings (for example QRS-duration 115ms during the first and 114ms during the second measurement) [8].

Despite a significant classification improvement, this approach was still sus-ceptible to inaccuracies of the determination of the QRS onset and QRS offset and feature extraction was not different from conventional time-domain analysis. Based on the conception that ventricular late potentials are high-frequency, low-amplitude signals overlapping the end of the QRS, time-domain VLP analysis tests only whether the QRS is prolonged and whether there is a low-amplitude terminal QRS portion of a certain length. Thus the initial and the mid portion of the QRS as well as the waveform of the signal are not utilized by this type of analysis. "Hidden" VLPs inside the QRS arising from the earlier excited an-teroseptal regions have been assumed from theoretical considerations and from empirical data (VLPs are more common following inferior myocardial infarc-tion), but they are difficult to measure. Partial spectral analysis of the initial, the whole, and the terminal QRS demonstrated significant spectral differences of the initial QRS between patients with and without anterior myocardial infarction

[9]. Moreover, using time-varying spectral analyses techniques (spectrotemporal mapping and spectroturbulence analysis) Haberl et al. [5] and Kelen et al. [10] demonstrated the importance of pathological signals inside the QRS. This, and as there were patterns which were always misclassified, lead to the conclusion that the three VLP parameters seemed to be inadequate. Therefore more elaborate features utilizing beat-to-beat recordings were extracted. Variability features of the amplitude were extracted on the slower repolarization phase of the cardiac cycle (T-wave) similar to the measurement of alternans [18]. With these features it was possible to gain analogous results of classification accuracy but with a much simpler model (3 hidden neurons).

This study showed exemplarily the mutual dependence of emerging medical knowledge and advanced classification techniques: The inadequacy of the three cut-off parameters of VLP analysis stimulated research of new classification techniques which again lead to the reconsideration of the features used so far. This again brings up new questions of classifier-combination and feature independence to be solved.

REFERENCES

1. E.J. Berbari and R. Lazzara. An Introduction to High-Resolution ECG Recordings of Cardiac Late Potentials. Arch Intern Med, 148:1859-1863, 1988.
2. G. Breithardt and M. Borggrefe. Pathophysiological mechanisms and clinical significance of ventricular late potentials. Eur Heart J, 7:364-385, 1986.
3. G. Breithardt, M.E. Cain, N. El-Sherif, N. Flowers, V. Hombach, M. Janse, M.B. Simson, and G. Steinbeck. Standards for analysis of ventricular late potentials using high resolution or signal-averaged electrocardiography. Eur Heart J, 12:473-80, 1991.
4. K. Fukunaga. Introduction to Statistical Pattern Recognition. Academic press, 2nd edition, 1990.
5. R. Haberl, G. Jilge, R. Pulter, and G. Steinbeck. Spectral mapping of the electrocardiogram with Fourier transform for identification of patients with sustained ventricular tachycardia and coronary artery disease. Eur Heart J, 10:316-322, 1989.
6. J. Hertz, A. Krogh, and R. G. Palmer. Introduction to the Theory of Neural Computation. Addison Wesley, New York, 1991.
7. M. Höher and V. Hombach. Ventrikulare Spatpotentiale - Teil I Grundlagen. Herz & Rhythmus, 3(3):1-7, 1991.
8. M. Höher, A. Peper, T. Eggeling, B. Thomas, and V. Hombach. Comparison of late potentials analysis of two signal averaging ECG-systems. Eur Heart J, 11:307, 1990. Abstract Suppl.
9. M. Höher, A. Peper, H. Sauer, E. Gross, T. Eggeling, M. Kochs, and V. Hombach. Fourier analysis of signal averaged ECG. Eur Heart J, 11:308, 1990. Abstract Suppl.

10. G. J. Kelen, R. Henkin, A. Starr, E. B. Caref, D. Bloomfield, and N. El Sherif. Spectral turbulence analysis of the signal-averaged electrocardiogram and its predictive accuracy for inducible sustained monomorphic ventricular tachycardia. Am J Cardiol, 67:965-975, 1991.

11. H. A. Kestler, F. Schwenker, M. Hoeher, and G. Palm. Adaptive Class-Specific Partitioning as a Means of Initializing RBF-Networks. In Proceedings of the International Conference on Systems, Man, and Cybernetics, pages 46-49. IEEE, 1995.

12. M. Kochs, T. Eggeling, and V. Hombach. Pharmacological therapy in coronary heart disease: prevention of life-threatening ventricular tachyarrhythmias and sudden cardiac death. European Heart Journal, 14:107-119, 1993. Supplement E.

13. T. Kohonen. The self-organizing map. Proc. IEEE, 78(9):1464-1480, 1990.

14. C.A. Micchelli. Interpolation of Scattered Data: Distance Matrices and Conditionally Positive Definite Functions. Constr. Appro ., 2:11-22, 1986.

15. J. Park and I. W. Sandberg. Approximation and Radial Basis Function Networks. Neural Computation, 5:305-316, 1993.

16. T. Poggio and F. Girosi. Networks for Approximation and Learning. Proc. IEEE, 78:1481-1497, 1990.

17. W.H. Press, B.P. Flannery, S.A. Teukolsky, and W.T. Vetterling. Numerical Recipes. Cambridge University Press, Cambridge, 1986.

18. D.S. Rosenbaum, L.E. Jackson, J.M. Smith, H. Garan, J.N. Ruskin, and R.J. Cohen. Electrical Alternans and Vulnerability to Ventricular Arrythmias. N Engl J Med, 330(4):235-41, 1994.

19. F. Schwenker, H. A. Kestler, G. Palm, and M. Höher. Similarities of LVQ and RBF learning - A survey of learning rules and the application to the the classification of signals from high-resolution electrocardiography. In Proceedings of the International Conference on Systems, Man, and Cybernetics, pages 646-651. IEEE, 1994.

20. M.B. Simson. Use of Signals in the Terminal QRS Complex to Identify Patients with Ventricular Tachycardia after Myocardial Infarction. Circulation, 64(2):235-242, 1981.

44. CARDIOVASCULAR SYSTEM IDENTIFICATION

THOMAS J. MULLEN, S.M. RAMAKRISHNA MUKKAMALA AND
RICHARD J. COHEN

INTRODUCTION

Cardiovascular System Identification (CSI) provides a novel, non-invasive technology for the quantitative characterization of cardiovascular regulation in an individual subject. CSI quantifies physiologic coupling mechanisms by mathematically analyzing the relationship between ongoing second-to-second fluctuations in non-invasively measured physiologic variables such as heart rate and arterial blood pressure (ABP). In this way, important physiologic coupling mechanisms, such as the heart rate baroreflex and other measures of autonomic function, can be quantitatively described. By characterizing each of the coupling mechanisms, one can construct an individualized model of closed-loop cardiovascular regulation for each subject. The CSI approach may be adapted to the number of physiologic signals available for analysis. In general, if one measures n physiologic variables from a subject, then $n(n-1)$ causal couplings can be identified. Thus, as more signals are made available, more physiologic coupling mechanisms may be characterized resulting in a more detailed model of closed-loop cardiovascular regulation.

H.-H. Osterhues et al. (eds.),
Advances in Noninvasive Electrocardiographic Monitoring Techniques, 453–461.
© 2000 *Kluwer Academic Publishers. Printed in the Netherlands.*

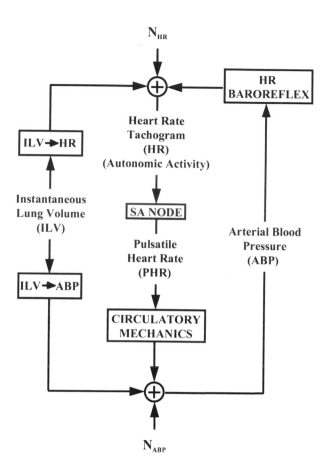

Figure 1. CSI model of short-term cardiovascular regulation relating HR, PHR, ABP, and ILV. See text for description. (Reproduced with permission from [7].)

SIMPLE CLOSED-LOOP MODEL

We have developed a CSI method to identify the couplings between second-to-second fluctuations in heart rate, ABP, and respiratory activity – in terms of time variations in instantaneous lung volume (ILV) [1,6,7,8]. The couplings between these variables that are identified are depicted in the closed-loop model of cardiovascular regulation in Figure 1. The model consists of five couplings – CIRCULATORY MECHANICS, HR BAROREFLEX, SA NODE, ILV→HR, and ILV→ABP – each of which represents a distinct physiologic mechanism.

CIRCULATORY MECHANICS represents the relationship between cardiac contraction and the generation of the ABP-waveform. The input to CIRCULATORY MECHANICS is pulsatile heart rate (PHR) which is defined to be a train of impulses occurring at the times of contraction of the ventricles (derived from the times of occurrence of the QRS-complexes in the ECG). The output from CIRCULATORY MECHANICS is the pulsatile ABP signal. The CIRCULATORY MECHANICS impulse response represents the ABP-wavelet generated with each cardiac contraction and is determined by the contractile properties of the heart as well as the mechanical properties of the great vessels and the peripheral circulation. It may also encompass reflex adjustment of vascular mechanical properties mediated by the α-sympathetic, β-sympathetic and renin-angiotensin systems.

HR BAROREFLEX represents the autonomically mediated baroreflex coupling between fluctuations in ABP and fluctuations in heart rate (HR). In this case, HR is defined to be a stepwise continuous process whose value corresponds to the reciprocal of the current inter-beat interval for the time period corresponding to the duration of that interval [2]. HR is closely related to the net autonomic input signal modulating sinoatrial node activity. SA NODE represents the coupling between HR and PHR. In this model, SA NODE is a nonlinear "integrate and fire" device which precisely relates the input HR to the output PHR.

ILV→HR represents the autonomically mediated coupling between respiration and HR and is responsible for mediating the respiratory sinus arrhythmia. ILV→ABP represents mechanical effects of respiration on ABP due to the alterations in venous return and the filling of intrathoracic vessels and heart chambers associated with the changes in intrathoracic pressure.

In addition to the five coupling mechanisms, the model incorporates two perturbing noise sources, N_{HR} and N_{ABP}. N_{HR} represents the fluctuations in HR not caused by fluctuations in ABP or ILV. Such fluctuations may result, for example, from autonomically mediated perturbations driven by cerebral activity. N_{ABP} represents fluctuations in ABP not caused by fluctuations in PHR or ILV. Such blood pressure fluctuations may result, for example, from fluctuations in peripheral vascular resistance as tissue beds adjust local vascular resistance in order to match local blood flow to demand or from beat-to-beat fluctuations in stroke volume.

SYSTEM IDENTIFICATION METHOD

In order to completely identify the CSI model, six minute segments of ECG, ILV and ABP data are obtained. Data are collected during a random interval

a)

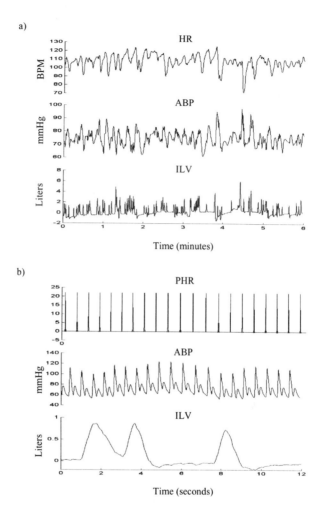

Figure 2. Representative 1.5- (a) and 90-Hz (b) data segments
from a single subject. PHR and HRT are derived from
measured ECG. ABP and ILV are decimated versions of
recorded signals. (Reprinted with Permission from [7])

breathing protocol [3] during which subjects breathe in response to auditory
cues at a comfortable mean rate of 12 breaths per minute but with inter-breath
intervals randomly varying between one and 15 seconds. Subjects adjust their
own tidal volumes thereby leaving blood gases unperturbed. The random
interval breathing protocol broadens the frequency content of the recorded

physiologic signals, thereby facilitating CSI. Representative segments of data are presented in Figure 2.

Using this data, each coupling (except for SA NODE which is a predefined, nonlinear "integrate and fire" device) and perturbing noise sources may be determined from the identification of a pair of linear, time-invariant autoregressive moving average (ARMA) difference equations of the form:

$$HR(t) = \sum_{i=1}^{m} a_i HR(t-i) + \sum_{i=1}^{n} b_i ABP(t-i)$$
$$+ \sum_{i=p'}^{p} c_i ILV(t-i) + W_{HR}(t) \tag{1}$$

$$ABP(t) = \sum_{i=1}^{q} d_i ABP(t-i) + \sum_{i=1}^{r} e_i PHR(t-i)$$
$$+ \sum_{i=s'}^{s} f_i ILV(t-i) + W_{ABP}(t) \tag{2}$$

where t is discrete time, and W_{HR} and W_{ABP} are noise terms referred to as residual errors. These equations include six sets of parameters, a_i, b_i, c_i, d_i, e_i, and f_i whose values may be determined by analysis of continuous records of the measured ECG, ABP and ILV signals. Once these parameters are determined, the transfer relations describing the input-output properties of the coupling mechanisms are fully defined, and the power spectra of the noise sources N_{ABP} and N_{HR} may be computed. Detailed methods are provided in [7,8,9].

It is important to note that this type of formulation allows one to impose causality on the HR BAROREFLEX and CIRCULATORY MECHANICS couplings and therefore, unlike nonparametric techniques, permits the unique identification of these distinct feedforward and feedback coupling mechanisms. In Equations (1) and (2), imposition of this causality condition is achieved by restricting the coefficients, a_i, b_i, d_i, and e_i to be zero for non-positive values of i. On the other hand, the coefficients, c_i and f_i, that relate to the ILV input which is not in the feedback loop, may be nonzero for a limited range of negative values of i. That is, p' and s' may be less than zero. One should also note that an additional requirement for identification of Equations (1) and (2) is that the noise terms, W_{HR} and W_{ABP}, be uncorrelated with each other except at the zero lag. Finally, in order to provide for accurate identification, the sampling rates of the ABP, ILV, PHR and HR signals may be selected to match the bandwidth of the specific transfer relations involved [7].

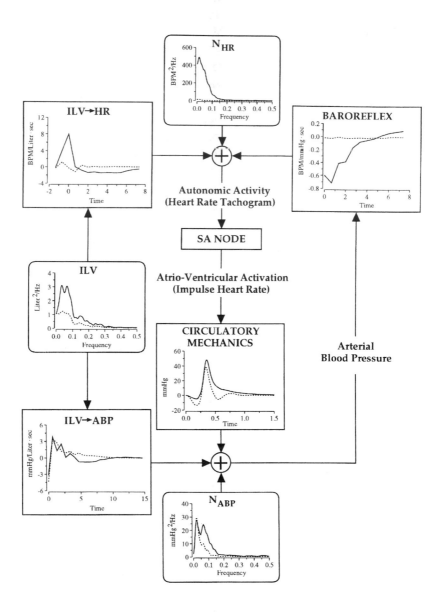

Figure 3. Group average CSI results for subjects in the supine posture before administration of any drugs (solid lines) and after parasympathetic and β-sympathetic autonomic blockade (dashed lines). (Reproduced with Permission from[7].)

APPLICATIONS

We evaluated this CSI method in 14 human subjects studied in the supine and standing postures under control conditions and under conditions of parasympathetic and β-sympathetic pharmacological blockade [7]. Figure 3 shows the group average CSI results for these subjects in the supine posture before (solid lines) and after (dashed lines) combined β-sympathetic and parasympathetic pharmacological blockade. Each coupling element is represented in terms of its impulse response function - the response of the system to a transitory perturbation of arbitrarily short duration. The perturbing noise sources are represented in terms of their power spectra (energy as a function of frequency).

Note that during combined β-sympathetic and parasympathetic blockade, the amplitude of the autonomically mediated physiologic coupling mechanisms (HR BAROREFLEX and ILV→HR) are both reduced essentially to zero as is the amplitude of the power spectrum of N_{HR}, which represents autonomically mediated perturbations to heart rate. Conversely, the amplitude of the mechanically mediated coupling mechanisms (ILV→ABP and CIRCULATORY MECHANICS) are preserved. There is a partial diminution in the power spectrum of N_{ABP}. The remaining power in N_{ABP} may reflect non-autonomically mediated perturbations to ABP resulting perhaps from local autoregulatory fluctuations in peripheral vascular resistance. There is also a reduction in amplitude of fluctuations in ILV representing decreased tidal volume. Perhaps this reduction is due to β-sympathetic mediated broncho-constriction. These results demonstrate that CSI correctly predicts the effect of pharmacological blockade on those couplings and noise sources that are autonomically mediated.

We have also applied this technique to evaluate autonomic neuropathy in patients with diabetes. Diabetic autonomic neuropathy is a progressive deterioration in sympathetic and parasympathetic nervous system function in patients with diabetes. We studied 60 diabetic subjects and 37 control subjects [5]. The diabetic subjects were divided into three groups with Minimal, Moderate, and Severe autonomic neuropathy on the basis of standard autonomic testing. The Minimal group was indistinguishable from the control group on the basis of this conventional testing. The results reveal a progressive diminution in the autonomically mediated physiologic coupling mechanisms with increasing degree of autonomic neuropathy across the four groups, while the mechanically mediated couplings are not affected. Interestingly, the CSI results reveal a statistically significant difference in autonomic function between the control and Minimal groups that was not revealed by standard autonomic testing. These results demonstrate that progressive changes in autonomic function can be quantitatively assessed by CSI.

Most recently, we have compared measures of baroreflex sensitivity derived noninvasively from CSI with those obtained from a traditional approach of calculating the slope of the systolic blood pressure versus preceding RR-interval regression line after administration of phenylephrine [10,11]. We found good agreement between the two techniques [10].

CONCLUSIONS

System identification provides a new means of investigating and monitoring cardiovascular function. It provides a detailed "snapshot" of cardiovascular regulatory function for the individual from whom the data was obtained. The system identification approach promises to provide a powerful noninvasive and quantitative means for evaluating closed loop cardiovascular regulatory dynamics. The technique is extensible (for example, to include additional signals and additional linear [8] or nonlinear couplings [4]) and may be applicable to a wide range of physiological systems and processes.

REFERENCES

1. Appel ML. Closed loop identification of cardiovascular regulatory mechanisms. Ph.D. Dissertation, Harvard University, Cambridge, MA. 1992.
2. Berger RD, Akselrod S, Gordon D, Cohen RJ. An efficient algorithm for spectral analysis of heart rate variability. *IEEE Trans Biomed Eng*, 33:900-4, 1986.
3. Berger RD, Saul JP, Cohen RJ, Assessment of autonomic response by broad band respiration, *IEEE Trans Biomed Eng*, 36(11):1061-5, 1989
4. Chon, K., T. J. Mullen, and R. J. Cohen. A dual-input nonlinear system analysis of autonomic modulation of heart rate. *IEEE Trans Biomed Eng*, 43: 530-544,1996.
5. Mukkamala, R, Mathias JM, Mullen TJ, Cohen RJ, Freeman R. System identification of closed-loop cardiovascular control mechanisms: Diabetic autonomic neuropathy, *Am. J Physiol*, 276(3p+2):r905-12,1999.
6. Mathias JM, Mullen TJ, Perrott MH, Cohen RJ, Heart rate variability: Principles and measurement, *ACC Curr J Rev*, 2(6):10-12, 1993.
7. Mullen TJ, Appel ML, Mukkamala R, Mathias JM, Cohen RJ. System identification of closed-loop cardiovascular control mechanisms: Effects of posture and autonomic blockade. *Am. J Physiol*, 272:H448-61, 1997.
8. Mullen TJ. A system identification approach to characterizing intermediate term hemo-dynamic variability, Ph.D. Thesis, Massachusetts Institute of Technology, Cambridge, MA, 1998.

9. Perrott MH, Cohen RJ. An efficient approach to ARMA modeling of biological systems with multiple inputs and delays. *IEEE Trans Biomed Eng* 43:1-14,1996.

10. Raeder EA, Mullen TJ, Mukkamala R, Toska K, Cohen RJ. Closed-loop analysis of baroreflex sensitivity: Comparison with pharmacologic assessment, *in preparation.*

11. Smyth HS, Sleight P, Pickering GW. Reflex Regulation of arterial pressure during sleep in man, *Circ Res*, 24:109-21, 1969

45. MAXIMUM LIKELIHOOD ANALYSIS IN ECG SIGNAL PROCESSING

LEIF SÖRNMO, MAGNUS ÉSTRÖM, ELENA CARRO, MARTIN STRIDH

1 INTRODUCTION

Electrocardiographic measurements from the body surface are often undesirably influenced by the presence of respiration-induced movements of the heart. Measures which quantify beat-to-beat variations in QRS morphology are particularly susceptible to this influence and special attention must therefore be given to this problem. The analysis of a vectorcardiographic (VCG) lead configuration has been found to reduce this problem. An important reason is that changes in the orientation of the electrical axis, caused e.g. by respiration, can to a certain degree be compensated for by VCG loop rotation. Such rotation can also improve the performance of serial VCG/ECG analysis in which two loops, recorded at different occasions, are compared in order to find pathological changes associated with e.g. myocardial infarction [1], [2].

In this paper, a statistical signal model is described which compensates for heart movements by means of scaling and rotation in relation to a "reference" VCG loop [3]. Temporal loop misalignment is also parameterized within the model framework. The maximum likelihood (ML) estimator of the parameters describing these transformations is found to possess a nonlinear structure and involves e.g. singular value decomposition. The optimal parameter estimates can be determined without the need for iterative optimization techniques. Although the model initially assumes that two loops are to be aligned, the method can easily be extended to the case of multiple loop alignment.

2 MAXIMUM LIKELIHOOD VCG LOOP ALIGNMENT

This section presents the essentials of the method for spatiotemporal alignment of VCG loops [3]. A statistical model is introduced in which a VCG loop is related

H.-H. Osterhues et al. (eds.),
Advances in Noninvasive Electrocardiographic Monitoring Techniques, 463–469.
© 2000 *Kluwer Academic Publishers. Printed in the Netherlands.*

to a reference loop by certain geometric transformations. Maximum likelihood (ML) estimation is then investigated for finding those parameter values of the transformations which provide the optimal fit between the two loops.

The signal model is based on the assumption that an observed VCG loop of the QRS complex, $\mathbf{Y}$, derives from a reference loop, $\mathbf{Y}_R$ but has been altered through a series of transformations. The matrix $\mathbf{Y} = [\, \mathbf{y}_1 \ \mathbf{y}_2 \ \mathbf{y}_3 \,]$ contains column vectors $\mathbf{y}_l$ with N samples for the l:th lead. The reference loop $\mathbf{Y}_R$ is $(N + 2\Delta)$-by-3 and includes 2Δ additional samples in order to allow for observations which constitute different consecutive subsets of N samples from $\mathbf{Y}_R$ indicates that $\tilde{\mathbf{Z}}$ has been augmented with samples. The following three transformations are considered for modeling activities of extracardiac origin: *Scaling* by the positive-valued, parameter α allows for loop expansion or contraction; *rotational* changes of the heart which are due to e.g. respiration are accounted for by the orthonormal, 3-by-3 matrix $\mathbf{Q}$. It should be noted that the rotation matrix is fixed during the entire QRS interval; *time synchronization* is introduced in the signal model by the shift matrix $\mathbf{J}_\tau$. Due to the larger size of $\tilde{\mathbf{Z}}_R$ the observed loop $\mathbf{Z}$ can result from any of the $(2\Delta+1)$ possible positions in $\tilde{\mathbf{Z}}_R$ The shift matrix $\mathbf{J}_\tau$ is defined by the integer time shift τ,

$$\mathbf{J}_\tau = [\, \mathbf{0}_{\Delta+\tau} + \mathbf{I} \ \mathbf{0}_{\Delta-\tau} \,] \tag{1}$$

where $\tau = -\Delta, \ldots, \Delta$. The dimensions of the left and right zero matrices in (1) are equal to $(\Delta + \tau)$-by-N and $(\Delta - \tau)$-by-N, respectively. One of the zero matrices vanishes when τ is $\pm\Delta$. The identity matrix $\mathbf{I}$ is N-by-N. By estimating the parameters which characterize these transformations, it will be possible to reduce the influence of extracardiac activities and thus to improve the alignment of $\mathbf{Y}$ to $\mathbf{Y}_R$.

The above scaling, rotation and time synchronization parameters are embraced by the following observation model

$$\mathbf{Y} = \alpha \, \mathbf{J}_\tau \, \mathbf{Y}_R \, \mathbf{Q} + \mathbf{W}. \tag{2}$$

The transformed reference loop is assumed to be additively disturbed by white, Gaussian noise represented by the N-by-3 matrix $\mathbf{W} = [\, \mathbf{w}_1 \ \mathbf{w}_2 \ \mathbf{w}_3 \,]$. Furthermore, the noise is assumed to be uncorrelated from lead-to-lead and with identical variance, σ_w^2, in all leads.

2.1 Maximum likelihood estimation

It can be shown that the joint maximum likelihood (ML) estimates of the parameters α, $\mathbf{Q}$ and τ are obtained by minimization of the Frobenius norm ε^2 between $\mathbf{Y}$ and $\mathbf{Y}_R$ [3],

$$\varepsilon_{\min}^2 = \min_{\alpha, \mathbf{Q}, \tau} \| \mathbf{Y} - \alpha \, \mathbf{J}_\tau \, \mathbf{Y}_R \mathbf{Q} \|_F^2, \tag{3}$$

where the Frobenius norm for an m-by-n matrix $\mathbf{X}$ is defined by

$$\|\mathbf{X}\|_F^2 = \text{tr}\,(\mathbf{XX}^{\mathrm{T}}) = \sum_{i=1}^m \sum_{j=1}^n |x_{ij}|^2, \tag{4}$$

and tr denotes the matrix trace.

The minimization in (3) is performed by first finding closed-form expressions for the estimates α and $\mathbf{Q}$ under the assumption that τ is fixed. The optimal estimates of α, $\mathbf{Q}$ and τ are then determined by evaluating the error ε^2 for all values of τ in the interval $[-\Delta, \Delta]$. The resulting ML estimate is given by [3]

$$\hat{\mathbf{Q}}_\tau = \mathbf{U}\mathbf{V}^{\mathrm{T}}, \tag{5}$$

where $\mathbf{U}$ and $\mathbf{V}$ are the left and right orthonormal matrices resulting from singular value decomposition of $\mathbf{Z}_\tau = \mathbf{Y}_R^{\mathrm{T}} \mathbf{J}_\tau^{\mathrm{T}} \mathbf{Y}$. The index τ has been attached in (5) since this estimate is optimal for only one particular value of τ. The estimate of α can be calculated when $\hat{\mathbf{Q}}_\tau$ is available,

$$\hat{\alpha}_\tau = \frac{\mathbf{Y}_R^{\mathrm{T}} \mathbf{J}_R^{\mathrm{T}} \hat{\mathbf{Q}}_\tau^{\mathrm{T}}}{\mathbf{J}_\tau \mathbf{Y}_R \mathbf{Y}_R^{\mathrm{T}} \mathbf{J}_\tau^{\mathrm{T}}} \tag{6}$$

The discrete-valued time synchronization parameter τ is estimated by means of a grid search for the allowed set of values,

$$\hat{\tau} = \arg\,\min_\tau \|\mathbf{Y} - \hat{\alpha}_\tau \mathbf{J}_\tau \mathbf{Y}_R \hat{\mathbf{Q}}_\tau\|_F^2. \tag{7}$$

Finally, the estimate $\hat{\tau}$ determines which of the estimates in the set of estimates $\hat{\alpha}_\tau$ and $\hat{\mathbf{Q}}_\tau$ that should be selected. It is noted that the above estimation procedure always yields the optimal estimates since τ belongs to a finite set of values.

Before demonstrating the effect of loop alignment, it should be pointed out that $\hat{\mathbf{Q}}$ can be used for retrieving information related to respiration. Such respiratory-related patterns are made more obvious by decomposing $\hat{\mathbf{Q}}$ into a product of three planar rotation matrices, where the angles φ_X, φ_Y and φ_Z define the rotation around each lead axis. These angles can be estimated by

$$\hat{\varphi}_Y = \arcsin\,(\hat{q}_{13}),$$

$$\hat{\varphi}_X = \arcsin\,(\frac{\hat{q}_{12}}{\cos\hat{\varphi}_Y}), \tag{8}$$

$$\hat{\varphi}_Z = \arcsin\,(\frac{\hat{q}_{23}}{\cos\hat{\varphi}_Y}),$$

where the estimate $\hat{q}_{kl}$ denotes the (k, l) element of $\hat{\mathbf{Q}}$.

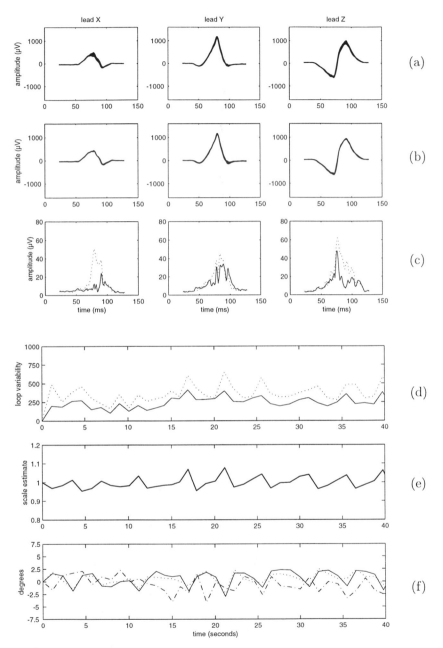

Figure 1: An example of fifty superimposed beats (a) before loop alignment, (b) after alignment, and (c) the corresponding ensemble standard deviation (dotted and solid line correspond to (a) and (b), respectively), (d) spatial variability before (dotted line) and after loop alignment ($\varepsilon_{\min}$) in (3); solid line), (e) the scaling estimate $\hat{\alpha}$ and (f) the angle estimates φ_X, φ_Y and φ_Z (solid, dotted and dashed/dotted line, respectively).

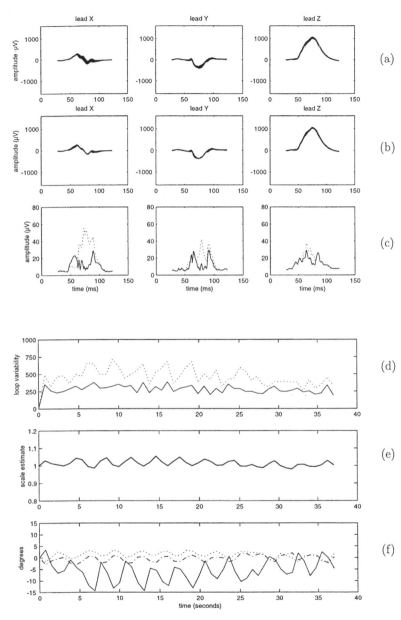

Figure 2: An example with large morphologic variability in which the ML loop alignment dramatically reduces the oscillatory component in ε. Again, fifty superimposed beats are shown (a) before loop alignment, (b) after alignment, and (c) the corresponding ensemble standard deviation (dotted and solid line correspond to (a) and (b), respectively), (d) spatial variability before (dotted line) and after loop alignment ($\varepsilon_{\min}$) in (3); solid line), (e) the scaling estimate $\hat{\alpha}$ and (f) the angle estimates φ_X, φ_Y and φ_Z (solid, dotted and dashed/dotted line, respectively).

3 LOOP ALIGNMENT AND MORPHOLOGIC VARIABILITY

The above ML loop alignment method can compensate for certain limitations associated with the analysis of subtle beat-to-beat variations in QRS morphology. This type of analysis has recently received clinical attention due to its potential value for diagnosing myocardial ischemia and acute infarction, see e.g. [5], [6], [7]. It has been hypothesized that subtle morphologic variations may reflect e.g. islets of ischemic tissue or variations in myocardial contraction patterns. Straightforward computation of the standard deviation for a time-aligned ensemble of beats has been suggested as a means for describing such morphologic beat-to-beat variability [8]. Unfortunately, few techniques have been presented in the literature which aim at reducing the undesirable influence of respiration. This is somewhat surprising since it is well-known that the electrical axis can vary as much as $10°$ in the transversal plane during inspiration [9].

The examples presented below illustrate the effect of ML loop alignment in terms of morphologic beat-to-beat variability. In each example, fifty consecutive sinus beats were selected from a high-resolution ECG recording using an orthogonal lead configuration (X, Y and Z). The sampling rate was equal to 1000 Hz and the amplitude resolution was 0.6 μV. The recordings were selected from a database of subjects with previous myocardial infarction and/or episodes of sustained ventricular tachycardia. Noisy and aberrant beats were excluded from further analysis. The reference beat was simply selected as the first one out of the fifty beats. Finally, the ensemble standard deviation was employed as a measure of morphologic variability and was computed both before and after loop alignment.

The effect of loop alignment is demonstrated by the example in Figs. 1a-c; the corresponding parameter estimates of $\alpha, \varphi_X, \varphi_Y, \varphi_Z, \varepsilon$ and $\varepsilon_{\min}$ are shown in Figs. 1d-f as functions of time. It is obvious from Figs. 1e-f that reduction in variability is related to scaling as well as to rotation of the loops. For ease of interpretation, the results in Figs. 1a-c are presented for individual leads although the alignment is an inherently spatiotemporal process.

Oscillatory patterns found in the error norm are likely to be related to respiratory activity. Such oscillations can be discerned in Fig. 1d both before and after loop alignment although the oscillations are less pronounced after alignment. However, in certain cases the model parameters are able to account very well for the oscillatory component in omin, see Fig. 2d. It is noted that the variability in lead X is essentially removed after loop alignment while the reduction in the other two leads is less dramatic (cf. the variation in the angle φ_X).

4 CONCLUSIONS

The problem of VCG loop alignment has been revisited by means of developing a statistical signal model to which ML estimation was applied. The resulting nonlinear estimation method is feasible from an implementational point of view while it still ensures that the optimal alignment parameter values (scaling, rotation and synchronization) are always found.

The loop alignment was applied to the analysis of subtle beat-to-beat variability in QRS morphology where the cancellation of respiratory-induced variations is important for accurate morphologic measurements. Two exemples illustrated that the effects of respiration on morphologic variability can be dramatically reduced by the new technqiue.

REFERENCES

1. J. Fayn, P. Rubel, P. Arnaud, C. Flaemens, M. Frachon, and S. Hacker, "New serial VCG comparison technqiues. Application to the detection of myocardial infarction after bypass surgery," in Proc. Computers in Cardiology, pp. 533- 536, IEEE Computer Society, 1986.
2. J. Fayn, P. Rubel, and N. Mohsen, "An improved method for the precise measurement of serial ECG changes in QRS duration and QT interval," J. Electrocardiology, vol. 24 (Suppl.), pp. 123-127, 1989.
3. L. Sörnmo, "Vectorcardiographic loop alignment and morphologic beat-to-beat variability," IEEE Trans. Biomed. Eng., vol. 45, pp. 1401-11413, 1998.
4. C. W. Therrien, Discrete random signals and statistical signal processing. Prentice-Hall, 1992.
5. S. Ben-Haim, A. Gil, Y. Edoute, M. Kochanovski, O. Azaira, E. Kaplinsky, and Y. Palti, "Beat to beat variation in healed myocardial infarction," Am. J. Cardiol., vol. 68, pp. 725- 728, 1991.
6. J. Nowak, I. Hagerman, M. Ylén, O. Nyquist, and C. Sylvén, "Electrocardiogram signal variance analysis in the diagnosis of coronary artery disease – A comparision with exercise stress test in an angiographically documented high prevalence population," Clin Cardiol, vol. 16, pp. 671-682, 1993.
7. H. Kestler, M. Hoeher, G. Palm, M. Kochs, and V. Hombach, "Time domain variability of high resolution beat-to-beat recordings classified by neural networks," in Proc. Computers in Cardiology, pp. 317-320, IEEE Computer Society, 1996.
8. K. Prasad and M. Gupta, "Phase-invariant signature algorithm. A noninvasive technique for early detection and quantification of Ouabain-induced cardiac disorders," Angiology, vol. 30, pp. 721-732, 1979.
9. J. Malmivuo and R. Plonsey, Bioelectromagnetism. Oxford: Oxford University Press, 1995.

46. WHAT CAN CARDIAC COMPUTER MODELS TELL US ABOUT ARRHYTHMOGENESIS?

HANS D. ESPERER, ANDREW B. FELDMAN AND
RICHARD J. COHEN

INTRODUCTION

Arrhythmogenic cardiac death remains a major clinical problem whose solution will require both effective risk stratification and therapy. Current understanding of the cardiovascular system has demonstrated that many problems in electrophysiology are inextricably linked to problems in the physics of excitable media, where one seeks to understand the propagation and stability of excitation waves (action potentials) through a highly complex structure, such as the heart. Arrhythmogenic cardiac death is known to be due to aberrant propagation of action potentials in the heart. Predicting such behavior and understanding how to prevent or interrupt it requires knowledge of the mechanisms underlying the genesis and maintenance of the arrhythmic electrical activity. Although theoretical models, like the reentry model of Mines (22), have contributed to the understanding of arrhythmic mechanisms from the very early days of electrophysiology, for the subsequent several decades, *in-vitro* studies of cellular electrophysiology and animal studies were the only models used. With the advent of computers it became possible to improve theoretical models and realize them in mathematical equations that can take specific advantage of digital computation for their rapid solution. In an era where computer power is progressively increasing, *in-silico* modeling of electrophysiological phenomena has become possible not only with respect to simulation of the behavior of a single cell, but also of larger structures, such as the atria, the ventricles, or even the whole heart. Whereas the first simple computer models allowed simulation of basic phenomena, such as excitation, propagation and refractoriness, over the past several decades more advanced models have been developed enabling the simulation of macroscopic phenomena, such as two-

H.-H. Osterhues et al. (eds.),
Advances in Noninvasive Electrocardiographic Monitoring Techniques, 471–480.
© 2000 *Kluwer Academic Publishers. Printed in the Netherlands.*

and three-dimensional wavefront propagation (17), as well as microsopic phenomena, such as the complex current flow in individual cells during stimulation by an external electric field [electric shock] (12). In numerous cases computer models have reproduced many important clinical phenomena related to arrhythmia initiation, maintenance, and termination. If the next generations of computer models prove more faithful and quantitatively reliable than their predecessors, they may open a new window for electrophysiologists, allowing for a more integrated approach to understanding the mechanisms underlying arrhythmogenesis. In this article we briefly review the different model types and describe a few instances that highlight the impact that modeling has had on clinical electrophysiology. The discussion of dipole models and the issue of direct and inverse modeling of the electrocardiogram is beyond the scope of this article.

THE VARIOUS COMPUTER MODELS

Computer models of cardiac electrical activity can generally be divided into two major classes: *local models*, which describe the electrical activity of a small patch of membrane (the area of which is significantly smaller than the surface area of a cell) in terms of its transmembrane currents and potential; and *distributed models,* which describe the electrical activity of a cell, macroscopic piece of tissue, heart chamber, or entire heart. Local models invariably consist of a set of coupled ordinary differential equations. By themselves, these models can only be used to simulate either a local membrane patch or a larger piece of membrane under space-clamp conditions, i.e., where there is no electrical current flow between neighboring membrane patches. Distributed models are useful for studying phenomena related to propagation, such as reentrant arrhythmias, and also electrotonic influences, such as the spatial smoothing of the action potential duration (APD) in tissue with spatial heterogeneities of electrical properties. The most commonly-used distributed models are the reaction-diffusion partial differential equation (PDE) models (of which the one-dimensional "cable" equation is a special case) in which the tissue is treated as a continuous medium (syncytium) with the intra- and extracellular electrical conductivities representing averaged values over many cells. The use of these models to study phenomena occuring on a spatial scale smaller than a few cells may not be justified under certain pathological conditions [e.g., when the pathology significantly reduces the gap junction conductivities](16), since under these conditions the smooth wave front realized in PDE models may be a poor approximation to reality and discreteness effects due to the anisotropic cellular structure (33) may become important in determining the behavior of the wave (e.g., "anisotropic reentry"). In this case, a distributed model in which the cells and the extracellular medium are subdivided and discretized into an equivalent electrical network (with current sources representing the membrane patches connected together with lumped resistive and capacitive elements) may be more appropriate for analysis. Such representations have been used recently to study electric field stimulation of individual cells (12).

The choice of membrane model to use depends on the specific scientific question under investigation. Simplified "two-variable" models such as the commonly-used FitzHugh-Nagumo (13) model employ a single "fast" excitatory current and a "slow" repolarizing current and have proved useful for understanding generic aspects of excitation, repolarization, and reentrant arrhythmias. Highly detailed membrane models, such as the Luo-Rudy (19) model require significantly more computational resources and are more suited for analysis of specific ionic mechanisms in a small region of tissue. For example, Shaw and Rudy (28) used such a model to study propagation in the presence of ischemia, where the activity of the individual ionic channels and the intracellular and extracellular ionic concentrations had to be incorporated.

A special class of distributed models are the cellular automata (CA) models. In CA models, the tissue is discretized into a set of elements that switch between a finite number of distinct states (e.g., resting, excited, and refractory) according to specific transition rules. The parameters of these models (i. e., the transition rules) may be computed such that the waves in the CA medium possess the major features of action potentials (APs) observed in myocardial tissue: the propagation speed, its dependence on the diastolic interval, and its dependence on the shape of the wave front (9). While the simplest CA models are computationally efficient, they suffer from drawbacks that have limited their usefulness in the context of cardiac electrophysiology (11). On the other hand, more sophisticated CA models can be both physiologically realistic and quantitatively reliable and can provide a useful tool for rapid and reliable simulation of cardiac electrophysiologic behavior under a variety of conditions (7, 10).

IMPACT OF MODELING ON CLINICAL ELECTROPHYSIOLOGY

In the late nineteenth century, the foundations of electrophysiology were laid by the experiments of Ringer and Nernst whose work helped to elucidate the physical basis for the resting membrane potential. The first ion-channel-based membrane model was developed by Hodgkin and Huxley (H&H) in the early 1950s (15). The H&H model described the local activity of the major transmembrane ionic currents (Na^+, K^+) in the giant squid axon via a set of ordinary differential equations. The solution of these equations yielded the ionic currents as a function of the transmembrane potential and time, with the parameters of the functions adjusted to fit the data obtained in voltage clamp experiments. H&H assumed that the gating (opening and closing) of the channels was controlled by the motion of a specific number of distinct charged particles in the membrane (with the numbers of each chosen to best represent the experimental data). A more recent channel model developed by Chernyak (7) suggests that the "particles" may represent electrical dipoles embedded in the channel protein structure. Hodgkin and Huxley were able to use their local model to simulate, for the first time, the spaced-clamped action potential and the variations of its morphology under various experimental conditions. In addition, they were able to embed their local model into a distributed (PDE) model and successfully predicted the propagation (including the numerical value of the propagation speed) of the action potential in the giant squid axon. The H&H formulation of the ion channel gating survives to this day in the more sophisticated membrane models for cardiac cells (5,19,20,23). Recent computer simulation studies (43) performed using the Luo-Rudy membrane model for the mammalian ventricular membrane have provided new insights into the ionic mechanisms underlying the AP abnormalities known as early after-depolarizations (EADs), which are involved in the genesis of some polymorphic ventricular tachycardias (PVTs). More modern versions of the activity of ion channels include voltage-gated multi-state models (18).

Computer modeling had, and still has, a significant impact on the evolution of the clinical concept of reentry, which is assumed to account for the overwhelming majority of arrhythmias occurring in the clinical setting. In 1946, Wiener and Rosenblueth (39), using a simple CA model of a two-dimensional slab of tissue, formulated the conditions governing stable reentrant circuits and also introduced the electrophysiologists' concept of the wavelength, which they defined as the product of the propagation speed and the duration of the action potential plateau. This differs from the definition for wavelength typically used in physics by the width of the "excitable gap" [see Ref. (42)]. From a modern point of view it is more useful to define the wavelength in terms of the duration of the physiologic effective refractory period (PERP), where the PERP is defined for the stimulus produced by an approaching AP front. If this wave length (speed x PERP) is less than the path length of the reentry circuit then a circulating wave front can be sustained. For a functionally reentrant circuit, the analysis of its stability is complicated by the fact that the wave front is curved and both its propagation speed and PERP will vary with the distance from the center of rotation due to electrotonic (diffusion) effects (4,38). Despite such limitations, the concepts of the wavelength and excitable gap have gained wide acceptance and still inspire experimental and clinical electrophysiology. The presence of an excitable gap is still used extensively as a diagnostic criterion in clinical electrophysiology, for example, for identifying a given tachycardia as being due to macro reentry or another mechanism.

It has long been suggested that one of the major contributing factors in the induction of reentrant arrhythmias is spatial variations in repolarization and in recovery of excitability ["Dispersion of Refractoriness" hypothesis] (14). Smith and Cohen (31), using a simple cylindrical CA model representing the ventricles, revealed that spatial dispersion of refractoriness is a sufficient condition to produce self-sustained reentry even in the absence of an anatomical obstacle, inhomogeneity in local conduction velocities, or the presence of ectopic foci. The dispersion of refractoriness hypothesis was subsequently supported by animal experiments (1). Applying percolation models from theoretical physics, Smith et al. (32) were the first to analytically describe and predict the width of the vulnerable period for the induction of ventricular fibrillation by a simulated stimulus (R on T phenomenon). Subsequent analysis using Smith and Cohen's model revealed that the presence of beat-to-beat alternations in the simulated electrocardiogram correlated significantly with the susceptibility to ventricular fibrillation. This provocative result led to a series of experiments that showed T-wave alternans to be a marker of malignant ventricular dysrhythmias. This is a beautiful example of how modeling results translated into a clinically very fruitful concept that is increasingly used for risk stratification for sudden cardiac death (27).

Computer simulation studies using sophisticated PDE models of myocardial tissue have led to new insights into the nature of functional reentry. Based on recent simulation results and mathematical computations, it appears that at the center of functionally reentrant circuits are objects known as rotors which give rise to spiral wave reentry in two dimensions and vortex filaments which give rise to scroll wave reentry in three-dimensional (3D) ventricular tissue (40,41). The models revealed that the 3D vortex filaments can twist and wander through the ventricular muscle in complicated ways that result in a variety of simulated ECG morphologies. These results motivated researchers to search for scroll waves in real life hearts and to examine the extent to which they contribute to PVTs and ventricular fibrillation (VF). Recent experiments by Baxter, et. al (3) in sheep confirmed through sophisticated techniques the existence of vortex filaments and scroll wave reentry in mammalian ventricular tissue. A recent study by Peeters, et. al. (24) has provided the first evidence supporting the conjecture that drifting scroll waves may underly PVTs in structurally normal human hearts. This is a striking example of the confluence of electrophysiologic theory, modeling, and animal experimentation with significant clinical implications.

IMPLICATIONS FOR CLINICAL TRIALS

Several computer modeling studies performed during the 1990's have now shed light on the possible mechanisms underlying the arrhythmogenic cardiac deaths in the verum-arm of the Cardiac Arrhythmia Suppression Trial [CAST] (37). In this study, Na^+-channel blockers were used to suppress premature ventricular depolarizations (PVDs) in post-myocardial infarction patients. Patients receiving Na^+-channel blockers in this study had an increased incidence of arrhythmic death even though their PVD's were significantly suppressed. The main effect of Na^+-channel blockade is to reduce the excitability of the tissue, which can give rise to several proarrhythmic phenomena. Computer models and experiments [see Ref. (26)] have shown that Class Ic antiarrhythmic drugs reduce AP propagation speed while clearly increasing the PERP (due to increased postrepolarization refractoriness), resulting in a new wavelength in the pharmacologically modified myocardial substrate. If the drug, for example, induces a 50% reduction in the propagation speed, the PERP would have to be doubled in order for the wavelength to remain the same as in the absence of the drug. If the speed reduction is not adequately compensated by an extension of the PERP, then reduced wavelengths and consequently reduced pathlengths for reentrant circuits would result, increasing the likelihood of sustaining episodes of VT.

A recent computer modeling study by Shaw and Rudy (29) and mathematical analysis of a simple PDE model by Starobin (35) both demonstrated that when the magnitude of the inward (excitatory) current is decreased, the vulnerable window (VW) for the induction of one-way block is increased. The VW is usually defined as the time interval within the relative refractory period during which a premature stimulus gives rise to an AP propagating in one direction only. This arrhythmogenic mechanism may be operative even in the absence of structural heart disease. These modeling results suggest that should a PVD occur in the presence of Na^+-channel blockade, it may, depending on the modified PERP, be more likely to initiate reentry than in the absence of the drug. An additional arrhythmogenic mechanism in poorly excitable tissue (or tissue subject to high frequency stimulation) hitherto not described in experimental models was revealed in computer simulations in the early 1990s by several investigators (2, 25, 36). The mechanism involves the detachment of a wave front from a fixed unexcitable obstacle, such as a scar in the tissue. If the excitability is sufficiently reduced, the wave front will detach from the obstacle rather than circumnavigate it and produce a pair of rotors or vortex filaments. Depending on the obstacle shape, the heart rate history, and the excitability, these functionally reentrant circuits can introduce additional wavelets into the medium or persist themselves giving rise to VT or VF. Interestingly, this mechanism does not require one-way block, but only a reduction of excitability (Na$^+$-channel blockade) and the presence of some structural heart disease. The detachment of wave fronts from obstacles in tissue with low excitability was recently observed in sheep hearts (6). This mechanism of arrhythmia could have played a significant role in the CAST study. Of interest, a recent mathematical and modeling study (34) has suggested that the physiologic mechanisms governing the detachment of the fronts from obstacles may also be related to that controlling the meandering of spiral and scroll waves.

CONCLUSIONS

For five decades, computer models have provided valuable information on arrhythmogenic mechanisms. Lately, a crossroads seems to have been reached where modeling technology is becoming sufficiently predictive qualitatively and quantitatively to play a more significant role in guiding arrhythmia research. The potential for mutual flow of information between the modeling, the experimental, and the clinical community constitutes a unique constellation that can accelerate progress in this field considerably. This "three-dimensional" approach has already contributed to the enhancment of our understanding of numerous clinical phenomena, such as unraveling the electro-cardiographic pleomorphism of atrial and ventricular tachycardias. In this regard, it is hoped that this approach may be helpful in future attempts to elucidate the arrhythmia mechanisms (30) responsible for sudden death in the failing heart and some recently defined clinical syndromes (21), such as idiopathic ventricular fibrillation, sudden unexplained nocturnal death syndrome, or the Brugada–Brugada syndrome, all of which are still puzzling clinicians. The growing number of publications related to quantitative models in clinical electrophysiology journals may be viewed as an expression of the growing interest and appreciation of clinicians regarding computer modeling results.

ACKNOWLEDGMENTS
This work was supported by a grant from the Otto-von-Guericke-University Magdeburg, FRG. (HDE), a grant from the U.S. National Space Biomedical Research Institute, NASA grant Nag5-4989, and NRSA Fellowship No. HL 09570 from NIH (ABF).

REFERENCES

1. Adam DR, Powell AO, Gordon H, Cohen RJ. Ventricular fibrillation and fluctuations in the magnitude of the repolarization vector. IEEE Comp Soc 1982;9:241-244
2. Agladze K, Keener JP, Muller SC, et al. Rotating spiral waves created by geometry. Science 1994;264:1746-1748
3. Baxter WT, Pertsov A, Berenfeld O, et al. Demonstration of three-dimensional reentry in isolated sheep right ventricle. PACE 1997;20: 1080-Abst. 121
4. Beaumont J, Davidenko N, Davidenko JM, Jalife J. Spiral waves in two-dimensional models of ventricular muscle: formation of a stationary core. Biophysical J 1998;75:1-14
5. Beeler GW, Reuter H. Reconstruction of the action potential of ventricular myocardial fibres. J Physiol 1977;268:177-210
6. Cabo C, Pertsov AM, Davidenko JM, et al. Vortex shedding as a precursor of turbulent electrical activity in cardiac muscle. Biophysical J 1996;70:1105-1111
7. Chernyak YB, A universal steady-state current-voltage relationship. IEEE Trans Biomed Eng 1995;45:1145
8. Chernyak YB, Feldman AB, Cohen RJ. Correspondence between discrete and continuous models of exitabile media: Trigger waves. Phys Rev E 1997;55:3215-3233
9. Feldman AB, Chernyak YB, Cohen RJ. A discrete element model of cardiac excitation wave fronts. To appear in Herzschr Elektrophysiol
10. Feldman AB, Chernyak YB, Cohen RJ. Wave-front propagation in a discrete model of excitable media. Phys Rev E 1998;57:7025-7040
11. Feldman AB. Chernyak YB, Cohen RJ. Spiral waves are stable in discrete element models of two-dimensional homogeneous excitable media. Int J of Bifurcation Chaos 1998;8, in press
12. Fishler MG, Sobie EA, Thakor NV, Tung L. Mechanisms of cardiac excitability with premature monophasic and biphasic field stimuli: a model study. Biophysical J 1996;70:1347-1362
13. FitzHugh R. Impulses and physiological states in theoretical models of nerve membrane. Biophysical J 1961;1:445
14. Han J, Moe GK. Nonuniform recovery of excitability in ventricular muscle. Circ Res 1964;14:44-60
15. Hodgkin AL, Huxley AF. A quantitative description of membrane current and its application to conduction and excitation in nerve. J Physiol 1952;177:500-544
16. Jalife J, Sicouri S, Delmar M, Michaels DC. Electrical uncoupling and impulse propagation in isolated sheep Purkinje fibres. Am J Physiol 1989;257:H179-189
17. Keener JP. An eikonal-curvature equation for action potential propagation in myocardium. J Math Biol 1991;29:629-651
18. Liebovich LS. Single channels: from Marcovian to fractal models. In: The classification of antiarrhythmic drugs. In: Zipes DP, Jalife J (eds) Cardiac Electrophysiology. From Cell to Bedside. Saunders Company, Second Edition, Philadelphia, 1995
19. Luo CH, Rudy Y. A dynamic model of the cardiac ventricular action potential. I. Simulations of ionic currents and concentration changes. Circ Res 1994;74:1071-1096
20. Luo CH, Rudy Y. A model of the ventricular cardiac action potential. Depolarization, repolarization, and their interaction. Circ Res 1991; 68:1501-1526

21. Marcus FI. Idiopathic ventricular fibrillation. J Cardiovasc Electrophysiol 1997;1075-1083
22. Mines GR. On dynamic equilibrium in the heart. J Physiol 1913;46:349
23. Noble D. A modification of the Hodgkin-Huxley equations applicable to Purkinje fibre action and pacemaker potentials. J Physiol (London) 1962:317-352
24. Peeters HAP, SippensGroenewegen A, Wever EFD, et al. Localization of polymorphic tachycardia in patients with primary electrical disease using body surface mapping: implications for the underlying mechanism of idiopathic ventricular arrhythmia. PACE 1998;21:855-Abs 263
25. Pertsov AM, Ermakova EA, Shnol EE. On the diffraction of autowaves. Phys D 1990;44:179-190
26. Rosen MR, Strauss HC, Janse MJ. The classificatrion of antiarrhythmic drugs. In: Zipes DP, Jalife J (eds) Cardiac Electrophysiology. From Cell to Bedside. Saunders Company, Second Edition, Philadelphia, 1995
27. Rosenbaum DS, Jackson LE, Smith JM, et al. Electrical alternans and vulnerability to ventricular arrhythmias. NEJM 1994;330:235-241
28. Shaw RM, Rudy Y. Electrophysiological changes of ventricular tissue under ischemic condions: a simulation study. IEEE Computers Cardiol 1994;641-644
29. Shaw RM, Rudy Y. The vulnerable window for unidirectional block in cardiac tissue: characterization and dependence on membrane excitable and intercellular coupling. J Cardiovasc Electrophysiol 1995;6:115-131
30. Singh BN. Antiarrhythmic Drugs: A Reorientation in Light of Recent Developments in the Control of Disorders of Rhythm. Am J Cardiol 1998;81(6A):3D-13D
31. Smith J, Cohen RJ. Simple finite-element model accounts for wide range of cardiac dysrhythmias. Proc Natl Acad Sc USA 1984;81:233-237
32. Smith JM, Ritzenberg AL, Cohen RJ. Percolation theory and cardiac conduction. IEEE Computers Cardiol 1984;175-178
33. Spach MS, Kootsey JM. The nature of electrical propagation in cardiac muscle. Am J Physiol 1983;244:H3-22
34. Starobin JM, Starmer CF. Common mechanism links spiral wave meandering and wavefront-obstacle separation. Phys Rev E 1997;55:1193-1196
35. Starobin JM, Zilbert YI, Starmer CF. Vulnerability in one-dimensional excitable media. Physica D 2994;70:321-341
36. Starobin JM, Zilbeter YI, Rusnak EM, Starmer CF. Wavelet formation in excitable cardiac tissue: The role of wavefront-obstacle interactions in initiating high-frequency fibrillatory-like arrhythmias. Biophys J 1995;70:581-594
37. The Cardiac Arrythmia Suppression Trial (CAST) Investigators: Preliminary Report: Effect of encainide and flecainide on mortality in a randomized trial of arrhythmia suppression after myocardial infarction. NEJM 1989;321:406-410
38. Tyson JJ, Keener JP. Singular perturbation theory of traveling waves in excitable media (a review). Physica D 1988;32:327-361
39. Wiener N, Rosenblueth A. The mathematical formulation of the problem of conduction of impulses in a network of connected excitable elements specifically in cardiac muscle. Archivos Latinoamericanos de Cardiologia y Hematologia 1946;16:205-236
40. Winfree AT. Electrical Turbulence in Three-Dimensional Heart Muscle. Science 1994;266:1003-1006

41. Winfree AT. Theory of spirals. In: Zipes DP, Jalife J (eds) Cardiac Electrophysiology. From Cell to Bedside. Second Edition, Saunders Company, Philadelphia, 1995

42. Winfree AT. Heart muscle as a reaction-diffusion medium: the roles of electric potential diffusion, activation front curvature, and anisotropy. In J Bifurcation Chaos 1997;7:487-526

43. Zeng J, Rudy Y. Early afterdepolarizations in cardiac myocytes: mechanism and rate dependence. Biophysical J 1995; 68:949-964

Index

Developments in Cardiovascular Medicine

109. J.P.M. Hamer: *Practical Echocardiography in the Adult.* With Doppler and Color-Doppler Flow Imaging. 1990   ISBN 0-7923-0670-8
110. A. Bayés de Luna, P. Brugada, J. Cosin Aguilar and F. Navarro Lopez (eds.): *Sudden Cardiac Death.* 1991   ISBN 0-7923-0716-X
111. E. Andries and R. Stroobandt (eds.): *Hemodynamics in Daily Practice.* 1991   ISBN 0-7923-0725-9
112. J. Morganroth and E.N. Moore (eds.): *Use and Approval of Antihypertensive Agents and Surrogate Endpoints for the Approval of Drugs affecting Antiarrhythmic Heart Failure and Hypolipidemia.* Proceedings of the 10th Annual Symposium on New Drugs and Devices (1989). 1990   ISBN 0-7923-0756-9
113. S. Iliceto, P. Rizzon and J.R.T.C. Roelandt (eds.): *Ultrasound in Coronary Artery Disease.* Present Role and Future Perspectives. 1990   ISBN 0-7923-0784-4
114. J.V. Chapman and G.R. Sutherland (eds.): *The Noninvasive Evaluation of Hemodynamics in Congenital Heart Disease.* Doppler Ultrasound Applications in the Adult and Pediatric Patient with Congenital Heart Disease. 1990   ISBN 0-7923-0836-0
115. G.T. Meester and F. Pinciroli (eds.): *Databases for Cardiology.* 1991   ISBN 0-7923-0886-7
116. B. Korecky and N.S. Dhalla (eds.): *Subcellular Basis of Contractile Failure.* 1990 ISBN 0-7923-0890-5
117. J.H.C. Reiber and P.W. Serruys (eds.): *Quantitative Coronary Arteriography.* 1991 ISBN 0-7923-0913-8
118. E. van der Wall and A. de Roos (eds.): *Magnetic Resonance Imaging in Coronary Artery Disease.* 1991   ISBN 0-7923-0940-5
119. V. Hombach, M. Kochs and A.J. Camm (eds.): *Interventional Techniques in Cardiovascular Medicine.* 1991   ISBN 0-7923-0956-1
120. R. Vos: *Drugs Looking for Diseases.* Innovative Drug Research and the Development of the Beta Blockers and the Calcium Antagonists. 1991   ISBN 0-7923-0968-5
121. S. Sideman, R. Beyar and A.G. Kleber (eds.): *Cardiac Electrophysiology, Circulation, and Transport.* Proceedings of the 7th Henry Goldberg Workshop (Berne, Switzerland, 1990). 1991
                                                                                      ISBN 0-7923-1145-0
122. D.M. Bers: *Excitation-Contraction Coupling and Cardiac Contractile Force.* 1991 ISBN 0-7923-1186-8
123. A.-M. Salmasi and A.N. Nicolaides (eds.): *Occult Atherosclerotic Disease.* Diagnosis, Assessment and Management. 1991   ISBN 0-7923-1188-4
124. J.A.E. Spaan: *Coronary Blood Flow.* Mechanics, Distribution, and Control. 1991 ISBN 0-7923-1210-4
125. R.W. Stout (ed.): *Diabetes and Atherosclerosis.* 1991   ISBN 0-7923-1310-0
126. A.G. Herman (ed.): *Antithrombotics.* Pathophysiological Rationale for Pharmacological Interventions. 1991   ISBN 0-7923-1413-1
127. N.H.J. Pijls: *Maximal Myocardial Perfusion as a Measure of the Functional Significance of Coronary Arteriogram.* From a Pathoanatomic to a Pathophysiologic Interpretation of the Coronary Arteriogram. 1991   ISBN 0-7923-1430-1
128. J.H.C. Reiber and E.E. v.d. Wall (eds.): *Cardiovascular Nuclear Medicine and MRI.* Quantitation and Clinical Applications. 1992   ISBN 0-7923-1467-0
129. E. Andries, P. Brugada and R. Stroobrandt (eds.): *How to Face "the Faces' of Cardiac Pacing.* 1992
                                                                                      ISBN 0-7923-1528-6
130. M. Nagano, S. Mochizuki and N.S. Dhalla (eds.): *Cardiovascular Disease in Diabetes.* 1992
                                                                                      ISBN 0-7923-1554-5
131. P.W. Serruys, B.H. Strauss and S.B. King III (eds.): *Restenosis after Intervention with New Mechanical Devices.* 1992   ISBN 0-7923-1555-3
132. P.J. Walter (ed.): *Quality of Life after Open Heart Surgery.* 1992   ISBN 0-7923-1580-4
133. E.E. van der Wall, H. Sochor, A. Righetti and M.G. Niemeyer (eds.): *What's new in Cardiac Imaging?* SPECT, PET and MRI. 1992   ISBN 0-7923-1615-0
134. P. Hanrath, R. Uebis and W. Krebs (eds.): *Cardiovascular Imaging by Ultrasound.* 1992
                                                                                      ISBN 0-7923-1755-6
135. F.H. Messerli (ed.): *Cardiovascular Disease in the Elderly.* 3rd ed. 1992   ISBN 0-7923-1859-5
136. J. Hess and G.R. Sutherland (eds.): *Congenital Heart Disease in Adolescents and Adults.* 1992
                                                                                      ISBN 0-7923-1862-5
137. J.H.C. Reiber and P.W. Serruys (eds.): *Advances in Quantitative Coronary Arteriography.* 1993
                                                                                      ISBN 0-7923-1863-3

Developments in Cardiovascular Medicine

138. A.-M. Salmasi and A.S. Iskandrian (eds.): *Cardiac Output and Regional Flow in Health and Disease.* 1993
ISBN 0-7923-1911-7
139. J.H. Kingma, N.M. van Hemel and K.I. Lie (eds.): *Atrial Fibrillation, a Treatable Disease?* 1992
ISBN 0-7923-2008-5
140. B. Ostadel and N.S. Dhalla (eds.): *Heart Function in Health and Disease.* Proceedings of the Cardiovascular Program (Prague, Czechoslovakia, 1991). 1992 ISBN 0-7923-2052-2
141. D. Noble and Y.E. Earm (eds.): *Ionic Channels and Effect of Taurine on the Heart.* Proceedings of an International Symposium (Seoul, Korea, 1992). 1993 ISBN 0-7923-2199-5
142. H.M. Piper and C.J. Preusse (eds.): *Ischemia-reperfusion in Cardiac Surgery.* 1993 ISBN 0-7923-2241-X
143. J. Roelandt, E.J. Gussenhoven and N. Bom (eds.): *Intravascular Ultrasound.* 1993 ISBN 0-7923-2301-7
144. M.E. Safar and M.F. O'Rourke (eds.): *The Arterial System in Hypertension.* 1993 ISBN 0-7923-2343-2
145. P.W. Serruys, D.P. Foley and P.J. de Feyter (eds.): *Quantitative Coronary Angio- graphy in Clinical Practice.* With a Foreword by Spencer B. King III. 1994 ISBN 0-7923-2368-8
146. J. Candell-Riera and D. Ortega-Alcalde (eds.): *Nuclear Cardiology in Everyday Practice.* 1994
ISBN 0-7923-2374-2
147. P. Cummins (ed.): *Growth Factors and the Cardiovascular System.* 1993 ISBN 0-7923-2401-3
148. K. Przyklenk, R.A. Kloner and D.M. Yellon (eds.): *Ischemic Preconditioning: The Concept of Endogenous Cardioprotection.* 1993 ISBN 0-7923-2410-2
149. T.H. Marwick: *Stress Echocardiography.* Its Role in the Diagnosis and Evaluation of Coronary Artery Disease. 1994 ISBN 0-7923-2579-6
150. W.H. van Gilst and K.I. Lie (eds.): *Neurohumoral Regulation of Coronary Flow.* Role of the Endothelium. 1993 ISBN 0-7923-2588-5
151. N. Sperelakis (ed.): *Physiology and Pathophysiology of the Heart.* 3rd rev. ed. 1994 ISBN 0-7923-2612-1
152. J.C. Kaski (ed.): *Angina Pectoris with Normal Coronary Arteries: Syndrome X.* 1994
ISBN 0-7923-2651-2
153. D.R. Gross: *Animal Models in Cardiovascular Research.* 2nd rev. ed. 1994 ISBN 0-7923-2712-8
154. A.S. Iskandrian and E.E. van der Wall (eds.): *Myocardial Viability.* Detection and Clinical Relevance. 1994 ISBN 0-7923-2813-2
155. J.H.C. Reiber and P.W. Serruys (eds.): *Progress in Quantitative Coronary Arteriography.* 1994
ISBN 0-7923-2814-0
156. U. Goldbourt, U. de Faire and K. Berg (eds.): *Genetic Factors in Coronary Heart Disease.* 1994
ISBN 0-7923-2752-7
157. G. Leonetti and C. Cuspidi (eds.): *Hypertension in the Elderly.* 1994 ISBN 0-7923-2852-3
158. D. Ardissino, S. Savonitto and L.H. Opie (eds.): *Drug Evaluation in Angina Pectoris.* 1994
ISBN 0-7923-2897-3
159. G. Bkaily (ed.): *Membrane Physiopathology.* 1994 ISBN 0-7923-3062-5
160. R.C. Becker (ed.): *The Modern Era of Coronary Thrombolysis.* 1994 ISBN 0-7923-3063-3
161. P.J. Walter (ed.): *Coronary Bypass Surgery in the Elderly.* Ethical, Economical and Quality of Life Aspects. With a foreword by N.K. Wenger. 1995 ISBN 0-7923-3188-5
162. J.W. de Jong and R. Ferrari (eds.), *The Carnitine System.* A New Therapeutical Approach to Cardiovascular Diseases. 1995 ISBN 0-7923-3318-7
163. C.A. Neill and E.B. Clark: *The Developing Heart: A "History' of Pediatric Cardiology.* 1995
ISBN 0-7923-3375-6
164. N. Sperelakis: *Electrogenesis of Biopotentials in the Cardiovascular System.* 1995 ISBN 0-7923-3398-5
165. M. Schwaiger (ed.): *Cardiac Positron Emission Tomography.* 1995 ISBN 0-7923-3417-5
166. E.E. van der Wall, P.K. Blanksma, M.G. Niemeyer and A.M.J. Paans (eds.): *Cardiac Positron Emission Tomography.* Viability, Perfusion, Receptors and Cardiomyopathy. 1995 ISBN 0-7923-3472-8
167. P.K. Singal, I.M.C. Dixon, R.E. Beamish and N.S. Dhalla (eds.): *Mechanism of Heart Failure.* 1995
ISBN 0-7923-3490-6
168. N.S. Dhalla, P.K. Singal, N. Takeda and R.E. Beamish (eds.): *Pathophysiology of Heart Failure.* 1995
ISBN 0-7923-3571-6
169. N.S. Dhalla, G.N. Pierce, V. Panagia and R.E. Beamish (eds.): *Heart Hypertrophy and Failure.* 1995
ISBN 0-7923-3572-4

Developments in Cardiovascular Medicine

Developments in Cardiovascular Medicine